Nutrition and Diet Therapy

REFERENCE DICTIONARY

Nutrition and Diet Therapy
REFERENCE DICTIONARY

❧ ❧

SECOND EDITION

ROSALINDA T. LAGUA, M.N.S.

Director of Nutritional Services, State University of New York–
Upstate Medical Center, Syracuse, New York

VIRGINIA S. CLAUDIO, Ph.D.

Quezon City, Rizal, Philippines

VICTORIA F. THIELE, Ph.D.

Professor of Nutrition, College for Human
Development, Syracuse University,
Syracuse, New York

SAINT LOUIS

THE C. V. MOSBY COMPANY

1974

SECOND EDITION

Copyright © 1974 by The C. V. Mosby Company

All rights reserved. No part of this book may be reproduced in any manner without written permission of the publisher.

Previous edition copyrighted 1969 in the Philippines by Rosalinda T. Lagua and Virginia S. Claudio

Printed in the United States of America

Distributed in Great Britain by Henry Kimpton, London

Library of Congress Cataloging in Publication Data

Lagua, Rosalinda T   1937-
  Nutrition and diet therapy.

  Bibliography: p.
  1. Diet in disease. 2. Nutrition. I. Claudio,
Virginia S., 1932-   joint author. II. Thiele,
Victoria F., 1933-   joint author. III. Title.
[DNLM: 1. Diet therapy—Dictionary. 2. Nutrition—
Dictionary. QU13 L181n 1974]
RM219.L26 1974   615'.854   74-612
ISBN 0-8016-2807-5

CB/CB/B   9   8   7   6   5   4   3   2   1

Contents

CONTENTS

Preface

This reference dictionary is a presentation of up-to-date and complete information on terms used in nutrition. Its outstanding feature is the thorough treatment of clinical nutrition and diet in disease. Written primarily for practitioners in the field of nutrition and dietetics, its contents are at the same time useful to physicians, nurses, professionals in other health care delivery services, educators, and students. To these varied groups, we have sought to furnish as much fingertip knowledge as can be offered in a brief and compact volume.

More than thirty-five hundred terms are presented alphabetically and treated in about a million and a quarter words of definition and other related data. In choosing the terms to be included, we used as criteria the frequency of use and importance of the terms in nutrition. For greater fullness of coverage, definitions are amplified by materials found in the appendices. Such additional information includes the chemistry of blood, urine, and body fluids, a summary of dietary management in selected disorders, and proprietary foods—composition, features, and uses.

First printed for use in the Philippines in 1969, this second edition has been redesigned for American and international use. Several new terms have been added and each definition has been updated and carefully reviewed.

Rosalinda T. Lagua
Virginia S. Claudio
Victoria F. Thiele

Guide to the use of the dictionary

Word entry The word or term to be defined is set in boldface and extends slightly to the left of the definition. All entries, including abbreviations and compounds of two or more words, have been entered in strict alphabetical order on sequence of the letters, regardless of space or hyphens that may occur between them. If two or more variant spellings of a single word exist, the one most frequently used is entered in boldface and the variant spellings are given in the definition. When usage is about evenly divided, both variant spellings are entered in boldface.

Subentries Groups or classes of definitions related by a common root term appear under that term: anemia, amino acid, dietitian, etc. The series is slightly indented and each subentry is set in the same boldface as the main word entry.

Definitions Innumerable definitions have been scrutinized, redefined, or expanded to conform to changing concepts of present-day knowledge. The definitions of a term are numbered when there is more than one distinct meaning or use. The most inclusive definition is presented first, followed by the more restricted meanings. Definitions restricted to specialized fields are preceded by field labels such as "In nutrition," "In medicine," etc. Advertently omitted are definitions in certain specialized fields that do not have any application in the field of nutrition. A semicolon after a definition generally means that the material that follows is not part of the definition proper but is additional information enlarging on the factual content.

Abbreviations Abbreviations with nutritional significance appear in their proper alphabetical sequence in the dictionary. They are defined in full in word entries for which such abbreviations stand.

Cross references The user is directed to additional or fuller information by such cross reference terms as **see** or **see under.** Cross references to related information are identified by the words **see also.** The word entry to which the user is directed is italicized; when a cross reference appears under a group entry, the user is instructed to look for the **subentry** under the **word entry** for definition of the specific term. Cross referencing to the Appendices is not italicized but written in the same type form as the definition; the user, however, is clearly directed to the Appendices for additional information.

Italics Some words are italicized either to lend emphasis or to indicate to the user that such words, in case they are not known to him, are defined elsewhere in the text. Cross reference words are also italicized.

Nutrition and Diet Therapy
REFERENCE DICTIONARY

A

AA Abbreviation for *adenylic acid* or *amino acid*.

Abdomen Large body cavity that contains the stomach, intestines, liver, spleen, pancreas, and kidneys. It is commonly called the belly.

Abomasum The fourth stomach of ruminant animals. It connects the omasum and duodenum through the pylorus.

Abort 1. To miscarry; to bring forth a fetus before it is capable of surviving. 2. To stop the development or progress of a disease.

Abortion The premature expulsion of a nonliving fetus. The term is used when the condition occurs during the first 3 months after conception.

Absorption Assimilation or taking up of fluids, gases, nutrients, or other substances by the skin, lacteals, mucous membranes, or absorbent vessels.

Acapnia Absence of carbon dioxide in the blood. The preferred term is *hypocapnia* (decrease in carbon dioxide content).

Accelerator globulin (Ac globulin or AcG) Factor that accelerates the conversion of prothrombin to thrombin, which is necessary in blood clotting. Formerly called accelerin.

Acceptable daily intake (ADI) Daily dose of a chemical used as a food additive that appears to be "without appreciable risk on the basis of all facts known at the time." This is an assurance that injury will not result even after a lifetime of exposure to the chemical.

Accessory food factors Earliest name given to vitamins by Hopkins, who demonstrated in 1906 that foods contain, in addition to the nutrients then recognized (i.e., carbohydrates, proteins, fats, minerals, and water), minute traces of unknown substances essential to health and life.

Acclimatization State of becoming accustomed to a new condition or climate.

Accommodation 1. Process by which any part or organ of the body adjusts to the environment. 2. Adjustment or adaptation of the eye to various distances.

Acerola A bright red fruit also known as West Indian cherry. It is claimed to be the richest natural source of vitamin C (2000 to 4000 mg/100 ml as compared to orange juice with 50 mg/100 ml). It grows abundantly in Puerto Rico.

Acetal Product formed when an aldehyde is allowed to react with two equivalents of alcohol.

Acetate Any salt of acetic acid. Active acetate is *acetylcoenzyme A*.

Acetic acid CH_3COOH; an organic acid commonly formed in the metabolism of sugars and related substances. As *acetylcoenzyme A*, it participates in a number of important metabolic processes.

Acetoacetate Compound formed by the condensation of two molecules of acetic acid. Active acetoacetate is *acetoacetylcoenzyme A*.

Acetoacetic acid Monobasic ketone acid formed in the course of normal fatty acid catabolism and oxidized further to acetic acid, which is utilized in various metabolic reactions. It accumulates in the blood when fatty acids are incompletely oxidized. The reduction of acetoacetic acid yields *beta-hydroxybutyric* acid, and its decarboxylation yields *acetone.* See also *Ketone bodies.*

Acetoin Acetylmethylcarbinol, precursor of *diacetyl,* produced by bacteria during the ripening of butter. It is also formed by the interaction of pyruvic acid and acetaldehyde in the presence of thiamin.

Acetolysis Breakdown of an organic compound by acetic acid.

Acetone Dimethylketone. A colorless liquid with a sweetish ethereal odor; formed by the decarboxylation of acetoacetic acid. It is normally present in minute quantities in blood and urine but may accumulate when fatty acid degradation is excessive or incomplete. See also *Ketone bodies.*

Acetone bodies See *Ketone bodies.*

Acetonemia Presence of large amounts of acetone (ketone bodies) in the blood.

Acetonuria Excretion of large amounts of acetone bodies in the urine. While normally present in trace amounts in the urine, their excretion may increase from 0.02 gm to as much as 6 gm/day in certain pathologic conditions.

Acetyl The two-carbon radical CH_3CO^-.

Acetylation Introduction of an acetyl group into a molecule.

Acetylcholine **(ACh)** Acetic acid ester of choline. It is released from nerve endings to initiate a series of reactions leading to the transmission of a nerve impulse. Its actions correspond to those of the cholinergic fibers, including a depressant effect on the blood pressure and stimulation of intestinal peristalsis.

Acetylcholinesterase **(ACh esterase)** Formerly called *cholinesterase;* an enzyme present in the blood and various tissues that catalyzes the hydrolysis of acetylcholine to choline and acetate. It plays an important role in the transmission of nerve impulses.

Acetylcoenzyme A **(acetyl CoA)** Acetyl derivative of coenzyme A. It is formed from the repetitive beta oxidation of fatty acids and from the oxidative decarboxylation of pyruvic acid; it can be synthesized from acetate in many animals, plants, and microorganisms. Acetyl CoA is an important member of the *Krebs cycle,* serves as a precursor for the biosynthesis of fatty acids and sterols, gives rise to acetoacetic acid, and is the biologic acetylating agent in the synthesis of acetylcholine.

Acetyl number Also called acid number; it refers to the number of milligrams of potassium hydroxide required to neutralize the acetic acid liberated by the hydrolysis of 1 gm of acetylated fat. It is a measure of the amount of free fatty acids.

AcG Abbreviation for *accelerator globulin.*

ACh Abbreviation for *acetylcholine.*

Achalasia Neuromuscular disorder of the esophagus that causes dyspepsia, esophageal regurgitation, and esophageal pain.

ACh esterase Abbreviation for *acetylcholinesterase.*

Achlorhydria Absence of hydrochloric acid in the gastric juice.

Acholic Without bile; suppression of biliary secretion.

Achroacyte A colorless cell; lymphocyte.

Achromacyte A decolorized erythrocyte.

Achromia Pallor; absence of normal color.

Achromotrichia Absence of pigment in hair; graying of hair. It is seen in rats as a result of *pantothenic acid* deficiency.

Achroodextrin A dextrin that is colorless with iodine. It is an intermediate product of the enzymic breakdown of starch to maltose.

Achylia Absence of *chyle.*

Achylia gastrica Complete absence of acid (HCl) and pepsin from the gastric juice.

Acid Compound capable of yielding hydrogen ion in solution. Also defined as a substance that produces or donates protons.

Acid-ash residue Inorganic radicals (chiefly chloride, sulfate, and phosphate) that form acid ions (anions) in the body.

Acid-base balance Equalization of total acid

and total base in body fluids at levels compatible with life. Normally the blood is kept within a narrow pH range of 7.35 to 7.45. Adjusting mechanisms come into play to neutralize or remove excess acid or base to maintain balance. These include the buffer systems of the blood, the excretion of carbon dioxide by the lungs, and the excretion of fixed acid or base by the kidneys.

Acidemia Increase in acid or decrease in blood pH. Any decrease in the pH of the blood, although still on the basic side, is called acidemia.

Acid-forming foods Foods in which the acidic residue exceeds the alkaline residue. These include meats, fish, poultry, eggs, and cereals. See *Acid-ash residue;* see also *Alkaline-forming foods.*

Acidity Amount of acid in any substance. The degree of acidity is usually expressed as actual acidity, free acidity, titratable acidity, or total acidity.

Actual a Concentration of hydrogen ions in solution, usually referred to as the pH of the solution.

Free a Amount of acid not combined with other substances present in solution.

Titratable a Concentration of hydrogen ions in solution plus those available for ionization although not actually ionized at the time, i.e., total hydrogen ion concentration both actually and potentially ionized.

Total a Amount of free acid in solution in addition to that present in acid salts and in combination with organic compounds. It is synonymous with titratable acidity.

Acidophilus milk See under *Milk.*

Acidosis An abnormal condition characterized by a fall in the pH of the blood or a decrease in the *alkali reserve* of the body. A reduction in blood bicarbonate (alkali reserve) indicates that an excess of fixed acids is being produced or retained in the body at a rate exceeding that of neutralization or elimination. Various acids retained in different conditions are the acidic ketone

bodies (as in diabetes mellitus), phosphoric, sulfuric, and hydrochloric acids (as in renal insufficiency), lactic acid (as in anoxia, ether anesthesia, and prolonged strenuous exercise), and carbonic acid (as in respiratory disease).

Acid tide Temporary increase in the acidity of urine and body fluids after eating while alkali is being secreted into the duodenum.

Ackee The fruit of a tree common in the West Indies and South America. Consumption of the unripe or bruised fruit, especially by undernourished people, causes an acute toxic hypoglycemia characterized by abdominal pains, severe vomiting, convulsions, and coma. Death occurs in the majority of cases. The fruit contains hypoglycin A and B, which may be responsible for the hypoglycemia.

Acne vulgaris Skin condition characterized by pimples or eruptions occurring most frequently on the face, back, and chest. An acne pimple is an obstructed and infected oil gland, and the pimples are more numerous where the oil glands are most abundant. For many years people have associated diets high in fat or carbohydrate (particularly chocolate, nuts, candies, carbonated drinks, and fried foods) with acne. There is no basis for such beliefs. Studies have shown that foods do not produce major flare-ups of acne.

Acral Pertaining to the limbs or extremities.

Acrodynia Condition seen in *pyridoxine*-deficient rats, characterized by edema and a form of dermatitis with thickening of the epidermis and denuding of the ears, paws, nose, mouth, and tail.

Acrolein Acrylic aldehyde, a substance resulting from the decomposition of glycerol. It gives the characteristic odor of burnt fat.

Acromegaly Chronic condition resulting from the hypersecretion of the growth hormone during adulthood. The characteristic features are overgrowth of the bones of the face and extremities, protrusion of the chin, enlargement of the hands, feet, and fingers, thickening of the scalp, bowing of the spine, glycosuria, and suppression of sexual function.

Acropathy Any disease of the extremities.

ACTH Abbreviation for *adrenocorticotropic hormone.*

Actin One of the two protein constituents of the muscle fibril. Together with myosin, as *actomyosin,* it is responsible for the contraction and relaxation of the muscles.

Activator A substance that renders another substance active, either by being part of the reaction system or by combining with the inactive substance. An enzyme activator is called a *cofactor.*

Active tissue mass See *Lean body mass.*

Active transport Also called biologic "pump." The process in which a substance is moved across a cell membrane from a lower to a higher electrochemical potential. It involves an expenditure of metabolic energy derived from the breakdown of adenosine triphosphate. Active transport appears to be mediated by a carrier molecule that combines with the substance to be transported.

Actomyosin The protein of muscle responsible for its contractile process; composed of myosin and F-actin.

Acuity Clearness or sharpness, such as clear vision and sharp hearing.

Acute Having a sudden beginning or onset, short course, or severe symptoms

Acyl R · CO; an organic radical derived from an organic acid without the hydroxyl group. *Acylation* is the introduction of an acyl radical into a compound.

ADA Abbreviation for *American Dietetic Association.*

Adaptation In biology, any modification in form, habit, or physiologic process to suit a new environment. Adaptation serves to maintain constancy despite changing environmental demands. It also brings about continuing or permanent changes to better meet environmental requirements. See *Nutritional adaptation.*

Addison's disease Metabolic disorder due to adrenal insufficiency. It is characterized by rapid loss of weight and appetite, weakness, emaciation, anemia, deep bronzing of the skin, low blood pressure, hypoglycemia, electrolyte imbalance with excessive loss of NaCl in the urine, and retention of potassium, usually ending in death.

Additive See *Food additive.*

Adenine One of the major purine bases of nucleic acids. As *adenosine phosphate,* it provides energy for muscular movement.

Adenohypophysis Anterior lobe of the *hypophysis* or pituitary gland. It secretes vital hormones that regulate other endocrine glands. These are the growth, thyrotropic, adrenocorticotropic, lactogenic, and gonadotropic hormones. See Summary of endocrine glands, Appendix K.

Adenoma Benign tumor of glandular origin.

Adenosine Mononucleoside composed of the base adenine and the sugar D-ribose. It is derived from the hydrolysis of adenosine monophosphate.

Adenosine phosphates Adenosine mono-, di-, and triphosphates are present in practically all tissues, especially in the muscles and liver. Adenosine monophosphate is important in the activation of *phosphorylase,* whereas the di- and triphosphates are important sources of *high-energy phosphate* for cellular activity.

Adenosine diphosphate (ADP) Compound composed of two molecules of phosphate and one molecule each of adenine and D-ribose.

Adenosine monophosphate (AMP) Also called adenylic acid; a compound composed of one molecule each of adenine, D-ribose, and phosphoric acid.

Adenosine triphosphate (ATP) Also called adenyl pyrophosphate; a compound composed of three phosphate molecules and one molecule each of adenine and D-ribose.

Adenyl cobamide One of the coenzyme forms of vitamin B_{12}. See *Cobamide.*

Adenylic acid (AA) Also called adenosine monophosphate. See under *Adenosine phosphates.*

Adenyl pyrophosphate Also called adenosine

triphosphate. See under *Adenosine phosphates.*

Adermin Former name for *vitamin B₆.*

ADH Abbreviation for *antidiuretic hormone.*

ADI Abbreviation for *acceptable daily intake.*

Adipic Pertaining to or belonging to fat.

Adipose tissue Fatty tissue that acts as depot fat for storage of energy and serves as insulation against heat loss and padding for protection and support of organs. It is found largely in subcutaneous tissues and around visceral organs. Like other body constituents, it is not inert but is in a *dynamic state.* Fat is constantly being formed and hydrolyzed in adipose tissue.

Adiposity See *Obesity.*

Adipsia Absence of thirst; avoidance of drinking.

Ad libitum (ad lib) As desired; freely.

ADP Abbreviation for *adenosine diphosphate.* See under *Adenosine phosphates.*

Adrenal glands Also called suprarenal glands; these two small endocrine glands are located at the upper end of each kidney. Each gland consists of two parts: the *cortex,* which elaborates estrogen, androgen, progesterone, and the adrenocortical hormones; and the *medulla,* which elaborates epinephrine and norepinephrine.

Adrenalin Trade name for *epinephrine.* It stimulates the heart muscle and increases the blood pressure and total output by the heart.

Adrenaline Now called epinephrine. See *Epinephrine.*

Adrenergic Having the characteristics of epinephrine or epinephrine-like substances.

Adrenocortical hormones These are the steroid hormones of the adrenal cortex, which are derivatives of pregnane (21 carbon atoms). These hormones are essential to life and play varied roles in water and electrolyte balance, metabolism of carbohydrate, protein, and fat, and protection against stress, allergy, and inflammatory processes.

Adrenocorticotropin See *Adrenocortical hormones.*

Adrenosterone Steroid hormone produced by the adrenal cortex; has androgenic activity. See *Androgen.*

Adsorption 1. Property or ability of a substance to attract and concentrate on its surface a thin layer of gas, liquid, or solid by adhesion. 2. Attachment of one substance to the surface of another.

Adulteration Addition, substitution, omission, or abstraction of any substance that may render food injurious to health, reduce its quality or strength, or make it appear better or of greater value than it is.

A/E ratio Number of milligrams of each essential amino acid per gram of total essential amino acids. This is a method of evaluating protein quality.

Aerobic Living or functioning in air or free oxygen.

Afferent Conveying or carrying toward the center. For example, afferent nerves carry impulses toward the central nervous system.

Affinity Tendency of a substance to combine with another substance. For example, hemoglobin has a greater affinity for carbon monoxide than for oxygen.

Aflatoxin Toxic substance produced by the common mold *Aspergillus flavus;* found in moldy peanuts, Brazil nuts, cottonseed, copra, and, to a lesser extent, cereal grains. It is carcinogenic and causes liver injury.

Afterbirth Placenta and fetal membranes expelled from the uterus after childbirth.

Agammaglobulinemia Condition characterized by extremely low levels of gamma globulins in the blood, resulting in frequent suppurative bacterial infections. The preferred term is hypogammaglobulinemia.

Agar Polysaccharide obtained from seaweed. It is not digested by man; hence it is a mild laxative. In the laboratory, agar is used as a culture medium for bacteria.

Aged Generally refers to "older" people age 65 years and over. Sixty-five is the age when Social Security benefits begin and is often the mandatory age for retirement. Medically it does not mean anything, since all individuals age differently. See *Aging.*

Agglutination Clumping together of cells; aggregation of suspended particles.

Agglutinin An antibody, present in normal plasma, that causes clumping or agglutination of a particulate antigen.

Agglutinogen A substance or antigen that induces the formation of a specific antibody or agglutinin.

Aging Theoretically aging is a continuous process from conception until death. But in the young and growing organism the building-up processes exceed the breaking-down processes, so that the net result is a picture of growth and development. Once the body reaches adulthood the process is reversed. Aging proceeds at different rates in different individuals. Environmental factors—chemical, physical, and biologic—influence the aging process. Certain physiologic functions show gradual decrement with age. These include basal metabolic rate, cardiac output, renal blood flow, and lung capacity. However, other physiologic functions remain quite stable over the entire life-span unless the individual is subjected to stress factors. For example, fasting blood glucose levels do not change significantly with age, and blood volume and red cell content remain relatively constant.

Aglycone Nonsugar portion of a glycoside.

Agranulocytosis A critical condition caused by a reduction in the number of polymorphonuclear leukocytes in the blood, leading to decreased resistance to infections. It may be due to infections or may result from a variety of chemicals used in the home, industry, or drug therapy.

A/G ratio See *Albumin/globulin ratio.*

AHF Abbreviation for *antihemophilic factor.*

AHG Abbreviation for *antihemophilic globulin.*

AID Abbreviation for *American International Development Agency.*

AIN Abbreviation for *American Institute of Nutrition.*

Alacta Powdered half skim milk product that is high in protein and moderately low in fat; used for low birth weight infants or those with digestive disturbances. (Mead Johnson.) See Proprietary foods: composition, features, and uses, Appendix P-1.

Alanine Alpha-aminopropionic acid, a nonessential amino acid readily formed from carbohydrate by its reversible conversion to pyruvic acid.

Beta-a Beta-aminopropionic acid, the only naturally occurring beta amino acid. It is found in pantothenic acid and in the naturally occurring peptides carnosine and anserine.

Albinism Inborn error of metabolism characterized by lack of pigmentation of the hair, skin, and eyes due to inability to form the pigment melanin. The condition is caused by lack of enzyme tyrosinase, which catalyzes the hydroxylation of tyrosine to dihydroxyphenylalanine (dopa) to form melanin.

Albumen 1. White of eggs, consisting chiefly of *albumin.* 2. *Oxford Dictionary* spelling of albumin.

Albumin A simple protein soluble in water and dilute salt solutions and coagulable by heat. Examples are lactalbumin in milk and ovalbumin in egg.

Albumin/globulin ratio Ratio of albumin to globulin concentration in the serum. The normal value ranges from 1.8 to 2.5.

Albuminoid Also called scleroprotein; simple protein characteristic of skeletal structures and protective tissues such as skin and hair. It is of three distinct types: *elastin* in tendons and ligaments, *collagen* in tendons and bones, and *keratin* in hair, nails, and hooves. See Classification of proteins, Appendix C-2.

Albuminuria Presence of albumin in the urine. It occurs in kidney disease, toxemia of pregnancy, and certain conditions when circulation to the kidney is inadequate. Normally the kidneys reabsorb plasma albumin, which filters out from the glomerulus into Bowman's capsule.

Alcohol 1. Aliphatic hydrocarbon derivative containing a hydroxyl (—OH) group. 2.

Group of organic compounds derived from carbohydrate fermentation. 3. Unqualified, it refers to ethyl alcohol in wines and liquors.

Alcoholism Chronic excessive use of alcohol, which eventually leads to irreversible disorders affecting the liver, digestive system, and nerves. Thiamin absorption is also impaired among alcoholics, causing alcoholic thiamin deficiency. The diet of most alcoholics is usually deficient in both calories and essential nutrients. As a consequence, malnutrition and liver *cirrhosis* result. Alcohol has also been reported to induce hypoglycemia in some insulin-dependent diabetics, leading to complications —even death.

Aldehyde Class of organic compounds derived from primary alcohols by oxidation. It contains the —CHO group. Examples are formaldehyde and acetaldehyde.

Aldohexose A hexose that contains an aldehyde group, e.g., glucose and mannose.

Aldopentose A pentose that contains an aldehyde group, e.g., ribose and arabinose.

Aldosterone An adrenocortical hormone formerly called electrocortin. It plays an important role in the regulation of electrolyte balance. Aldosterone acts on the distal convoluted tubules of the kidneys to reabsorb sodium and water and excrete potassium.

Aldosterone-stimulating hormone (ASH) A specific hormone believed to be the immediate effector of aldosterone production by the adrenal cortex.

Aleukia Absence or extremely decreased number of leukocytes in circulating blood.

Algae Group of plants that have chlorophyll but do not have true stems, roots, or leaves. Certain algae are single-celled and form scum, whereas others are large, such as seaweed. Some algae are good sources of nutrients. See *Chlorella*.

Alginate Any of several salt derivatives of alginic acid, a colloidal acid polysaccharide obtained from seaweed. It is used as thickener and stabilizer in food products, sizing material for paper, and dental impression material.

Alicyclic Term given to organic compounds that have the "closed ring" arrangement of carbon atoms.

Alimentary Pertaining to food, nutrition, or diet.

Alimentary toxic aleukia (ATA) Fatal blood disorder caused by a toxin produced by a soil fungus growing on damaged grain.

Alimentary tract The digestive tract; extends from the mouth to the anus.

Aliment de sevrage Mixture of millet flour, peanut flour, skim milk powder, sugar, added vitamins A and D, and calcium. Developed in Senegal and used as a source of protein.

Aliphatic 1. Term given to organic compounds that have the "open-chain" structure. 2. Pertaining to fat or oil.

Aliquot A definite part of a whole; a known fraction of a sample.

Alkalemia Increase in pH or alkalinity of the blood.

Alkali Also called base. 1. Any substance that accepts or acquires protons. 2. A substance that dissociates in aqueous solution to yield —OH ions. 3. Class of compounds that saponify fats, form salts with acids, and form soluble carbonates.

Alkaline-ash residue Inorganic elements, chiefly sodium, potassium, calcium, and magnesium, that form basic ions (cations) in the body.

Alkaline-forming foods Foods in which the alkaline residue exceeds the acidic residue. These include milk, vegetables, and fruits (except cranberries, plums, and prunes). Most fruits, despite their acidity, exert a basic effect on the body since the organic acids in them, such as citric acid and malic acid, may be completely oxidized to carbon dioxide and water, leaving the salts to contribute to the supply of basic elements. Cranberries, plums, and prunes, however, contain benzoic and quinic acids, which are not oxidized in the body.

Alkaline tide Temporary increase in alkalinity of the urine and blood during digestion; due to the removal of hydrochloric acid from the blood.

Alkali reserve Buffer compounds in the blood, e.g., sodium bicarbonate, dipotassium phosphate, and proteins, that are capable of neutralizing acids. Sometimes called *blood bicarbonate* since bicarbonate is the chief alkali reserve of the body.

Alkaloid Naturally occurring basic nitrogenous compound, usually of plant origin. It is insoluble in water but soluble in organic solvents and can precipitate proteins. Many alkaloids from plants such as cocaine, strychnine, morphine, and quinine are useful in medicine.

Alkalosis An abnormal condition characterized by a rise in the pH or a fall in the hydrogen ion concentration of the blood. The condition results from excessive loss of acids from the body without comparable loss of base or the formation or supply of base at a rate faster than its neutralization or elimination. Alkalosis is commonly due to persistent vomiting and excessive intake of sodium bicarbonate; it may also be due to hyperventilation.

Alkaptonuria Inborn error of metabolism characterized by excretion of urine that darkens on contact with air due to the presence of abnormal amounts of homogentisic acid. Phenylalanine and tyrosine are not completely oxidized because of a lack of hepatic homogentisic acid oxidase. The precise dietary treatment is not known, although restriction of dietary protein to reduce homogentisic acid formation may be of some value.

Alkene Unsaturated aliphatic hydrocarbon having one double bond and represented by the general formula C_nH_{2n}.

Alkyl Saturated hydrocarbon radical with the general formula C_nH_{2n+1}. Examples are methyl (CH_3) and ethyl (C_2H_5).

Allantoin Final excretory product of purine metabolism in mammals, except primates. This results from the oxidation of uric acid by uricase, an enzyme lacking in primates.

Allele Also called allelomorph; the alternative form of the same gene. Alleles can occupy the same position on homologous chromosomes.

Allergen An agent or substance capable of producing an allergic reaction. Common allergens are inhalants (pollen, dust, hay), ingestants (food, beverage, condiment, drug), contactants (cosmetics, medicine, environment), and injectants (vaccine, serum, drug). It is also possible to have physical (heat, cold, sunlight) and emotional (feelings, moods) forms of allergy. See also *Food allergen*.

Allergy Unusual or exaggerated susceptibility to a substance (allergen) that is harmless in similar amounts to most people. See *Allergen* and *Food allergen*.

Allied health professions Those professions dedicated to the full delivery of comprehensive health care through assistance to the medical and dental professions.

Alligator skin See *Xeroderma*.

Alliithiamin Compound of thiamin and a substance found in onion and garlic oil. It enhances the absorption of thiamin.

Allopurinol Analog of hypoxanthine; a potent inhibitor of *xanthine oxidase*. It is widely used in treating hyperuricemia and gout.

All-or-none law 1. Response of an individual nerve or muscle fiber to an adequate stimulus is always maximal, i.e., a stimulus either causes a full-size impulse or it fails to set up an impulse. 2. Tissue synthesis occurs only when all the necessary amino acids are present in the proper amounts and proportion at the site of tissue formation. Absence of even one amino acid will prevent synthesis, and unless a tissue protein can be synthesized all at once, it is not synthesized at all.

Alloxan A red crystalline substance produced by the oxidation of uric acid. It can cause necrosis of the islets of Langerhans in the pancreas. Alloxan has been used in cases of hyperinsulinism due to pancreatic tumors, but it is toxic in high amounts.

Alloxan diabetes Experimental diabetes following the administration of alloxan, which preferentially damages the beta cells of the pancreas.

Alopecia Baldness or loss of hair. This is seen in experimentally induced *biotin* deficiency in rats, which begins with dermatitis around the eyes and progresses to general loss of hair. Alopecia in man is not corrected by administration of biotin. It is due to various causes, including seborrheic dermatitis, dandruff, effect of certain drugs or chemicals, syphilis, and other bacterial, fungal, or viral infections. It is also seen in *myxedema* and others cases of pituitary insufficiency.

Alpha First letter of the Greek alphabet. It is used with the name of a chemical compound to indicate the first of a series of isomers or the carbon atom next to the carboxyl group.

Alpha particle Positively charged particle given off by certain radioactive elements. It contains two protons and two neutrons. Alpha particles are known as alpha rays when ejected in a stream.

Aluminum A nonessential mineral found in trace amounts in the lungs, probably by inhalation with atmospheric dust. Its function in metabolism is not known, although aluminum in vitro promotes the reaction between cytochrome *c* and its reductant. It is very poorly absorbed. Large intakes, however, are known to produce gastrointestinal irritation and rickets. Aluminum combines with the phosphates present in food to form insoluble aluminum phosphate, which is excreted in the feces. But contrary to earlier beliefs, trace amounts of aluminum from cooking utensils are harmless and do not cause chronic poisoning.

Alveolus Pl. alveoli. Air sac in the lungs formed by terminal dilatations of the bronchioles. In the adrenal glands the small saclike structure is also referred to as the alveolus.

Amama A *multipurpose food* used in Nigeria, Kenya, and Uganda. It is a protein supplement for infants composed of a mixture of peanut flour, casein, and added vitamins and minerals.

Amaurosis Partial or total blindness.

Amblyopia Dimness of vision.

Amebiasis Infestation or infection with pathogenic amoebas, particularly *Entamoeba histolytica*. The parasite is commonly transmitted through cyst-containing feces, infected food, insects, and animals.

American Dietetic Association (ADA) Professional organization whose objectives are to improve the nutrition of human beings, to advance the science of dietetics and nutrition, and to promote education in these and allied areas. It publishes monthly the *Journal of the American Dietetic Association*.

American Institute of Nutrition (AIN) Professional organization founded in 1928 to develop and extend nutrition knowledge and to promote personal contact between researchers in nutrition and related fields. Only those who have published research and who are currently engaged in the field of nutrition may be elected to membership.

American International Development Agency (AID) Agency that helps developing countries in their various food, agricultural, and educational programs. See Agencies concerned with nutrition in the United States, Appendix L.

American Society for Clinical Nutrition (ASCN) Division of the *American Institute of Nutrition (AIN)* that aims to promote education about human nutrition in health and disease, to promote the presentation and discussion of research in human nutrition, and to publish a journal devoted to experimental and clinical nutrition. Members of AIN who have publications in the field of clinical nutrition may become members.

Amethopterin A potent metabolic antagonist of *folic acid*, a member of the vitamin B complex. It interferes with the conversion of folic acid to its active form, folinic acid.

Amidase Enzyme that catalyzes the hydrolysis of nonpeptide C—N linkages. It is a de-amidizing enzyme.

Amide Organic compound containing the radical —CO · NH$_2$. It is formed by replacing the hydrogen of ammonia with an acyl radical, R · CO—, to form R · CO · NH$_2$ or by replacing the —OH of the —COOH group of an acid with —NH$_2$.

Amine Compound that has the characteristic amino (NH$_2$) group. It is formed by replacing one or more of the hydrogen atoms of ammonia with one or more organic radicals. Amines are classified as *primary, secondary,* or *tertiary,* depending on whether one, two, or three hydrogens are replaced.

Amino acid (**AA**) Fundamental structural unit of protein with the general formula

$$NH_2-\underset{\underset{H}{|}}{\overset{\overset{R}{|}}{C}}-COOH.$$ Amino acids may be

acidic, basic, or neutral, depending on the number of acidic or basic groups in the molecule. According to structure, amino acids may be aliphatic, aromatic, or heterocyclic. Of the more than 20 amino acids considered to be physiologically important, eight are known to be essential for the human adult. The others are dietary nonessential amino acids.

Antiketogenic AA See *Glucogenic amino acid* under *Amino acid.*

Dispensable AA See *Nonessential amino acid* under *Amino acid.*

Essential AA (**EAA**) Also called indispensable amino acid; an amino acid that cannot be synthesized by the body from materials readily available at a speed commensurate with the demands for normal growth. It must therefore be supplied preformed in the diet. The eight essential amino acids for human adults are *isoleucine, leucine, lysine, methionine, phenylalanine, threonine, tryptophan,* and *valine.* In addition, *histidine* is essential for growing children.

Glucogenic AA An amino acid that can be converted to an alpha keto acid, a carbohydrate former. Examples are glycine, alanine, serine, threonine, aspartic acid, and glutamic acid.

Indispensable AA See *Essential amino acid* under *Amino acid.*

Ketogenic AA An amino acid that can be converted to acetate or acetoacetate, a ketone body. Examples are leucine, isoleucine, and lysine.

Limiting AA The essential amino acid that is most deficient in a protein, in comparison with the amino acids of a standard protein. Lysine is the limiting amino acid in rice and other cereals; tryptophan is limiting in corn; and methionine and cystine are limiting in beans.

Nonessential AA Also called dispensable amino acid; an amino acid that can be synthesized in the body provided there is an adequate source of nitrogen. It need not be supplied preformed in the diet. Examples are alanine, arginine, asparagine, aspartic acid, cystine, cysteine, glycine, glutamic acid, glutamine, hydroxyproline, proline, serine, and tyrosine.

Semidispensable AA See *Semiessential amino acid* under *Amino acid.*

Semiessential AA Also called Semidispensable amino acid; an amino acid that, when present in the diet, reduces the need for an essential amino acid. For example, cystine reduces the need for methionine, and tyrosine reduces the need for phenylalanine.

Amino acid antagonism Also called amino acid toxicity; applies to the "adverse effects resulting from the administration of excessive amounts of an amino acid."

Amino acid balance-imbalance Various amino acids are required by the body in certain definite proportions and amounts. Proteins that contain the right amounts of amino acids are said to be balanced. Any change in the proportion of amino acids, such as an excess or deficiency in one or more, creates an imbalance with respect to amino acids. Such an imbalance produces a protein that is said to be unbalanced. Intake of more of this unbalanced protein to meet the stated requirement for the deficient amino acid would create an excess of other amino acids, causing an antagonism that is more severe than the original amino acid deficiency or imbalance.

Amino acid pool Reservoir or metabolic pool of amino acids that come from the diet (exogenous source), that are synthesized in cells, and that are derived from the breakdown of tissue proteins (endogenous sources). The size of the pool is the quantity of the constituents instantaneously present and available for all of the reactions leading into and from the pool (i.e., anabolic and catabolic reactions).

Amino acid reference pattern The ideal combination of amino acids in total quantity and proportion to meet all physiologic requirements. The Food and Agriculture Organization reference pattern was derived from the minimal daily requirements for the essential amino acids for infants and adults. Other reference patterns have been based on the amino acids present in egg and human milk.

Amino acid toxicity See *Amino acid antagonism.*

Aminoaciduria Increase in the urinary excretion of amino acids due to elevated concentrations of amino acids in the plasma. The condition is caused by a defect in the renal tubular reabsorption of amino acids. The renal defect may be congenital in nature, or it may be acquired as a result of toxic agents, metabolic disorders such as acidosis and hypercalcemia, and deficiencies of vitamins B, C, and D.

Amino alcohol Compound containing both an amino group and an alcoholic hydroxyl group.

Aminogram Amino acid pattern showing the quantitative relationship between the essential amino acids in a dietary protein and those found in egg protein. Since egg is an unreasonably high protein standard for world supply, the Food and Agriculture Organization uses a theoretical ideal aminogram as the protein standard.

Aminopeptidase Enzyme occurring in the intestinal mucosa that catalyzes the hydrolysis of peptide linkages adjacent to the free alpha amino groups of a peptide.

Aminopterin Folic acid antagonist used clinically in the treatment of leukemia and other neoplastic diseases.

Amino sugar Sugar in which a hydroxyl group has been replaced by an amino group. Amino sugars known to occur in nature are all derivatives of aldohexoses, with the amino group on carbon atom 2. Examples are glucosamine and galactosamine.

Ammonia 1. Volatile alkaline gas soluble in water. 2. By-product of protein metabolism by deamination of amino acids. In the body, ammonia may be used in the reductive amination of alpha keto acids to form new amino acids, or it may be used in the synthesis of purines and pyrimidines. Ammonia is toxic in large concentrations and normally not allowed to accumulate in the cells. It is either excreted directly in the urine or eliminated via glutamine or urea formation. See Utilization of proteins, Appendix D-2.

Ammonium The univalent radical NH_4^+. It exists only in combination and forms salts such as the alkaline metals.

Amniotic fluid Fluid of the fetal membrane that serves as protection for the embryo.

AMP Abbreviation for *adenosine monophosphate.* See under *Adenosine phosphates.*

Amphetamine Synthetic drug used as a central nervous system stimulant and appetite depressant. It produces a sense of well-being and early satiety feeling during meals.

Ampholyte Amphoteric electrolyte capable of reacting either as a weak base or as a weak acid. Amino acids are amphoteric because they contain both the carboxyl or acidic group and the amino or basic group.

Amylase Enzyme that catalyzes the hydrolysis

of starch to sugar. There are two types: *alpha-amylase,* which splits 1,4-alpha-glucosidic bonds in random fashion, and *beta-amylase,* which attacks polysaccharide chains by successive removal of maltose units from the nonreducing end. An increased level of amylase in the blood is diagnostic of acute pancreatitis.

Amylo-1,6-glucosidase A glycogen debranching enzyme that hydrolytically removes glucose present in alpha-1,6 linkages at the branch points of a glycogen molecule. See also *Debranching enzyme.*

Amylolytic Pertaining to digestion of starch or its conversion to maltose.

Amylopectin A branched-chain starch component consisting of alpha-1,6 branch linkages in addition to alpha-1,4 linked glucose units. It gives a purple color with iodine.

Amylopsin Pancreatic enzyme that changes starch to maltose. It is an alpha-amylase with an optimal pH of about 7.1. Now called pancreatic amylase.

Amylose A starch component consisting of alpha-1,4 linked glucose units in a long, unbranched (linear) chain. It gives a blue color with iodine.

Amylo-(1,4-1,6)-transglucosylase A glycogen branching enzyme that cleaves fragments of the glycogen chain at alpha-1,4 linkages and transfers them to the alpha-1,6 linkages of the same or another glycogen molecule. See also *Branching enzyme.*

Amyotrophic lateral sclerosis Disease suspected of being associated with the consumption of flour prepared from the kernels of *Cycas circinalis.* It has been seen in cattle, sheep, and humans. Afflicted individuals progressively become paralyzed in their arms and legs and die about 5 years after the onset of symptoms.

Anabiotic Apparently lifeless but capable of revival or bringing to life.

Anabolism Synthesis; process by which simple substances are converted by living cells into more complex substances.

Anacidity Absence of hydrochloric acid in the stomach.

Anadipsia Intense thirst.

Anaerobic Occurring in the absence of oxygen.

Analgesia Absence of or insensibility to pain. An *analgesic* is a substance capable of abolishing the sensitivity to or feeling of pain.

Anaphylaxis Hypersensitivity or increased susceptibility to a foreign protein or substance. It is characterized by exaggerated reactions and widespread systemic involvement.

Anastomosis Surgical joining or formation of a passage between two organs, blood vessels, or nerves.

Anatomy Study of the structure of the body.

Androgen Generic name for the hormones secreted by the testes that are responsible for the development of male accessory sex organs and secondary sex characteristics. Androgenic hormones also have anabolic influence on nitrogen and calcium metabolism. The two major naturally occurring androgens are androsterone and testosterone.

Androsterone Hormone secreted by the testes. See *Androgen.*

Anemia Reduction in size or number of the red blood cells, of the quantity of hemoglobin, or of both, resulting in decreased capacity of the blood to carry oxygen. The symptoms are varied, e.g., breathlessness on exertion, easy fatigue, pallor, dizziness, insomnia, and lack of appetite. Anemias may be classified according to cell size, which may be large (macrocytic), small (microcytic), or normal (normocytic). Another classification is based on the color index of the blood, which may be high (hyperchromic), low (hypochromic), or normal (normochromic). Anemia may be due to excessive loss of blood, to excessive blood destruction as a result of chemical poisons such as lead or specific infections such as malaria, or to congenital abnormalities of the red cells, as in sickle cell anemia. Anemias may also be due to a defect in blood formation. This may be nutritional in origin or the defect may be due to aplasia of the bone marrow, toxic inhibition, or diseases that affect the bone marrow, spleen, liver, or lymph nodes.

Anemia, nutritional Anemia due to a deficiency of nutrients necessary in the formation of blood. Iron, protein, folic acid, vitamin B_{12}, and vitamin C are the major nutrients essential in blood formation. Copper and cobalt are also essential, but the amounts needed are so small that they are more than amply supplied by the normal adequate diet. The deficiency in these nutrients may be caused by inadequate intake, defective absorption, imperfect utilization, increased requirement, or increased excretion. See also *Hemopoiesis* and Dietary management of selected disorders, Appendix O.

Iron-deficiency a Form of anemia characterized by small (microcytic) and pale (hypochromic) erythrocytes. It is generally due to chronic blood loss, as in excessive or prolonged menstruation, repeated pregnancies, and parasitic infestation; faulty iron intake; impaired iron absorption, as in achlorhydria and chronic diarrhea; and increased blood volume, which occurs during infancy and pregnancy.

Protein-deficiency a Macrocytic type of anemia seen in association with protein malnutrition. Patients with this type of anemia also show signs of multiple nutritional deficiencies, especially folic acid, vitamin B_{12}, and iron.

Vitamin B_{12}– and folic acid–deficiency a Deficiency in either vitamin B_{12} or folic acid interferes with the normal development of erythrocytes, characterized by megaloblastic arrest in the bone marrow and the production of an insufficient number of large erythrocytes that carry a normal complement of hemoglobin (i.e., megaloblastic macrocytic normochromic anemia). Vitamin B_{12} deficiency may be due to inadequate intake of animal protein foods, lack of intrinsic factor, reduced absorptive capacity of the ileal mucosa, and competition for the vitamin by intestinal parasites. Folic acid deficiency may be due to inadequate dietary intake, increased demand for folic acid, as in pregnancy and chronic blood loss, malabsorption syndromes, and administration of drugs that are folic acid antagonists.

Vitamin C–deficiency a Macrocytic type of anemia seen in severe cases of vitamin C deficiency (scurvy). Vitamin C is necessary for the absorption of iron and the conversion of folic acid to its biologically active form, folinic acid.

Anesthesia Loss of feeling or sensation. It may be intentional through the use of various agents (anesthetics) or may be caused by disease.

Aneurine Former name for thiamin or vitamin B_1.

Aneurysm Localized dilatation or outpouching of a segment of an artery or wall of the heart due to weakness in the wall.

Angina pectoris A sudden, severe pain radiating from the heart region to the left shoulder and down the arm into the fingers. It tends to occur suddenly following emotional stress, physical exertion, and other conditions subjecting the heart to heavy strain. Angina occurs more frequently among men over the age of 40 years.

Angiogram X-ray film of the blood vessels after injection of an indicator substance that is opaque to x-rays.

Angiotensin A vasoconstrictor substance present in the blood. It is formed from an alpha$_2$ globulin by the action of the enzyme *renin,* which originates from the kidney. This substance was formerly called hypertensin or angiotonin.

Angiotensinogen Inactive precursor of angiotensin; formerly called hypertensinogen.

Angiotonase Enzyme that inactivates angiotonin (angiotensin). It is now called angiotensinase.

Angiotonin A vasoconstrictor substance in the blood. It is now called *angiotensin.*

Angstrom (Å) A unit for measuring light wavelengths. One angstrom is 0.1 mμ or 1×10^{-8} cm.

Anhydrase Enzyme that catalyzes reactions involving removal of water.

Anhydride Compound derived from a substance from which a molecule of water has been abstracted.

Animal protein factor (APF) Name given to a nutrient found in cow manure and fish meal that is required for rapid growth of animals. This is now known to be vitamin B_{12}. See *Vitamin B_{12}*.

Animal starch See *Glycogen*.

Anion A negatively charged ion.

Ankylosis The growing together of tissues in a joint with resulting stiffness and immobility.

Anode The positive pole or terminal of an electrode.

Anomaly 1. An abnormality or deviation from the usual. 2. Any part or organ existing in an abnormal form, location, or structure. The term is often used to describe development occurring before birth.

Anomers Pair of stereoisomers related to each other, as are alpha and beta D-glucose.

Anopia Absence of sight or defect in vision.

Anorexia Lack or loss of appetite.

Anorexia nervosa A mental state characterized by severe rejection of food, resulting in extreme loss of weight, low basal metabolic rate, exhaustion, and sometimes loss of hair. Death may occur from starvation. See Dietary management of selected disorders, Appendix O.

Anorexigenic drug An appetite depressant; used in weight reduction programs.

Anoxemia More correctly called hypoxemia; anoxemia is a decrease in the oxygen content of the blood. It may be due to heart failure, low partial pressure of oxygen, or high altitude.

Anoxia More correctly called hypoxia; anoxia is a condition of oxygen lack in the tissues or body. It may be caused by the failure of tissues to receive or utilize enough oxygen because of decreased blood capacity to carry oxygen (anemic anoxia), defective oxygenation of the blood in the lungs (anoxic anoxia), slow movement of blood through the capillaries as a result of shock or arterial obstruction (stagnant anoxia), or inability of body cells to utilize oxygen following certain types of poisoning (histotoxic anoxia).

Anserine Naturally occurring dipeptide of methyl histidine and beta-alanine universally distributed in muscles. It was first isolated from goose muscle.

Antacid A substance that neutralizes or counteracts acidity.

Antagonist An agent or substance that counteracts or blocks the effect of another. See also *Antimetabolite* and *Antivitamin*.

Anthelmintic Remedy for worms; a chemical destructive to worms.

Anthranilic acid Product resulting from the hydrolysis of *kynurenine* by the enzyme kynureninase with pyridoxal phosphate as a cofactor. In pyridoxine deficiency, hydrolysis of kynurenine results instead in the production of *xanthurenic acid*, which is excreted in the urine.

Anthropometry Scientific measurement of the various parts of the body. This includes the measurement of body weight, height, shoulders, chest, arms, head, and other body parts. Anthropometry is a useful aid in assessing nutritional status of individuals and groups.

Antiberiberi factor Former name for thiamin or vitamin B_1.

Antibiotic A substance elaborated by certain microorganisms that has the capacity to destroy or inhibit the growth of bacteria and other microorganisms. Examples are penicillin, aureomycin, terramycin, and neomycin.

Antibiotics and nutrition Antibiotics can enhance growth by altering intestinal microflora or by combating actual infection. However, under certain conditions antibiotics inhibit growth by interfering with normal physiologic function or by producing toxic metabolites. Therapeutic doses of tetracycline interfere with normal bone growth and protein synthesis, causing negative nitrogen balance. Neomycin is known to induce malabsorptive disorders similar to those seen in idiopathic steatorrhea.

Antibiotics in animal feeds Antibiotics are used in livestock and poultry feeds to prevent or treat diseases and to stimulate growth. Data on residues of antibiotics in meat, milk, and eggs from treated animals have raised questions about the potential hazards for man. If residues are not destroyed during food preparation or digestion, individuals sensitive to antibiotics might suffer adverse allergic reactions. Also, continued exposure to minute amounts of antibiotic residues in food could sensitize some individuals to these drugs.

Anti-black tongue factor Former name for niacin or nicotinic acid, a member of the vitamin B complex. See also *Black tongue.*

Antibody A specific substance produced in the body in response to invasion by a foreign or antagonistic substance known as an *antigen.* Antibodies are serum proteins elicited by the lymphoid cell system. These proteins, called *immunoglobulins* (Ig), protect the body by reacting as *agglutinins, lysins, precipitins,* or *antitoxins.*

Anticatalyst A substance that can retard the action of a *catalyst* by directly acting on the catalyst itself.

Anticholinergic Pertaining to the blocking of nerve impulses to the parasympathetic nervous system.

Anticholinesterase A substance that inhibits the action of cholinesterase (acetylcholinesterase), an enzyme needed in the transmission of nerve impulses. Anticholinesterase preparations serve as the active principle in some insecticides and in the so-called nerve gases.

Antichromotrichia factor Obsolete name for *pantothenic acid,* a water-soluble vitamin.

Anticoagulant A substance that inhibits or prevents blood coagulation by interfering with the clotting mechanism. Examples are *Dicumarol* and *heparin,* which inhibit prothrombin formation, and *oxalate* and

citrate, which combine with calcium. See *Blood clotting.*

Antidermatitis factor Obsolete name for *vitamin B_6.*

Antidiuretic An agent or drug that reduces urine formation.

Antidiuretic hormone (ADH) A hormone produced by the posterior portion of the pituitary gland (neurohypophysis). It has a marked antidiuretic action by increasing the rate of reabsorption of water from the kidney tubules, thus decreasing water excretion. A deficiency in this hormone results in a condition known as *diabetes insipidus.*

Antidote Drug or agent that counteracts the action of poison.

Anti-egg white injury factor Obsolete name for *biotin,* a member of the B complex vitamins.

Antienzyme An enzyme inhibitor. Various antienzymes are found in natural foodstuffs, among which are those that inactivate vitamins (such as thiaminase and ascorbic acid oxidase) and those that interfere with the activity of hydrolases in the intestinal juice (e.g., the antiproteinases and trypsin inhibitors).

Antigen A foreign substance that induces the production of an antibody when introduced directly into the body, as into the bloodstream.

Anti-gray hair factor Obsolete name for *pantothenic acid,* a water-soluble vitamin.

Antihemophilic globulin (AHG) Also called antihemophilic factor (AHF); factor necessary for the production of the plasma thromboplastic activity that is lacking in hemophilia. It is concerned with the conversion of prothrombin to thrombin. See *Blood clotting.*

Antihemorrhagic vitamin Former name for *vitamin K.*

Antiketogenic factor See *Ketogenic/antiketogenic ratio.*

Antimetabolite Structurally related compound that interferes with the metabolism or function of a chemical compound (metabolite) in the body. Also called metabolic antagonist.

Antineuritic vitamin See *Vitamin B₁* and *Thiamin*.

Antinutritive substance Chemical agent of natural origin whose action is contrary to optimum nutrition. It may act by decreasing nutrient solubility or hindering its utilization; increasing body requirement for certain nutrients; inactivating or destroying a nutrient; or reducing nutrient quantity or availability. Some of the well-known antinutritive substances are phytic acid, oxalic acid, avidin, Dicumarol, thiaminase, and the enzyme inhibitors.

Antioxidant A substance that delays or prevents oxidation. The more common ones are alpha-tocopherol, ascorbic acid, propyl gallate, butylated hydroxyanisole (BHA), butylated hydroxytoluene (BHT), and lecithin.

Anti-peptic ulcer factor See *Vitamin U*.

Antipernicious anemia principle One of the early names given to *vitamin B₁₂*. See also *Pernicious anemia*.

Antipyretic Agent or drug that relieves or reduces fever.

Antipyrine A chemical used as an antipyretic and analgesic; also widely used in total body water determinations. See *Water determination, body*.

Antirachitic factor See *Vitamin D*.

Antiscorbutic factor See *Vitamin C*.

Antiseptic A substance that prevents or inhibits the growth of microorganisms without necessarily killing them.

Antispasmodic Drug or agent that relieves spasms.

Antisterility vitamin See *Vitamin E*.

Antithrombin A substance present in blood plasma that inactivates *thrombin*, thus preventing coagulation of the blood.

Antithyroid agents A large number of substances that inhibit normal thyroid function either by inhibiting the synthesis of thyroid hormones or by preventing their release from the thyroid gland. Examples are thiourea, thiouracil, and goitrogens in foods.

Antitoxin A specific antibody that has the power of neutralizing the effect of a specific toxin.

Antivitamin A substance that interferes with the normal functioning of a vitamin by competitive inhibition, by inactivation, or by chemical destruction. Some of the most common antivitamins are Dicumarol (vitamin K), thiaminase (vitamin B₁), Atabrine (vitamin B₂), deoxypyridoxine (vitamin B₆), aminopterin (folic acid), and avidin (biotin).

Anuria Suppression of renal secretion; absence of urinary excretion. It may occur in the final stages of glomerulonephritis or after severe trauma, surgery, or transfusion of incompatible blood. Sometimes anuria is nervous in origin.

Anus Outlet of alimentary canal; the terminal portion of the rectum.

AOAC Abbreviation for *Association of Official Agricultural Chemists*.

Aorta Largest artery in the body, arising from the left ventricle and branching into every part of the body. Inflammation of the aorta is called *aortitis*.

AP Abbreviation for *as purchased*.

Apathetic Undemonstrative; indifferent.

Aperture An opening or orifice.

Apex The top or point of a conical part; the point of greatest response to stimuli.

APF Abbreviation for *animal protein factor*.

Aphagia Loss of ability or power to swallow.

Aphasia Loss of power of expression by speech.

Aphonia Loss of voice.

Aplasia Incomplete or defective formation of a tissue.

Apnea Temporary cessation of breathing.

Apoenzyme The protein component of an enzyme. See *Enzyme*.

Apoerythein Original name suggested for *intrinsic factor*.

Apoferritin The protein component of *ferritin*, an iron-protein complex.

Apoplexy Paralysis caused by a vascular lesion in the brain, such as hemorrhage or thrombosis.

Aposia Lack or absence of thirst.

Apositia Aversion for food; lack of desire for food associated with disgust.

Apparent digestibility Difference between the measured intake of food and the portion recovered in the feces. Expressed as a percentage, apparent digestibility is called *coefficient of digestibility.*

Appetite Natural desire or craving for food.

Applied Nutrition Program A practical nutrition program aimed at strengthening the national nutrition services and group feeding practices of a country; sponsored by the specialized agencies of the United Nations—WHO, FAO, and UNICEF. Applied nutrition programs are administered through these three international agencies in cooperation with the national and governmental agencies of the country.

Aqueous humor Clear watery fluid that fills the anterior chamber of the eye. It maintains the intraocular tension desirable for optical function. Increased secretion of the aqueous humor raises the intraocular pressure, giving rise to *glaucoma.*

Araban A pentosan that yields mixtures of L-arabinose.

Arabinose A pentose sugar widely distributed in root vegetables and plants, usually as a component of a complex polysaccharide. It has no known physiologic function in man, although it is used in studies of bacterial metabolism.

Arachidonic acid Unsaturated fatty acid containing 20 carbon atoms and four double bonds. It is an important constituent of lecithin and cephalin and occurs in the lipids of the brain, liver, and other organs. This fatty acid is considered one of the essential fatty acids. See *Essential fatty acid* under *Fatty acid.*

Arachidoside See *Goitrogens.*

Arachin A simple protein of the globulin type found in peanuts.

Areola A colored or pigmented circular area surrounding a central point, such as a pustule or nipple.

Argentaffin cells Cells found in the gastric glands of the stomach. They produce serotonin, which is secreted directly into the blood. The name means "silver-loving," indicating that these cells take up a silver stain.

Arginine Aminoguanidovaleric acid; a dibasic amino acid that is essential to growing chickens and rats. Its major metabolic roles include the synthesis of urea and creatine. Arginine is hydrolyzed to ornithine and urea by the enzyme *arginase,* found chiefly in the liver.

Arginosuccinic acid Intermediate product in the conversion of citrulline to arginine. It is formed by the condensation of citrulline and aspartic acid in the presence of adenosine triphosphate and magnesium.

Arginosuccinic aciduria Inborn metabolic defect due to a lack of the enzyme *arginosuccinase.* The condition is characterized by increased excretion of arginosuccinic acid in the urine, hair abnormalities, intermittent ataxia, seizures, coma, mental retardation, and ammonia intoxication. A diet moderately low in protein with arginine supplementation has been recommended.

Ariboflavinosis Term given to *riboflavin* deficiency. It is characterized by inflammation of the lips with cracking at the angles (cheilosis), sore mouth with purplish red tongue (glossitis), and dermatitis around the folds of the nostrils. Visual symptoms include photophobia, lacrimation, burning and itching of the eyes, and dimness of vision.

Arlac A protein-rich mixture developed in Nigeria; contains peanut flour, skim milk powder, salts, thiamin, riboflavin, vitamin B_{12}, and vitamin D.

Aromatic Carbon compound originating from benzene.

Arrest Cessation or stopping, as in cardiac arrest.

Arrhythmia Any irregularity in the normal rhythm of the heartbeat.

Arsenic A nonessential trace element found in the human body chiefly in the red blood cells, nails, and hair. Its biologic value is not known, although it is used therapeutically for treating syphilis. Arsenic is toxic even in small amounts, producing digestive disturbances, conjunctivitis, polyneuritis, stomatitis, and laryngitis. It is fatal in large amounts. Although naturally present in foods, the amount is too minute to cause toxicity.

Arteriole A very small arterial branch.

Arteriosclerosis Hardening, thickening, and loss of elasticity of the walls of the arteries. It is generally a part of the aging process, although factors other than advancing age are believed to hasten the condition. Among these are high blood pressure, diabetes mellitus, excessive nerve strain, certain infectious diseases, and several other factors not definitely known nor clearly understood. See also *Atherosclerosis*.

Artery Vessel conveying blood from the heart to the various parts of the body.

Arthritis Acute or chronic inflammation of a joint. It occurs in varying forms according to severity, location, deformity, and cause. The most common are *rheumatoid arthritis* (also called arthritis deformans and atrophic arthritis), *osteoarthritis* (also called degenerative or hypertrophic arthritis), and *gouty arthritis*. See Dietary management of selected disorders, Appendix O.

Articulation Junction or place of union between two or more joints.

Artificial feeding Introduction of food by an unnatural method, such as by *tube feeding, parenteral feeding,* and *gastrostomy feeding*. In infant feeding it refers to the nourishment of the baby other than by breast feeding. See *Infant feeding*.

Artificial kidney Device that removes blood from the artery of an arm, pumps it through a dialyzing membrane that allows accumulated toxic materials to pass into a surrounding bath, and returns clean blood to a vein. It is used in acute and chronic renal failure.

Ascites Accumulation of fluid in the peritoneal cavity due to portal hypertension, low blood protein levels, or sodium retention. The condition is often associated with cirrhosis of the liver, cardiac failure, and renal insufficiency. See Dietary management of selected disorders, Appendix O.

ASCN Abbreviation for *American Society for Clinical Nutrition*.

Ascorbase Ascorbic acid oxidase, a metalloenzyme that catalyzes the oxidation of free ascorbic acid to dehydroascorbic acid and other compounds with reduced or negligible vitamin activity.

Ascorbic acid Reduced form of *vitamin C*. See *Vitamin C;* see also *Dehydroascorbic acid*.

Aseptic Free from disease-producing germs.

Aseptic sterilization In infant feeding a process of formula preparation wherein the ingredients and equipment are separately sterilized. The sterile formula is then measured into sterile bottles, nippled, capped, and stored under conditions that will prevent contamination. See also *Terminal sterilization*.

ASH Abbreviation for *aldosterone-stimulating hormone*.

Ash Incombustible mineral residue remaining after all the organic matter has been burned or oxidized.

Asparagine The beta amide of aspartic acid present in most tissues and occurring abundantly in higher plants. It participates in transamination reactions. The enzyme *asparaginase* has anticancer activity in guinea pigs but produces side effects in humans. It depresses protein synthesis and causes nausea, anorexia, and loss of body weight.

Aspartic acid Aminosuccinic acid. A nonessential glucogenic amino acid involved in transamination reactions and the formation of urea, purines, and pyrimidines. It is hydrolyzed by the enzyme *aspartase* to fumaric acid and ammonia.

Asphyxia Loss of consciousness from too little oxygen and too much carbon dioxide in the blood. It may be brought about by suffocation or inhalation of toxic gases.

Aspiration 1. Inspiration or the act of

breathing. 2. Sucking in of fluids and gases from cavities.

As purchased (AP) The form in which food is offered for sale on the retail market; also refers to food before removing or trimming inedible parts. See also *Edible portion.*

Assay Analysis of a substance for determination of purity or content.

Assimilation Process of transforming food into a simpler form suitable for absorption and conversion into body tissues.

Association of Official Agricultural Chemists (AOAC) Voluntary organization of chemists that sponsors the development and testing of methods for analyzing nutrients, foods, food and color additives, animal feeds, liquors, beverages, drugs, cosmetics, pesticides, and many other commodities.

Asthenia Extreme weakness; loss of strength.

Asthma Chronic disorder characterized by wheezing, sneezing, and difficult breathing. It is usually an allergic reaction to pollens, feathers, food, or even bacteria.

Astrophysiologic dietetics Regulation of diet consistent with the normal functioning of an organism beyond the earth environment. See *Nutrition, space feeding.*

Asymptomatic Without symptoms.

ATA Abbreviation for *alimentary toxic aleukia.*

Atabrine Antimalarial drug; a riboflavin antagonist.

Ataxia Inability to coordinate bodily or muscular movements. It is generally due to a disorder in the brain or spinal cord, or it may be due to nutritional deficiencies, especially of the B complex vitamins.

Atelectasis 1. Airless or nearly airless state of the lung; collapse of the lung. 2. Incomplete expansion of the lung seen in the newborn.

Atheroma Fatty degeneration of the walls of the arteries.

Atherosclerosis Term denoting a number of different processes resulting in patchy deposition of various materials in the intima of the arteries. These deposits are produced by an accumulation of fatty substances (cholesterol, phospholipids, and triglycerides), complex carbohydrates, calcium and calcific plaques, fibrin, and the formed elements of the blood. Areas of thickening in the intima of affected arteries lead to narrowing and diminution of blood-carrying capacity. Atherosclerosis is the result of an interplay of several factors, including elevated blood lipids, high blood pressure, cigarette smoking, sedentary living, obesity, psychologic tensions, and endocrine disorders. Foods influence many of these risk factors. A diet high in saturated fat and cholesterol increases cholesterol and blood lipid levels; habitual overeating coupled with inactivity leads to obesity. Thus the recommended dietary modification for the general public in the prevention of atherosclerotic diseases involves three things, i.e., adjustment in caloric intake to achieve and maintain optimal weight; reduction in dietary cholesterol intake to 300 mg/day or less; and control of saturated fat intake to less than 10% of total calories. See *Diet, cholesterol-restricted, fat-controlled;* see also *Hyperlipoproteinemia.*

Athetosis Condition occurring chiefly in children and characterized by constant but slow recurrent movements of the hands, feet, and other parts of the body. It usually results from a lesion in the central part of the brain.

Athrepsia Malnutrition; severe undernutrition.

Atony Lack or absence of normal muscle tone.

ATP Abbreviation for *adenosine triphosphate.* See under *Adenosine phosphates.*

Atria Pl. of atrium. Upper chambers of the heart that receive blood from the veins.

Atrophy Wasting away; reduction in size of cell, tissue, organ, or part.

Attenuation Weakening or reduction of the virulence of pathogenic microorganisms.

Attrition 1. Abrasion or chafing of the skin or any surface. 2. Wearing away of tooth enamel by prolonged mastication of hard foods or because of clasp friction.

Atwater respiration calorimeter Apparatus for measuring total energy expenditure of the body by confining the subject inside the chamber. The original Atwater apparatus was later modifed by Rosa and Benedict. See *Direct calorimetry* under *Calorimetry*.

Atwater values Average physiologic fuel values of carbohydrate, protein, and fat based on experiments conducted by Atwater. He approximated that on a typical American diet each gram of carbohydrate, fat, and protein will yield 4, 9, and 4 calories, respectively. The Atwater values are used extensively in dietary calculations and food analysis. See also *Food, energy value*.

Aura Premonitory symptom or sensation that precedes the onset of a convulsive seizure. These are varied and may be a sensation of dizziness, abdominal discomfort, or numbness or spasm of an extremity.

Aureomycin Trade name for *chlortetracycline,* an antibiotic.

Auricle 1. Term commonly used for atrium of the heart. 2. Outer flap or pinna of the ear.

Auscultation Listening to sounds in the body to determine a condition, particularly of the heart, lungs, and abdomen.

Autoclasis Breakdown or destruction of a part developing within itself.

Autoclave Apparatus for sterilizing by steam under high pressure.

Autodigestion Self-digestion, as in the digestion of the walls of the stomach by the gastric juice.

Autoimmunity Self-immunity; the development of antibodies that react in vivo with a body constituent. These autoantibodies may arise as a result of individual contact with a substance related in structure to the body constituent. Recent interest in autoimmunity is focused on its possible role in the development of *diabetes mellitus*.

Autolysis Destruction or disintegration of tissues or cells by the action of specific enzymes; self-digestion of tissues within the body.

Auxin Natural or synthetic substance capable of stimulating growth in plants. The natural materials are found in the tips or roots of growing plants. Three of several that have been identified in foods are *3-indolacetic acid (IAA), gibberellin,* and *kinin.*

Avidin A specific protein in egg white that combines firmly with *biotin,* making it unavailable to the body. This results in a biotin deficiency syndrome known as *egg white injury*. Avidin in raw egg white is inactivated by heat and other agents that denature proteins.

Avitaminosis Literally, it means without vitamin. A better term to use is probably hypovitaminosis. The condition may be due to inadequate intake of vitamins, deficient absorption, increased body requirement, or ingestion of antivitamins.

Axerophthol See *Vitamin A.*

Axon Filament that conducts impulses away from a nerve cell.

Azaserine Diazoacetyl-1-serine; a compound that delays tumor growth in experimental animals and inhibits purine biosynthesis by retarding glutamine utilization. It is also used in the treatment of acute leukemia.

Azotemia Retention of urea and other nitrogenous substances in the blood. It is a manifestation of kidney disease.

B

Bacillus Pl. bacilli. One of the three major forms of *bacteria.* It is rod shaped and may be slender, short, straight, or slightly bent.

Bacitracin Antibiotic obtained from *Bacillus subtilis,* a gram-positive, spore-forming organism; it disrupts the structure and/or function of bacterial cell walls.

Bacteremia Presence of bacteria in the blood.

Bacteria Simple, one-celled microorganisms that multiply by simple division or by fission into two parts; visible only under the microscope. Bacteria are grouped as *cocci* (round shaped), *bacilli* (rod shaped), and *spirilla* (spiral shaped). Some are pathogenic, whereas others are harmless and beneficial (e.g., synthesize vitamins and other nutrients).

Bactericidal Capable of killing bacteria.

Bacterioclasis Breaking up or destruction of bacteria.

Bacteriolysis Dissolution of bacteria within or outside the living organism.

Bacteriophage Agent capable of injuring bacteria. The agent may be a living organism, e.g., a virus, or it may be an enzyme.

Bacteriostatic Hindering or checking the growth of bacteria.

Bag of waters Amniotic sac and its fluid that protects the fetus during pregnancy and helps dilate the cervix during delivery.

Bal-ahar A protein-rich food mixture used in India; made of mixed wheat flour, vegetables and defatted oil seed flour, vitamins, and calcium.

Balance study Quantitative method of measuring the amount of a nutrient ingested and the amount of the same nutrient or its metabolic end product(s) excreted in order to determine whether there has been a gain (positive balance) or loss (negative balance) in the body. At equilibrium, nutrient intake equals output. Balance studies are generally classified into two types, i.e., *balance of matter* (those dealing with nutrients that can be weighed) and *balance of energy* (those dealing with heat and energy). See *Energy balance, Nitrogen balance,* and *Water balance.*

Balm A healing or soothing medicine; a resinous, semifluid aromatic juice obtained from certain trees.

Band cells Those cells in which the nucleus appears as a curved, coiled, or twisted band without segmentation.

Barbiturate A sedative; a derivative of barbituric acid.

Barfoed's test Test for monosaccharides, which give a red precipitate of cuprous oxide when mixed with Barfoed's solution (copper acetate in acetic acid) and heated in a boiling water bath.

Barium 140 A relatively short-lived radioisotope with a half-life of about 13 days. Its metabolism is similar to that of calcium, being deposited mainly in the bones.

Barium test meal Meal consisting of a pint of fluid, either buttermilk or malted milk, into which a small amount of barium sulfate or bismuth is added. It is given after a 12-hour fast, usually in the morning before breakfast. The meal makes the stomach and intestinal tract opaque to x-rays and allows examination of the shape and movements in the gastrointestinal tract to determine the character and extent of any defect or abnormality.

Barlow's disease Scurvy in children. See *Scurvy.*

Basal metabolic rate (BMR) Amount of energy expended per unit of time under basal conditions. The adult basal metabolic rate is approximately 1 *calorie*/kg body weight per hour. The rate is affected by size, shape, and weight of the individual, body composition (amount of active protoplasmic tissue), age (highest during infancy with a gradual decline with advancing age), activity of the endocrine glands, state of nutrition, rate of growth, and pregnancy. Clinically the BMR is reported as percent above or below normal.

Basal metabolism Energy expended in the maintenance of "basal metabolic" processes or involuntary activities in the body (respiration, circulation, gastrointestinal contractions, and maintenance of muscle tonus and body temperature) and the functional activities of various organs (kidneys, liver, endocrine glands, etc.). It is taken under "basal" conditions, i.e., at complete physical and mental rest, in the postabsorptive state (12 to 16 hours after taking food), and in a temperature within the zone of thermal neutrality.

Basal metabolism determination Amount of heat produced by the body may be measured in two ways: *directly,* by measuring the amount of heat given off with the use of an apparatus called a *calorimeter;* or *indirectly,* by measuring the amount of oxygen consumed over a given period of time with the use of a *respirometer.* Basal metabolism may also be determined by using various prediction formulas developed by Boothby, DuBois, Berkson, and Dunn (based on *body surface area*); Harris and Benedict (based on body weight and standing height); and Kleiber (based on *metabolic body size*). Other prediction formulas include those of Brody, Fleisch, Robertson and Reid, and Young.

Base Same as alkali. See *Alkali.*

Basic food groups Classes of foods listed together under one heading because of their similarities as good sources of certain nutrients. The groupings may vary in different nations depending on the food habits, food economics, and dietary needs of a country. The basic food groups are used in planning and evaluating diets for nutritional adequacy. See the Four basic food groups and the Food grouping system in different countries, Appendices B-1 and B-2.

Basic-forming foods See *Alkaline-forming foods.*

Basophil 1. Basic-staining cell or tissue such as a basophil leukocyte. 2. Type of beta cell found in the *adenohypophysis.*

Basophilia Abnormal increase of basophils in the blood. It occurs in leukemia, severe anemia, lead poisoning, and other toxic states.

Batina A synthetic food resembling rice; made from vegetable sources. The major components are cereal flours (mostly wheat with some oats, barley, and corn), toasted legume flour (soy), wheat germ, dehydrated yeast, and vitamin and mineral supplements.

BCG *Bacillus of Calmette and Guerin;* a preparation of attenuated bovine tubercle bacilli culture used for immunization against tuberculosis.

Beer-Lambert law Fundamental law in spectrophotometry that states that the light absorbed by a solution is directly proportional to the thickness of the sample being analyzed and the concentration of the solute in the sample.

Behenic acid Saturated fatty acid containing 22 carbon atoms; found in seed oils.

Bence Jones protein Type of protein that appears in the urine in most cases of multiple myeloma, a disease involving the bone marrow.

Benedict-Roth spirometer Closed-circuit apparatus for measuring oxygen consumption over a period of time to determine basal metabolism. Body heat production is calculated by multiplying the volume of oxygen consumed by 4.825, the caloric equivalent of 1 L of oxygen. The Benedict-Roth spirometer is widely used in hospitals for basal metabolic rate tests. See also *Indirect calorimetry* under *Calorimetry*.

Benedict's test Semiquantitative test of the amount of reducing sugar present in solution (such as urine). Heating with Benedict's reagent (copper sulfate, sodium citrate, and sodium carbonate) gives a green, yellow, or orange-red precipitate, depending on the amount of reducing sugar (such as glucose) present in solution. This is a useful test for the presence of sugar in the urine.

Benign Not malignant; not fatal; not endangering life. The term is generally used to describe a growth that is not cancerous.

Benzidine test A sensitive test for blood. It gives a blue or green color in a saturated solution of benzidine in glacial acetic acid and hydrogen peroxide.

Benzimidazole cobamide One of the coenzyme forms of vitamin B_{12}. See *Cobamide*.

Benzinger apparatus An instrument that measures body heat by direct calorimetry. It is very sensitive to temperature changes and has a high degree of precision. See *Direct calorimetry* under *Calorimetry*.

Benzoic acid 1. An organic acid detoxified in the liver by combining with glycine, forming hippuric acid. 2. An antibacterial preservative in pickles, soft drinks, and sauces.

Beriberi Nutritional disease due to lack of thiamin (vitamin B_1). It is characterized by loss of appetite, general weakness, progressive edema, polyneuritis, and enlarged heart. There are three forms: *dry beriberi,* a form in which polyneuropathy and progressive paralysis are the essential features; *wet beriberi,* a form characterized by pitting edema and enlarged heart (beriberi heart disease); and *infantile beriberi,* seen in infants breast-fed by mothers suffering from beriberi. Cyanosis, tachycardia, and

cardiac failure are the advanced features of infantile beriberi. See *Thiamin* and *Vitamin B₁*.

Beta Second letter of the Greek alphabet. It is used with the name of a chemical compound to indicate the second of a series of isomers or to indicate the position of substituting atoms or groups in certain compounds.

Betaine Trimethylglycine, a methyl donor in the synthesis of choline and creatine. See also *Lipotropic agent* and *Methylating agent*.

Beta oxidation Also called Knoop theory of fatty acid degradation. Beginning at the carboxyl end or beta carbon of the chain, successive two-carbon fragments are removed, leaving a fatty acid two carbon atoms shorter than the original.

Beta particle Negatively charged particle identical with the electrons found in the outer structure of atoms. Nearly weightless, it may be emitted at high speed from a radioactive nucleus during beta decay, or it may be generated in a cyclotron or a high-voltage accelerating machine. When ejected in a stream, beta particles are called beta rays.

Bial's test Test for *pentoses,* which give a green flocculent precipitate of furfural when heated in a strongly acidified solution of orcinol.

Bicarbonate Salt of carbonic acid, characterized by the radical $—HCO_3$. Blood bicarbonate is the chief *alkali reserve* of the body. It plays a key role in the maintenance of constant hydrogen ion concentration in body fluids.

Bifidus factor Collective term for growth factors needed by *Lactobacillus bifidus* var. *pennsylvanicus* found in human milk and growing in the intestines of breast-fed infants. It is believed to be beneficial to young infants in preventing the growth of less desirable bacteria that cause intestinal putrefaction.

Bile Fluid produced and secreted by the liver, stored and concentrated in the gallbladder, and poured into the duodenum at intervals, particularly during fat digestion. It is greenish yellow to golden brown in color, bitter tasting, and alkaline in reaction. It aids in the emulsification and absorption of fat, activates the pancreatic lipase, and prevents putrefaction. Among its constituents are *bile acids, bile salts, cholesterol, lecithin,* and *bile pigments.*

Bile acids Glycocholic and taurocholic acids formed by the conjugation of glycine or taurine with cholic acid.

Bile pigments Principally bilirubin and biliverdin, which are responsible for the color of bile. Fresh bile manufactured in the liver is golden yellow because of its bilirubin content (an orange pigment). Bladder bile becomes greenish because of the oxidation of bilirubin to biliverdin. Bile pigments are derived from the breakdown of hemoglobin in the cells of the *reticuloendothelial system;* especially the liver.

Bile salts Chiefly sodium glycocholate and sodium taurocholate, which are the sodium salts of bile acids.

Biliary Pertaining to bile or the gallbladder.

Biliary dyskinesia Condition characterized by vague abdominal and colicky pains. It is due to improper or slow emptying of the gallbladder that is not associated with stone formation or inflammation.

Bilineurine See *Choline.*

Biliousness Digestive ailment commonly attributed to disorders of bile secretion. It is characterized by indigestion, headache, constipation, coated tongue, and general malaise.

Bilirubin Principal orange pigment of bile formed by the reduction of biliverdin, a product of hemoglobin breakdown. It is normally present in the feces and sometimes in the urine. Its accumulation in the blood results in jaundice. See *Jaundice.*

Bilirubin-globin The complex form in which bilirubin is transported in the blood. The globin portion is separated in the liver, and bilirubin is subsequently excreted into the bile canaliculi.

Bilirubin test Liver function test. Test is based on the ability of the liver to remove injected bilirubin from the blood. More than 5% bilirubin retention in the blood after 4 hours is indicative of impaired excretory function of the liver.

Bilirubinuria Presence of bilirubin in the urine. The urine is unusually dark, and the condition accompanies jaundice.

Biliverdin The green pigment of hemoglobin that undergoes reduction to bilirubin in the liver; one of the *bile pigments.*

Bioassay Also called biologic assay; measurement of the activity of a drug, substance, or nutrient by noting its effect on test animals or organisms.

Biocatalyst Biochemical catalyst or *enzyme.*

Biochemical test One method of assessing nutritional status. See Methods of research in nutrition: biochemical tests, Appendix M-4.

Biochemistry Study of the chemical composition of living matter and the changes that occur in it. Such changes may be *physiologic* (those existing under normal conditions) or *pathologic* (those occurring under abnormal conditions).

Biocytin Biotinyl lysine; a naturally occurring complex of biotin and lysine that can be isolated from yeast. It is a source of biotin for some microorganisms but is unavailable for other uses unless previously hydrolyzed.

Bioenergetics Study of the transformation of energy in biologic functions.

Bioflavonoid One of a group of naturally occurring substances belonging to the flavin and flavonoid compounds. It was originally called *vitamin P* and was first isolated from the peel of citrus fruits. The bioflavonoids (citrin, hesperidin, rutin, quercetin) are widely distributed among plants. They are thought to reduce capillary fragility and maintain normal conditions in the walls of the small blood vessels.

Biogenesis The origin of life; the theory that living organisms come only from living organisms.

Biologic assay See *Bioassay.*

Biologic oxidation Also called physiologic

oxidation; the cellular reactions in liberating energy by the transfer of electrons via the *redox systems.*

Biologic value (BV) Relative nutritional value of individual proteins as compared to a standard protein. It is the percentage of the true digestible protein utilized by the body, i.e., digested and absorbed nitrogen (protein) that is utilized by the body and not excreted in the urine. As expressed by the Thomas-Mitchell equation, the BV may be calculated as follows:

$$\%BV = \frac{100 \times N \text{ intake} - [(FN - MN) + (UN - EN)]}{N \text{ intake} - (FN - MN)}$$

where N = nitrogen, FN = fecal nitrogen, MN = metabolic nitrogen, UN = urinary nitrogen, and EN = endogenous nitrogen.

Biology Study of living cells in plants (botany) and animals (zoology).

Biometrics Statistical study of biologic problems.

Biomicroscopy Microscopic study of living cells in the body.

Biophotometer Instrument designed to measure *dark adaptation* ability.

Biopsy Microscopic examination of an excised piece of living tissue for purposes of diagnosis.

Bios Term given to a substance that stimulates the growth of yeast, which was later shown to be composed of two fractions: bios I (inositol) and bios II (biotin).

Biosterol Obsolete name for *vitamin A.*

Biosynthesis Synthesis or building up of a substance in a living organism.

Biotin A member of the B complex vitamins. It is essential for the activity of many enzymes in bacteria, animals, and man. Biotin is involved in *carbon dioxide fixation* reactions and in the synthesis of fatty acids and purines. Dietary biotin deficiency is unlikely to occur; the vitamin is widely distributed in nature. However, deficiency can be induced by large intakes of raw egg white, producing a syndrome charac-

terized by scaly dermatitis, muscle pains, general malaise, and depression. Former names given to this vitamin are vitamin H, bios II, coenzyme R, anti-egg white injury factor, and factors S, W, and X. For further details, see Summary of vitamins, Appendix I-1. See also *Avidin.*

Bitot's spot A small, triangular, silvery patch of epithelial degeneration, sometimes with a foamy surface, on the conjunctiva. Its exact cause is not known but it frequently occurs in persons with definite signs of vitamin A deficiency.

Biuret Compound derived from heating two molecules of urea, liberating ammonia.

Biuret reaction Test for *peptide* bond. Compounds with two or more peptide linkages give a blue-violet color with dilute copper solution in strong alkali.

Bivalent Having a valence of two; having the ability to combine with or displace two atoms of hydrogen or their equivalent.

Black tongue Nutritional disease in dogs analogous to human pellagra; due to *niacin* deficiency.

Bladder 1. Hollow organ in the anterior part of the pelvic cavity that serves as a reservoir for urine. 2. Any sac or receptacle for fluids or gases.

Blastoma A tumor.

Bleeding time Time required for bleeding to stop following puncture of the earlobe or ball of the finger. It is normally 1 to 4 minutes.

Blood Fluid medium that carries oxygen and nutritive materials to the tissues, removes carbon dioxide and waste products for elimination by the excretory organs, and distributes other substances (such as clotting factors, regulatory agents, and body defense mechanisms) throughout the body for utilization or action. It consists of *formed elements* (erythrocytes, or red blood cells; leukocytes, or white blood cells; and thrombocytes, or blood platelets) and a pale yellow portion, *plasma,* which contains a large number of organic and inorganic substances in solution. See Normal constituents of blood, Appendix Q.

Blood clotting An extremely complicated process that takes place in several phases. For simplicity, the process may be divided into three phases: first, the formation of thromboplastin by the sequential action of factors V, VII, XII, XI, IX, VIII, and X in the presence of calcium ion; second, the conversion of the inactive prothrombin into its active form, thrombin, by the action of thromboplastin in the presence of calcium ion and factors V, VII, and X; and third, the conversion by thrombin of the soluble fibrinogen into insoluble fibrin, which forms the meshwork of the clot. At least 12 factors are involved in blood clotting. These factors are designated by Roman numerals: I (fibrinogen), II (prothrombin), III (thromboplastin), IV (calcium), V (proaccelerin; also called accelerator globulin, labile factor, and prothrombin accelerator), VII (proconvertin) VIII (antihemophilic factor, AHF), IX (Christmas factor or plasma thromboplastin component, PTC), X (Stuart factor), XI (plasma thromboplastin antecedent, PTA), XII (Hageman factor), and XIII (fibrin stabilizing factor).

Blood grouping Classification of human blood into four groups based on the presence or absence of two major substances, A and B, in the erythrocytes. These substances may be found separately, or together, or both may be missing. Thus the four blood grouping or types are A, B, AB, and O. Another grouping of blood is based on the presence of MN factors, with three blood groups—M, N, and MN.

Blood lipids Principally cholesterol, phospholipid, and triglyceride. These lipids circulate in the plasma bound to proteins. As lipoprotein complexes, the otherwise insoluble lipids are solubilized, thus enabling their transport in and out of the plasma. Four major types of lipoproteins have been identified by electrophoresis and ultracentrifugation: *beta lipoprotein* (or low den-

sity lipoprotein, LDL), *prebeta lipoprotein* (or very low density lipoprotein, VLDL), *alpha lipoprotein* (or high density lipoprotein, HDL), and *chylomicron*. Each type contains phospholipid, triglyceride, cholesterol, and protein in varying proportions. Most of the lipid in the blood is in the beta lipoprotein form. See *Hyperlipoproteinemia*.

Blood platelet Also called thrombocyte; one of the three formed elements of the blood that is necessary in the clotting of blood. Blood platelets are thought to liberate small amounts of thromboplastin, which activates the proenzyme prothrombin to its active form, thrombin, the enzyme that catalyzes clot formation. See *Blood clotting*.

Blood pressure (BP) Pressure of the blood on the walls of the arteries. The human heart pumps intermittently by means of a sudden contraction of the entire ventricular musculature, followed by a period of relaxation. The pressure during the contraction phase is called systolic pressure and the pressure during the resting phase is called diastolic pressure. In recording blood pressure the systolic pressure is written first followed by the diastolic pressure.

Blood sugar level (BSL) Normal level of sugar (glucose) per 100 ml of blood is about 70 to 100 mg by the Somogyi method or 80 to 120 mg by the Folin-Wu method. Among several factors that *maintain* blood sugar level are glycogen-glucose interconversion in the liver, conversion of carbohydrate to fat, formation of muscle glycogen and its utilization, and glucose excretion in the urine (renal threshold). Conditions that *increase* blood sugar level include diabetes mellitus, hyperfunction of the anterior pituitary gland, hyperfunction of the adrenal cortex, epinephrine, insufficient insulin production, hyperfunction of the thyroid gland, head injury, fright, and anger. Conditions that *decrease* blood sugar level include functional hyperinsulinism, anterior pituitary deficiency, adrenal insufficiency, hypothyroidism, prolonged undernutrition, tumor of the pancreas, and abnormal kidney function (renal glycosuria).

Blood type Generally refers to the ABO system of blood grouping. See *Blood grouping*.

Blue baby Newly born infant suffering from *cyanosis*.

BMR Abbreviation for *basal metabolic rate*.

Boas test meal Test meal for *gastric analysis*. One pint of thin oatmeal gruel is given on an empty stomach, usually in the morning, to stimulate the secretion of gastric juices. See *Gastric analysis* under *Gastric*.

Bodansky unit A measure of *alkaline phosphatase* activity; the quantity of phosphates equivalent to the actual (or calculated) liberation of 1 mg phosphorus as phosphate ion during the first hour of incubation at 37° C and at a pH of 8.6 with the substrate hydrolysis not exceeding 10%. See *Alkaline phosphatase* under *Phosphatase*.

Body composition Representative percentage composition of a human adult is about 16% protein, 20% fat, 0.5% carbohydrate, 4.5% ash, and 60% water. These body components are distributed through four separate compartments designated as lean body mass, extracellular fluid, mineral skeleton, and adipose tissue. Complete chemical analyses of the human cadaver are few and not sufficient to give the range of variations in people of different ages and sex.

Body composition determination The living body can be partitioned into essentially two compartments: the fat-free portion and the fat portion, or adipose tissue. The fat-free weight of an individual remains relatively constant; variability in total weight is attributed to varying degrees of fatness. Several methods have been employed in determining human body composition. These include body density and specific gravity measurements; basal oxygen consumption; urinary creatinine excretion; soft tissue x-ray films; skin-fold, skeletal, and anthropometric measurements; and total body water determinations.

Body surface area Area covered by the exterior of the body. The surface area of the body was first determined by wrapping the body with a gauze tape, removing the tape, and measuring the area covered. Body surface area can now be estimated by plotting a person's height and weight on a standard chart developed by DuBois.

Body water See *Water compartment, body*.

Boiling point Temperature at which the vapor pressure of a liquid is equal to the prevailing atmospheric pressure. Water boils at 100° C at sea level when the atmospheric pressure is 760 mm Hg.

Bolus Mass of food ready to be swallowed.

Bomb calorimeter Apparatus that measures directly the energy value of foods. It consists of an inner chamber that holds the food sample and a double-walled insulated jacket that holds a can containing water. An electric connection ignites the weighed sample of food. A differential thermometer records the rise in the temperature of the water surrounding the chamber. The bomb calorimeter was devised by Berthelot and modified by Atwater.

Bone Also called osseous tissue; a mineralized connective tissue consisting of an organic matrix in which inorganic elements (mineral salts) are precipitated in a crystal lattice structure similar to that of the naturally occurring mineral *hydroxyapatite*. The organic matrix consists largely of *collagen* in a gel of cementing substance. The mineral fraction is composed largely of calcium phosphate, carbonate, fluoride, and citrate. Specialized bone cells (osteoblasts, osteoclasts, and osteocytes) control the relationship between the organic matrix and the bone salts.

Boron A nonessential mineral found in most tissues, especially the brain, liver, and body fat. Although required by all plants, its role in human nutrition is not known. Dietary lack in man has not been demonstrated.

Botulism Food poisoning caused by the toxin produced by *Clostridium botulinum*. The spores produced by the bacillus are relatively heat resistant, and they develop under anaerobic conditions, such as found in improperly canned foods. Botulinal poisoning is usually fatal. The toxin affects the nervous system, causing double vision, difficulty in swallowing, and respiratory failure.

Bourquin-Sherman unit Amount of riboflavin that will give an average weekly weight gain of 3 gm, using rats as test animals.

Bout An attack.

Bovine Pertaining to cattle.

Bowel The intestines.

Boyle's law Volume of a gas is inversely proportional to the pressure at constant temperature.

BP Abbreviation for *blood pressure*.

Bracken fern poisoning Type of "poisoning" observed in horses and cattle that graze on ferns that contain thiaminase, an enzyme that destroys thiamin (vitamin B_1). Bracken fern also contains a large amount of a cancer-producing chemical.

Bradycardia Abnormally slow heartbeat.

Brain Part of the nervous system contained in the cranial cavity; it consists of the *cerebrum, cerebellum, pons,* and *medulla oblongata,* which are connected to the spinal cord by the brain stem.

Branching enzyme Amylo $(1,4 \rightarrow 1,6)$ transglycosylase; an enzyme that transforms alpha-1,4 linkages to alpha-1,6 linkages to make the necessary branching points for amylopectin and glycogen.

Bremil Commercial product for routine infant feeding; made of nonfat milk with vegetable oil (corn, coconut, and peanut oils) and added lactose. (Borden.) See Proprietary foods: composition, features, and uses, Appendix P-1.

Bromelin Proteolytic enzyme found in pineapple; commercially used as a meat tenderizer.

Bromsulphalein Trade name for sulfobromophthalein sodium, a chemical used in liver function tests.

Bromsulphalein test Liver function test. Test is based on the ability of the liver to remove injected Bromsulphalein from the blood. Normal retention of this dye is less than 5% after 30 minutes. Delayed removal indicates liver damage or dysfunction.

Bronchi Pl. of bronchus. The branches of the trachea that are the air conduits supplying the right and left lungs. Each bronchus divides repeatedly until the branches become fine tubes known as bronchioles.

Bronchitis Acute or chronic inflammation of the membrane lining the bronchial tubes. Acute bronchitis may be due to extension of infection from the upper respiratory tract. Chronic bronchitis may be caused by irritants in polluted air, particularly smoke or gas fumes.

Bronsted theory According to Bronsted, an *acid* is any substance in ionic or molecular form that produces or donates protons, while a *base* is any substance that accepts or acquires protons. This is a broader definition of acid and base. The older established definitions restricted an acid to a substance producing hydrogen ions and a base to a substance producing hydroxide ions in water solution.

Bronsted-Lewis theory Lewis' modification of the *Bronsted theory* is more general. This theory states that "an acid is any substance which acts as an electron-pair acceptor in a chemical reaction, and a base as an electron-pair donor."

Brownian movement Random and zigzag motion of particles in solution, especially those of colloidal dimensions, due to the collision or bombardment of one molecule with another.

Brucellosis Also called undulant fever; a general infection with acute or insidious onset caused by one of the species of *Brucella*. It is characterized by intermittent fever, headache, weakness, profuse sweating, chills, and general aching. The disease is usually transmitted by contact with infected animals or by ingestion of milk and dairy products from infected animals.

BSL Abbreviation for *blood sugar level.*

BSP Abbreviation for *Bromsulphalein.*

Buccal Pertaining to the cheek.

Buffer Agent that resists marked changes in hydrogen ion concentration with the addition of acids or bases. In general, buffer action is exhibited by ions of weak acids or weak bases and their salts, by proteins, and by amino acids. Buffers play a vital role in the regulation of acid-base balance in the body. The principal buffer systems in the blood are the plasma proteins, carbonic acid, sodium bicarbonate, mono- and disodium phosphate, mono- and dipotassium phosphate, oxyhemoglobin, and reduced hemoglobin.

Bufotenin A methylated derivative of *serotonin* that is fairly widely distributed among amphibians. It can cause marked central nervous system damage in mammals.

Bulimia Excessive hunger; insatiable appetite.

Bulk The indigestible portion of carbohydrates that is not hydrolyzed by enzymes of the human gastrointestinal tract. See also *Crude fiber.*

Bulking agent A metabolically inert substance, such as nonfibrous cellulose, added to food to increase its volume without any calorie contribution.

BUN Abbreviation for *blood urea nitrogen.* See *Urea* and Normal constituents of blood, Appendix Q.

Bunion Inflammation in the synovial *bursa* of the great toe with thickening of the overlying skin.

Burn Tissue injury or destruction caused by excessive heat, caustics (acids or alkalis), friction, electricity, or radiation. On the basis of the extent of injury, burns are divided into three degrees: *first degree,* with simple redness of the affected parts; *second degree,* with the appearance of blisters in addition to redness; and *third degree,* with actual destruction of the skin and underlying tissues. Nutritional management following burns consists of immediate fluid and electrolyte replacement followed by a diet high in protein, calories, and vitamins, especially vitamin C.

Burning feet syndrome Nutritional deficiency disease due to lack of protein and the B complex vitamins, especially pantothenic acid. There is a burning or throbbing sensation in the feet that intensifies, with sharp, stabbing pains as the condition becomes worse.

Bursa Small sac filled with viscid fluid situated between tissues or parts where friction would otherwise develop. *Bursitis* is the inflammation of a bursa.

Butyric acid Short-chain saturated fatty acid containing four carbons. It is present as triglyceride in butterfat and milk; other fats contain very small amounts of butyric acid. It is a mobile liquid, is miscible with water, alcohol, and ether, and can easily volatilize with steam.

Butyryl CoA A butyryl derivative of *coenzyme A* (CoA); an intermediate product in the biosynthesis of fats.

BV Abbreviation for *biologic value.*

C

Cachexia Weakness, extreme weight loss, and severe wasting of tissues due to long-standing chronic diseases, malnutrition, or terminal illnesses. It is often associated with cancer.

Cadaver A corpse; a dead body.

Cadaverine Diaminopentane, a compound formed by the decarboxylation of lysine. It is produced during the decomposition of protein and occurs occasionally in the urine of patients with cystinuria.

Cadmium Mineral believed to be related to fat metabolism and the development of hypertension and atherosclerosis. High levels of cadmium are present in the kidneys of hypertensive patients.

Caffeine Trimethyl xanthine, theine, and methyltheobromine; an alkaloidal purine found in coffee, tea, and cola drinks. It is a cardiac and renal stimulant producing varying pharmacologic effects in people.

Cal Abbreviation for *calorie*.

Calcareous Containing calcium; of the nature of limestone.

Calcemia Presence of large amounts of calcium in the blood; more appropriately called *hypercalcemia*.

Calcifediol 25-Hydroxycholecalciferol (25-HCC), the functional, hormonal form of vitamin D_3 responsible for stimulating intestinal calcium transport. This compound is very effective in treating vitamin D–resistant rickets.

Calcification Deposition of calcium salts within the tissues of the body. It is a normal process in bone formation or may be abnormal, as in pathologic calcification in soft tissues, particularly arteries, kidneys, lungs, pancreas, and stomach. Deposition of calcium salts also occurs in areas of fatty degeneration and in dead or chronically inflamed tissues. Thus areas of necrosis, infarcts, scar tissues, and caseous tuberculous areas have calcium deposits.

Calcitonin Hormone secreted by the thyroid gland that is concerned with the regulation of calcium ions in the blood. Its action is opposite that of *parathormone*. When the blood calcium level is high, calcitonin is secreted and somehow "shuts off" the release of calcium from bones.

Calcium A major mineral constituent of the body that makes up 1.5% to 2% of body weight. Of this amount, 99% is present in bones and teeth; the remaining 1% is found in soft tissues and body fluids and serves a number of functions not related to bone structure. Calcium is important in blood coagulation, transmission of nerve impulses, contraction of muscle fibers, myocardial function, and activation of enzymes. It is a dietary essential. Good food sources are milk, cheese, and other milk products (except butter) and some green leafy vegetables. Calcium deficiency results in *rickets* in children and *osteomalacia* in adults. For further details, see Summary of minerals, Appendix H.

Calcium rigor State of tonic contraction of muscles due to elevated blood calcium levels. It is probably due to dysfunction of the parathyroid gland.

Calculus Pl. calculi. An abnormal stony mass in the body, found principally in ducts, passages, hollow organs, and cysts. It is more commonly called a stone, such as a kidney stone and a gallbladder stone.

Calibration Measurement of the caliber of a tube or performance of a device so that it may be used for subsequent measuring procedures.

Caliper Instrument for measuring linear dimensions. Calipers may be fixed, adjustable, or movable. The three types that are often used in nutrition surveys are the skin-fold, sliding, and spreading calipers.

Callus A horny thickened area of the epidermis often found on the palms of the hands and the soles of the feet. It may be of the same nature as corns, although sometimes a fungus is associated with it.

Calorie A heat unit. The amount of heat required to raise the temperature of 1 kg of water 1 degree centigrade. This is the large Calorie, or kilocalorie (spelled with a capital C), which is 1000 times as large as the small calorie (spelled with a small c). In nutrition, the kilocalorie is used, and this is generally understood whether the word is written with a capital C or a small c. The small calorie is used in physics. See also *Joule*.

Calorimeter Apparatus for measuring the amount of heat produced by an individual or a substance.

Calorimetry Measurement of heat absorbed or given out by a system or body. The measurement is carried out in either of two ways: *direct* or *indirect* calorimetry.

Direct c Direct measurement of heat loss from the body by placing the subject in an insulated boxlike chamber and noting the rise in temperature of the water circulating in the tubes surrounding the chamber. Examples of equipment used for direct calorimetry are the Atwater calorimeter and Benzinger's apparatus.

Indirect c Measurement of heat produced by a subject by calculating oxygen consumption and carbon dioxide elimination over a given period of time. A certain amount of heat is liberated per liter of oxygen used in oxidizing each of the major foodstuffs (known as the calorific value of 1 L of oxygen). Also, a specific ratio or *respiratory quotient* exists between the amount of carbon dioxide liberated and the oxygen used to oxidize each foodstuff. Under basal conditions the calorific value of 1 L of oxygen is 4.825 and the respiratory quotient is constant at 0.82. The *Kofranyi-Michaelis respirometer* uses the principle of indirect calorimetry.

CAMP Abbreviation for *computer-assisted menu planning*. See *Computer*.

Camu-camu A small red sour fruit known for its high ascorbic acid content (about 2000 mg/100 gm). It grows abundantly in Peru.

Cancer Common term for a malignant cellular growth that tends to spread. The cause(s) of human cancer is not definitely established, although contributing or predisposing factors are known in many cases.

Cancrum oris An infective gangrene of the mouth that erodes the lips and cheeks, giving the appearance of harelip. This has been reported chiefly in South Africa and is presumably caused by a combination of malnutrition and infection. See *Synergism*.

Canker A small area of ulceration of the mouth and lips, usually associated with various infections or stomach upsets.

Capillary A minute blood vessel connecting arteries with veins. It exists as part of a vast network throughout the body.

Capillary resistance test Test to determine the tendency of blood capillaries to break down and produce petechial hemorrhages. This is done by applying enough pressure to obstruct venous blood return on an arm and noting the number of *petechiae* produced after 5 minutes.

Capric acid Solid fatty acid with 10 carbon atoms in its chain. It is found in coconut oil, butter, and other animal fats.

Caproic acid Liquid fatty acid with six carbon atoms in its chain. It occurs as a glyceride in butter and coconut fat.

Caprylic acid Solid fatty acid with eight carbon atoms in its chain. It is found in coconut oil, butter, and human fat.

Caratatoxin A toxic substance isolated from the ordinary carrot. Large doses can produce neurotoxic symptoms in mice. However, it is unlikely that the normal consumption of carrots would ever lead to toxic effects in humans.

Carbaminohemoglobin Compound of hemoglobin and carbon dioxide; the principal form in which carbon dioxide is transported from the tissues to the lungs.

Carbamylphosphate Product formed by the reaction between carbon dioxide and ammonia in the presence of adenosine triphosphate. It is the active carbamylating compound in the biosynthesis of pyrimidine and in the formation of citrulline from ornithine.

Carbanion Ion containing a negatively charged carbon. It is also called a nucleophil because it has a pair of unshared electrons.

Carbohydrases Collective term for enzymes that hydrolyze higher carbohydrates into simple sugars. See Summary of enzymes, Appendix J-2.

Carbohydrate Polyhydroxy aldehyde, ketone, or any substance that yields one of these compounds. The term was originally designated for compounds of hydrates of carbon having the general formula $C_x(H_2O)_y$. Now it includes other compounds having the properties of carbohydrate even though they do not have the required 2:1 ratio of hydrogen to oxygen. Some carbohydrates contain nitrogen and sulfur in addition to carbon, hydrogen, and oxygen. The most important carbohydrates are sugar, starch, and cellulose. Carbohydrate is the major source of energy and provides 45% to 50% of the calories of the American diet. It occurs in the body chiefly as glucose ("physiologic sugar") and glycogen ("animal starch"). For further details, see Classification of carbohydrates and Utilization of carbohydrates, Appendices C-1 and D-1.

Carbohydrate by difference In the *proximate analysis* of food this is the difference ob-

tained by subtracting from 100 the sum of the percentages of water, protein, fat, and ash content. Included in this value, in addition to the sugars and starches, which the body can utilize almost completely, are the *crude fiber* and some organic acids that the body cannot utilize.

Carbohydrate function Carbohydrate is the primary source of heat and energy. It has a protein-sparing effect and serves as carbon skeleton for the synthesis of nonessential amino acids. Glucose is the major energy source of the brain and nervous tissues, lactose increases absorption of calcium from the intestinal tract and provides a medium for the growth of favorable intestinal bacteria, and the indigestible carbohydrates stimulate peristaltic movement and help prevent constipation.

Carbohydrate intolerance (malabsorption) Carbohydrate or sugar malabsorption comprises a group of conditions in which the absorption of one or more nutritionally important carbohydrates is caused by a deficiency in one or more of the intestinal disaccharidases (lactase, maltase, isomaltase, invertase, and trehalase) or by blockage in the transport mechanism across the gut. Disaccharidase deficiency may be a congenital defect, or it may be acquired in association with certain diseases (celiac disease, enteritis, kwashiorkor, and malnutrition) due to unspecific lesions in the intestinal mucosa. The chief clinical manifestation is diarrhea, which occurs when the sugar that cannot be absorbed is introduced into the diet.

Carbohydrate metabolic index (CMI) Formula developed by Horwitt and Kreisler for determining the thiamin requirement and detecting early thiamin deficiency states. Healthy persons have a CMI value below 15; thiamin-deficient persons have a CMI value above 15.

Carbon A nonmetallic element occurring in all organic compounds and widely distributed in nature. Its tetrahedral atom enables it to link with a wide variety of chemical combinations. Radioactive carbon is widely used as a tracer element in metabolic studies.

Carbon dioxide–combining power Carbon dioxide capacity of the plasma. It is measured by exposing a sample of plasma to an atmosphere of carbon dioxide under conditions existing in the body and by determining the volumes of gas that are combined with bicarbonate. Normal values range from 53 to 75 vol%. It is increased in alkalosis and decreased in acidosis.

Carbon dioxide fixation Process of utilizing carbon dioxide to synthesize more complex molecules. It takes place in photosynthesis whereby plants, in the presence of solar energy, use carbon dioxide from the atmosphere to build carbohydrates and other organic compounds. The ability to fix carbon dioxide is now known to be possessed also by animal tissues even without radiant energy but with chemical energy and the aid of the vitamin *biotin*. This carbon dioxide fixation in the body is referred to as dark-reaction photosynthesis. See *Photosynthesis*.

Carbonic acid H_2CO_3; a weakly ionized acid formed by the dissolution of carbon dioxide in water. It is a good buffer and its salt is the chief alkali reserve of the body. See *Buffer* and *Alkali reserve*.

Carbonic anhydrase Zinc-containing enzyme that catalyzes the reversible hydration of carbon dioxide. It is found in the tissues and erythrocytes and facilitates the transfer of carbon dioxide from the tissues to the blood and then to the lungs for elimination.

Carbonium Ion containing a positively charged carbon. It is also called an *electrophil,* since it is deficient in electrons and has an affinity for them.

Carboxyhemoglobin (**HbCO**) Hemoglobin combined with carbon monoxide, which has a stronger affinity for hemoglobin than oxygen. Carbon monoxide displaces oxygen, causing asphyxia and carbon monoxide poisoning.

Carboxylase Enzyme that catalyzes the decomposition of organic acids with the liberation of carbon dioxide. It is found in higher animals, plant cells, and microorganisms. *Carboxylation* is the introduction of carbon dioxide into a molecule.

Carboxypeptidase An exopeptidase synthesized by the pancreas in the form of a zymogen that is converted to the active enzyme by trypsin. It catalyzes the hydrolysis of polypeptides having a carboxyl group at the end of the chain, forming smaller peptide units and amino acids with a free carboxyl group.

Carcinogen Cancer-producing agent or substance. Carcinogenic compounds such as *aflatoxin* and *cycasin* have been identified in some plants. A variety of chemical agents have been used to induce malignancy in animals, but not all of them show the same capability in humans.

Carcinoma Malignant tumor made up of epithelial cells that tend to infiltrate the surrounding tissues.

Cardia The heart. The term also refers to the opening or entrance between the esophagus and the stomach.

Cardiac Pertaining to the heart. *Cardiac failure* is a set of symptoms resulting from the inability of the heart to function as a pumping organ. It may be of sudden or slow onset and may be left sided, right sided, or a mixture of the two, depending on which side of the heart is mostly affected. Difficult breathing is the most prominent symptom if the left side of the heart is affected. Edema and engorgement of body organs with blood characterize right heart failure, often referred to as congestive heart failure.

Cardiac output Volume of blood pumped per minute by the left ventricle.

Cardiograph Instrument placed over the heart that traces cardiac movement graphically.

Cardiology Branch of medicine devoted to the study, diagnosis, and treatment of the heart and its diseases. A heart specialist is called a *cardiologist*.

Cardiovascular disease (**CVD**) Collective term denoting a large group of diseases affecting the heart and blood vessels. The most important of these diseases from the public health point of view are arteriosclerotic heart disease, cerebrovascular disease, and hypertensive disease.

Cardiovascular system Those structures, such as the heart, arteries, veins, and capillaries, that provide channels for the flow of blood.

Caries Molecular decay of bones and teeth, making them soft and porous. See *Dental caries.*

Cariogenic Conducive to dental caries.

Carminative A substance that relieves or expels gas from the stomach and intestines.

Carmine A red coloring substance derived from cochineal by the addition of alum. It is used as a histologic stain for microscopic studies and as a marker for feces in balance and digestibility studies.

Carnaubic acid Fatty acid with 24 carbon atoms. It is found in wool fat and carnauba wax.

Carnitine A betaine derivative that is a constituent of muscle extract. It is an essential nutritional factor for the mealworm *Tenebrio molitor.*

Carnosine Beta-alanylhistidine, a dipeptide found in vertebrate muscle tissue. Its biochemical function is not known. A protease, *carnosinase,* that attacks the peptide bond of carnosine is present in the liver, pancreas, and kidneys.

Carnosinemia Inborn error of amino acid metabolism characterized by excretion of large amounts of *carnosine* in the urine, even when all dietary sources of this dipeptide are excluded. The condition is also associated with unusually high concentrations of homocarnosine in the cerebrospinal fluid and with progressive neurologic disorder characterized by severe mental defect and myoclonic seizures. The defect may be due to a deficiency in the enzyme carnosinase.

Carotene Carotenoid present in green leafy and yellow vegetables. It exists in several forms, of which alpha-, beta-, and gamma-carotene are provitamins A. Beta-carotene is the most active of these three forms. Carotene is converted in the body to *vitamin A.*

Carotenemia Presence of large amounts of carotene in the blood, resulting in a yellowish discoloration of the skin. The condition is harmless and should not be mistaken for jaundice. The conjunctivae and urine are not discolored in carotenemia.

Carotenoids Fat-soluble pigments with marked yellow to orange-red color; widely present in plants, usually along with chlorophyll in the lipid material. Carotenoids are unsaturated hydrocarbons with the general formula $C_{40}H_{50}$. The most important are *carotene* and *cryptoxanthin,* which are precursors of vitamin A.

Carotid Principal large artery on each side of the neck.

Carrageenan A mixed polysaccharide found in seaweed. It is used as a thickening, clarifying, and stabilizing agent in such products as chocolate milk, frozen desserts, gels, and salad dressings.

Carrier 1. A person who, without showing symptoms of a communicable disease, harbors and transmits disease-producing germs. 2. A substance that transports another substance or compound, as fat is a carrier of fat-soluble vitamins. 3. A naturally occurring element added to a pure substance of minute quantity for ease in handling. 4. In physiologic oxidation it is a compound that can accept hydrogen or electrons from a substrate and transfer them to another compound in the transport system. See *Respiratory carriers.*

Carr-Price reaction Development of a blue color when vitamin A or its precursor is treated with antimony trichloride in chloroform. The resulting blue color has a specific spectral absorption that is useful for the identification and quantitative determination of the vitamin.

Cartilage Form of connective tissue consisting of cells embedded in a dense matrix of collagenous fibers. Chemically it resembles the organic matrix of the bone. It is commonly called gristle because of its firm, resilient texture.

Casal's necklace Type of dermatitis seen in *pellagra* as a result of niacin deficiency. The lesions on the face and areas of the neck exposed to the sun are so distributed that they often appear as a necklace.

Casec Proprietary milk formula high in protein and calcium and low in fat. It is used as a high protein, high calcium formula for premature infants or those with gastrointestinal disorders. (Mead Johnson.) See Proprietary foods: composition, features, and uses, Appendix P-1.

Casein A phosphoprotein; the principal protein of milk. It is converted to calcium caseinate or milk curd by the enzyme *rennin* in the presence of calcium, leaving a residual clear fluid called *whey*.

Castle's extrinsic factor See *Extrinsic factor*.

Castor oil A purgative; the oil obtained from the castor oil bean. When digested by lipase in the intestines, it is converted to *ricinoleic acid*, which is irritating to the intestinal mucosa, causing purgation.

Catabolism Destructive metabolism; the breakdown of complex substances by living cells into simpler compounds with the liberation of energy. It is the opposite of *anabolism*. Together catabolism and anabolism constitute *metabolism*.

Catalase Enzyme present in tissues that splits hydrogen peroxide to water and oxygen. It functions as a physiologic safeguard by preventing peroxide accumulation in the body.

Catalin Obsolete term for *vitamin*.

Catalyst A substance that hastens the speed of a chemical reaction without itself undergoing a change. Catalysts in living cells (biocatalysts) are called *enzymes*.

Cataract Eye disease in which the crystalline lens becomes opaque, causing partial or total blindness; of several types and severity depending on the cause. Cataract formation is seen in *galactosemia*, an

inherited disorder in carbohydrate metabolism.

Catarrh Inflammation of a mucous membrane with a free discharge, especially in the air passages of the nose and throat.

Catatorulin test Test for vitamin B_1 or thiamin. It measures in vitro the uptake of oxygen by brain tissue from avitaminotic pigeons. Addition of thiamin proportionally increases the amount of oxygen consumed.

Catecholamines Substituted diorthophenols synthesized in the brain, sympathetic nerve endings, peripheral tissues, and adrenal medulla. They are discharged into the circulation under conditions of stress, rage, and fear. Catecholamines (chiefly epinephrine and norepinephrine) are pressor substances and can mobilize sources of rapidly utilizable energy from the body's storage depot to "prepare the animal for flight or fight." See *Epinephrine* and *Norepinephrine*.

Cathartic Medicine that aids in the evacuation of the bowels; a purgative.

Cathepsin An intracellular proteolytic enzyme found in most animal tissues, presumably responsible for the autolysis of the tissues after death. It may function in the continual breakdown of tissue protein.

Cathode Negative electrode or pole of a battery.

Cation Ion having a positive charge.

Cautery Destruction of tissues by the use of an agent that causes charring.

CCF Abbreviation for *cephalin-cholesterol flocculation*.

CDP Abbreviation for *cytidine diphosphate*. See *Cytidine phosphates*.

Cecum A blind pouch; the first part of the large intestine from which the appendix is suspended.

Celiac Abdominal; pertaining to the abdomen.

Celiac disease Form of malabsorption syndrome primarily affecting the proximal portion of the small intestines. It occurs in both children and adults and is believed to be due to sensitivity to gluten in cereals. The principal abnormality is the failure of the jejunal mucosa to adequately absorb digested substances because of villus atrophy and resultant reduction in the number of functioning absorptive cells. As a consequence, there is general malabsorption of fat, carbohydrate, protein, vitamins, and minerals. The condition is characterized by loss of weight, nausea and vomiting, abdominal pains, weakness, and diarrhea consisting of pale, bulky, frothy, foul-smelling stools. Anemia, cheilosis, glossitis, peripheral edema, tetany, rickets, and hypoprothrombinemia with a tendency to bleed develop secondary to nutritional malabsorption. The condition is completely relieved if *gluten*, derived chiefly from wheat, oat, and rye, is excluded from the diet. See *Diet, gliadin-free.*

Cell Basic structural and functional unit of an organism. Cells vary in size, type, and shape but the basic structure of most cells contains a central *nucleus* embedded in the *cytoplasm* and various specialized *organelles*, the whole being encased in a filmlike covering or *membrane*. Organelles that are common to most cells include the mitochondria, endoplasmic reticulum, ribosomes, Golgi apparatus, and lysosomes. Animal cells contain a centriole; plant cells have chloroplasts and cell walls. Other cells with specific specialized functions possess other organelles, e.g., flagella and cilia.

Cell membrane Boundary of a cell that serves as a selective permeable membrane for all nutrients, secretions, and waste products. It maintains the biochemical equilibrium of the intracellular fluids.

Cellobiose Disaccharide formed by the partial hydrolysis of *cellulose*. It consists of two glucose units linked in beta-1,4 configuration.

Cellulase Enzyme capable of hydrolyzing cellulose; present in bacteria and certain mammals, particularly those with a rumen or large cecum.

Cellulose Polysaccharide that acts as a supporting structure for plant tissues. It yields glucose on complete hydrolysis; partial hydrolysis yields the disaccharide *cellobiose*. It is generally not digested by man and merely provides bulk or roughage. Ruminants can utilize cellulose, which is digested by the microorganisms that inhabit their alimentary tract. See also *Crude fiber.*

Cell wall Outermost nonliving covering of a plant cell composed chiefly of cellulose. It is found only in plant cells.

Cementum Bony tissue covering chiefly the root of the tooth.

Centrifugal Moving away from the center.

Centriole A cytoplasmic organelle peculiar to animal cells located adjacent to the nucleus. It is a dark-staining cylindric structure composed of nine sets of triple fibers. It controls the formation of the spindle during cell division.

Centripetal Moving toward the center.

Cephalin Phosphatide (phospholipid) that yields on hydrolysis phosphoric acid, glycerol, a mixture of saturated and unsaturated fatty acids, and either ethanolamine or serine. It is found in the brain, nerve tissues, and lipid portion of glandular organs. It participates in *blood clotting* as thromboplastin, a cephalin-protein complex. It is also thought to participate in the manufacture of the protoplasm and cell membrane.

Cephalin-cholesterol flocculation test (CCF) Liver function test. An emulsion of cephalin and cholesterol is added to the serum and allowed to stand from 24 to 48 hours. Normal serum remains clear, whereas the serum from a patient with liver disease shows flocculation.

Cerebellum The smaller lower back portion of the brain that controls body balance and muscular coordinations.

Cerebral cortex Outer covering of the brain.

Cerebral palsy Variety of neurologic dysfunctions secondary to brain damage as a result of birth injury, cerebral hemorrhage, or prematurity. Two general types of motor disability are known: *athetosis*, which is characterized by constant uncontrollable movements, and *spastic paralysis*, which is characterized by limited activity. The motor dysfunction varies in severity and distribution, affecting one or more extremities or the trunk, head, and neck. Descriptive terms such as monoplegia, hemiplegia, and paraplegia are used to specify the distribution of the dysfunction. See also Dietary management of selected disorders, Appendix O.

Cerebronic acid A saturated fatty acid containing 24 carbon atoms; found in *sphingomyelin*.

Cerebroside Orgalactyl ceramide; a glycolipid that yields on complete hydrolysis one molecule each of fatty acid, 4-sphingenine, and galactose. It occurs in the brain and myelin sheaths of nerves.

Cerebrum The main part of the brain that occupies the entire upper part of the skull and is divided into a right and left hemisphere. It is the "center" of consciousness.

Ceroid An insoluble brown substance found in atheromatous plaques and in fat deposits of certain forms of liver disease. It is associated with disorders in lipid metabolism.

Cerotic acid Saturated fatty acid containing 26 carbon atoms; found in beeswax and wool fat.

Ceruloplasmin The transport form of plasma copper bound to alpha globulin. It is important in the regulation of copper absorption by reversibly binding and releasing copper at various sites of the body. Low plasma ceruloplasmin concentration is associated with *Wilson's disease*.

Cervix Neck or constricted portion, as cervix of the uterus.

Cesium-137 Radioactive isotope with a half-life of 30 years. It is distributed in fat-free tissues.

Cevitamic acid Obsolete name for *vitamin C*.

CF Abbreviation for *citrovorum factor*.

cH Concentration of hydrogen ions in solution.

Charles' law Volume occupied by a fixed weight of gas is directly proportional to the absolute temperature at constant pressure.

Charting Writing of information on a patient's chart or record. The dietitian's contribution to medical records may include diet order details, nutritional history, daily food intake, acceptance or rejection of food or diet, problems in meeting the dietary prescription, dietary calculations, and dietary instructions.

Chastek paralysis Type of spastic paralysis characterized by rigidity and retraction of the head. It was originally seen in foxes feeding on raw fish, which contain the enzyme *thiaminase*.

Chaulmoogric acid Unsaturated cyclic fatty acid found chiefly in chaulmoogra oil. Its ethyl ester is used in the treatment of leprosy.

CHD Abbreviation for *coronary heart disease*.

Cheilitis Inflammation of the lips.

Cheilosis Cracks and fissures at the corners of the mouth characteristic of *riboflavin* deficiency. The lesions of the lips begin with redness and denudation along the line of closure or may appear as pale macerations at the angles of the mouth. The lips look dry and chapped, and shallow ulcerations or crusting may occur in severe deficiency. Nonnutritional factors such as cold and wind may also cause cheilosis.

Chelate Compound formed by the binding of an atom (usually a metal) by an organic molecule, with the formation of a heterocyclic ring structure. The ability to form chelate compounds is common to many metal cations. Metal chelates, e.g., the iron-binding porphyrin group of hemoglobin, are found in many biologic systems.

Chemical score The essential amino acid of

a protein that shows the greatest percentage deficit in comparison with the amino acids contained in the same quantity of another protein selected as a standard. The concept of chemical score for proteins was introduced by Mitchell, who expressed the concentration of the essential amino acids in food as a percentage of the concentration of the same amino acid in whole egg, taken as the standard. Since the limiting amino acid determines the value of the dietary protein, the lowest percentage obtained was taken as the chemical score of the protein in that food.

Chemoautotrophs Organisms capable of deriving their energy for growth by oxidizing simple inorganic compounds.

Chemoreception Response of organisms to a change in chemical environment. The chemical senses, through the specialized taste receptors, play an important role in nutrition and feeding. Acceptance or rejection of food depends on its taste, and disorders affecting taste also influence food intake.

Chick antidermatitis factor Former name for *pantothenic acid,* a B complex vitamin.

Chief cells Cells in the gastric glands of the stomach that secrete the digestive enzymes pepsinogen, rennin, and lipase.

Child Nutrition Act A legal measure enacted in 1966 that appropriated monies for schools to start and expand school lunch programs and to feed preschool children. A pilot school breakfast program was also initiated.

Chitin Polysaccharide with glucosamine as the repeating unit. It is the principal constituent of the shells of insects and crustaceans.

Chloramphenicol Antibiotic isolated from *Streptomyces venezuelae* and marketed under the trade name Chloromycetin. It is useful in combating certain gram-negative infectious and rickettsial diseases but inhibits protein synthesis in the body.

Chlorella A unicellular green alga that forms scum on the surface of many ponds. It can synthesize protein, carbohydrate, and fat out of carbon dioxide, water, and inorganic nitrogen. The primary interest in chlorella is its use as a food source for protein and other essential nutrients.

Chloride An essential mineral found largely in the extracellular fluids. It is important in acid-base balance, regulates osmotic pressure, and is a constituent of gastric juice as hydrochloric acid. For further details, see Summary of minerals, Appendix H.

Chloride shift Exchange of chloride ion for bicarbonate ion between the intracellular fluid without a corresponding movement of cations. Bicarbonate ions diffuse into the plasma when its concentration in red blood cells is high. To maintain ionic equilibrium, chloride ions diffuse from the plasma into the red cells, where they combine with the base. Similarly bicarbonate ions also combine with sodium released from chloride to form plasma bicarbonate.

Chlorine Element universally found in biologic tissues as the *chloride* ion. As free chlorine, it is a disinfecting, bleaching, and purifying agent. Chlorinated water contains 1 part chlorine per 1 million parts water.

Chloroform Trichloromethane; used as an organic solvent and as an anesthetic and antispasmodic agent.

Chloromycetin Trade name for *chloramphenicol.*

Chlorophyll The green pigment in plants capable of absorbing radiant energy from the sun necessary for light-reaction *photosynthesis.* It has four different forms—a, b, c, and d. The first two forms are found in higher plants; the latter two are found in certain algae and diatoms.

Chloroplast Plant cell organelle that contains chlorophyll and all the enzymes needed for carbon dioxide fixation in photosynthesis. It has several "stacks" of membranes called grana, composed of proteins, modified fats, chlorophyll, and other pigments arranged in a layered structure.

Chlorosis Form of hypochromic microcytic anemia common in young women. It is characterized by a greenish tinge to the skin.

Chlorpropamide An oral hypoglycemic agent used in the treatment of diabetes mellitus. It belongs chemically to the arylsulfonylurea drugs and is sold under the trade name Diabinese.

Chlortetracycline (CTC) A broad-spectrum antibiotic first obtained from the soil bacterium *Streptomyces aureofaciens*. It is effective against various gram-positive and gram-negative bacterial infections as well as certain rickettsial and viral diseases. It is used commercially as a food additive for delaying spoilage in meat, fish, and poultry and is marketed under the trade name Aureomycin.

CHO Abbreviation for *carbohydrate*.

CHO-free A carbohydrate-free, milk-free liquid preparation fortified with vitamins and minerals; contains soy oil and soy protein isolates. It is used in cases of intolerance to milk and/or carbohydrate. (Syntex.)

Cholagogue Any agent that stimulates the gallbladder to release bile. Fat and egg yolk are food cholagogues.

Cholangitis Inflammation of the bile ducts.

Cholecalciferol Activated 7-dehydrocholesterol or vitamin D_3. See *Vitamin D*.

Cholecystitis Acute or chronic inflammation of the gallbladder. It is commonly due to imprisoned bile, bacterial infection, or obstruction of the cystic duct by stones, tumor, fibrosis, or adhesion. Acute cholecystitis is characterized by epigastric pain that radiates to the shoulder and lower abdominal region, nausea and vomiting, chills and fever, and jaundice. Sensitivity to fatty foods, colicky pain, belching, and flatulence are the general features of the chronic type. See Dietary management of selected disorders, Appendix O.

Cholecystogram X-ray film of the gallbladder.

Cholecystokinin Hormone that regulates the contraction of the gallbladder. It is secreted in the upper portion of the small intestine when fat enters the duodenum and is carried by the bloodstream to the gallbladder, causing it to contract.

Choleglobin Also called verdohemoglobin; a compound of globin and an open-ring iron porphyrin. It is an intermediate product in the formation of bile pigment and a precursor of *biliverdin*.

Choleic Pertaining to bile.

Cholelith Gallstone or biliary calculus.

Cholelithiasis Presence of stones or calculi in the gallbladder or bile duct. Gallstones are formed from the constituents of bile, and their composition and structure vary. Stones contain cholesterol, lecithin, bile pigments, inorganic salts of calcium, and other elements found in the bile. In the absence of inflammation, gallstones are silent and give no localizing symptoms. In the presence of inflammation or obstruction of the biliary passages, they give rise to dyspeptic symptoms such as flatulence, epigastric pain after eating, abdominal distention, nausea, and vomiting. See Dietary management of selected disorders, Appendix O.

Cholera A food-borne infectious disease caused by the *Vibrio comma* organism and transmitted through such vectors as flies, mice, and cockroaches, polluted water, and food contaminated with cholera germs. The disease is characterized by severe diarrhea, vomiting, and muscular cramps. It is usually fatal unless the fluid and electrolyte balance are immediately corrected.

Choleretic Agent that increases bile secretion by the liver.

Cholestanol Compound formed by the reduction of the double bond of cholesterol. It is a minor constituent of blood sterols and some tissues. It is found in greater concentration in the feces.

Cholesterol The chief sterol in the body found in all tissues, especially the brain, nerves, adrenal cortex, and liver. It is also a constituent of bile and serves as precursor of vitamin D. Cholesterol in the body comes from two sources: *exogenous* or dietary cholesterol, chiefly from egg yolk, liver, and other organ meats; and *endogenous* cholesterol synthesized by the liver and other organs, e.g., the adrenal cortex, skin, and intestines. Cholesterol circulates in the blood as lipoprotein in combination with protein and other blood lipids. Part of the sterol has the hydroxyl group free (free cholesterol) and part occurs as esters of fatty acids (esterified cholesterol). Normal cholesterol value in human blood plasma ranges from 150 to 250 mg/100 ml; of this amount, two-thirds is esterified and the rest exists as free sterol. Cholesterol is related in some unknown fashion to hardening of the arteries, high blood pressure, stone formation, and other diseases. See *Atherosclerosis* and *Hypercholesterolemia*. See also *Diet, cholesterol-restricted*.

Cholestyramine Drug that can lower serum lipids indirectly by sequestering bile acids in the intestines. It is an ion-exchange resin that binds bile acids and sterols in the gut and causes greater fecal excretion, resulting in less available sterols for conversion to cholesterol in the liver. The drug is also claimed to be capable of dissolving gallstones.

Cholic acid A trihydroxycholinic acid; the most abundant bile acid in human bile. It is conjugated with the amino acids glycine and taurine and occurs as glycocholic and taurocholic acids, respectively.

Choline An important dietary factor necessary for fat transport in the body. It occurs in all plant and animal cells as free choline, acetylcholine, or a constituent of lecithin and sphingomyelin. Choline can be readily synthesized in the body from the amino acid glycine, providing another source of methyl group is available. Thus choline is not considered a vitamin since the body is not solely dependent on a dietary source of either choline or its direct

precursor. Fatty liver is the most common manifestation of choline deficiency in experimental animals. Other manifestations of choline deficiency include liver cirrhosis, hemorrhagic degeneration of the kidneys, adrenal glands, heart, and lungs, and *perosis* in chicks. Choline deficiency has not been demonstrated in man. Good food sources are egg yolk, liver, brain, kidney, heart, milk, legumes, and nuts. See also *Lipotropic agent*.

Cholinergic Term applied to nerve fibers that liberate acetylcholine when a nerve impulse is transmitted.

Cholinesterase Enzyme present in the blood and various tissues that hydrolyzes acetylcholine into choline and acetic acid. It plays an important role in the transmission of nerve impulses.

Chondroitin Mucopolysaccharide that yields on hydrolysis glucuronic acid and galactosamine. As chondroitin sulfate, it is found in small quantities in the eyes, skin, and connective tissues.

Chorea A nervous disorder characterized by irregular and involuntary muscle movements of the face, arms, and legs.

Christmas factor Plasma component concerned in thromboplastin formation. A deficiency in this factor results in a hemophilia B type of disease called Christmas disease. See also *Blood clotting*.

Chromatin Granular or netlike cell constituent that stains readily with basic dyes. It is composed chiefly of nucleoproteins and forms the *chromosomes* during cell division.

Chromatography Analytic technique for the separation and identification of the components of a mixture or compound.

Adsorption c Separation of components by the use of solid adsorbents (e.g., aluminum oxide, silica gel, and magnesium oxide) that have specific affinities for the components. The sample is dissolved in a suitable solvent and then poured on a column containing an adsorbent. Addition of an eluting solvent separates each adsorbed substance according to its adsorbing affinity.

Gas c Separation of gaseous or volatile material by injection into a column containing a liquid adsorbent supported on an inert solid. The basis for the separation of the components of the volatile material is the difference in the partition coefficients of the components as they are carried through the column by an inert gas such as helium. Gas chromatography is used in the analysis of fat, fatty acids, flavor components, gaseous mixtures, and any compound that can be converted into a volatile material.

Ion-exchange c Separation of ionic substances on a polyelectrolyte surface, such as synthetic resin polymers and cellulose derivatives. The basic principle involves an electrostatic interaction with the exchanging ion and normal charge on the surface of the resin. By adjusting the ionic strength and pH of the eluting solvent, the electrostatically held ions are eluted differentially to yield the desired separation.

Paper c A strip of paper is used as the porous solid supporting a stationary water phase. The substances to be separated are spotted on one end of the paper, which is then placed in a jar containing a mobile organic solvent. The solvent either ascends (ascending paper chromatography) or descends (descending paper chromatography) onto the paper, which is later removed and sprayed with a chemical developing agent. The R_f value, or the ratio of the distance traveled by the compounds to the distance traveled by the solvent front from the original spot, is a constant in various compounds.

Thin-layer c Separation of components through a thin adhesive layer of cellulose or similar inert material, e.g., silica gel G, supported on a glass or plastic plate. This gives a sharper separation of components, and the analysis can be done in a very short time. Thin-layer chromatography is widely used for analysis of amino acids, peptides, and related compounds.

Chromium An essential trace mineral occurring in minute amounts in the blood and various tissues. It is present at birth at higher concentrations, and there appears to be a steady decline in tissue concentration with age, depending on the dietary habits and the amount of chromium in water supplies. It plays a role in carbohydrate metabolism by increasing the effectiveness of insulin, hence facilitating the transport of glucose into the cells. Chromium deficiency in rats leads to the development of diabetes and vascular lesions similar to atherosclerosis. This mineral is also implicated in the development of kwashiorkor and marasmic types of protein-calorie malnutrition.

Chromoprotein A conjugated colored protein such as hemoglobin and flavoprotein.

Chromosome Threadlike structure in the cell nucleus that contains the genes of the cell in its deoxyribonucleic acid (DNA) component.

Chronic Of long duration; not acute.

Chyle The milky white emulsion of fat globules formed in the small intestine and transported into the lymph.

Chylomicron The largest and lightest of the *blood lipids;* approximately 1μ in diameter and consisting chiefly of triglyceride and smaller amounts of cholesterol, phospholipid, and protein. Chylomicrons are normally synthesized in the intestines and serve to transport absorbed dietary triglycerides to sites of utilization in the tissues. They are responsible for the turbid and milky appearance of normal plasma after a fatty meal. Their presence in the plasma 12 to 16 hours after eating is abnormal.

Chyme Thick semifluid mass into which food is converted after gastric digestion. It is in this form that food passes into the small intestine.

Chymotrypsin Endopeptidase secreted by the pancreas as an inactive proenzyme, chymotrypsinogen. It possesses milk-clotting action and preferentially attacks peptide linkages of the aromatic amino acids tyrosine and phenylalanine. Administration of chymotrypsin has a marked therapeutic effect in the control of certain cases of insulin-resistant diabetes.

Circulation Movement of blood from the heart to the body tissues and back to the heart; the process of transporting nutrients, internal secretions, gases, and wastes among the tissues and organs of the body.

Circulatory system Includes both the cardiovascular and lymphatic systems. The former consists of the heart, blood vessels, and circulating fluid (blood); the latter consists of lymph channels (lymphatics), nodes, and fluid lymph, which empties into the bloodstream.

Cirrhosis Chronic, progressive disease of the liver in which fibrous connective tissue replaces the functioning liver cells. There are many types of cirrhosis caused by a number of conditions such as chronic alcoholism, various infections such as syphilis and malaria, obstruction of the bile duct, and nutritional deficiency. It is thought that alcoholic cirrhosis is due to deficiencies in nutrient intake, particularly protein and vitamins. There is loss of appetite, polyneuritis, cheilosis, low serum albumin levels, and edema due to protein lack. In advanced cases, ascites and esophageal varices complicate the condition, often ending in liver failure and hepatic coma. See Dietary management of selected disorders, Appendix O.

Cis Latin, meaning "on this side." A prefix used to designate geometric isomers with a double bond between two carbon atoms. The isomer is called *cis* when a given atom or radical is positioned on the same side of the carbon axis.

Citral Constituent of orange oil that can cause damage to blood vessels when taken in large amounts. It is present in such food products as marmalade, fruit juices, and fruit drinks flavored with orange oil. This raises the question as to whether excessive consumption of such foods might not cause damage to blood vessels and hence be a contributory cause of cardiovascular disease.

Citric acid Tribasic acid present chiefly in lemon, lime, and other citrus fruits. It is used as acid flavoring in beverages and confectionery. Citric acid is completely metabolized in the body.

Citric acid cycle See *Krebs cycle*.

Citrin A crystalline substance from the peels of citrus fruits thought to be necessary for the integrity and permeability of capillaries. It was originally described as vitamin P. See *Bioflavonoid*.

Citrovorum factor (CF) Growth factor for the organism *Leuconostoc citrovorum;* has been given the name *folinic acid,* a biologically active form of the vitamin folic acid.

Citrulline An amino acid first isolated from watermelon, although it does not appear to be a constituent of common proteins. It is closely related to arginine and is involved in the *urea cycle*.

Citrullinemia Inborn error of metabolism believed to be due to lack of arginosuccinic acid synthetase, which is involved in the biosynthesis of urea. It is characterized by elevated levels of citrulline in the blood, urine, and cerebrospinal fluid, increased concentration of ammonia in the blood, persistent vomiting, generalized convulsions, and progressive mental retardation. The exact dietary treatment is not known, although protein restriction is recommended to control blood ammonia.

Clarification Process of clearing a liquid from turbidity or suspended particles. It may be accomplished by filtration, centrifugation, or addition of a substance that precipitates suspended particles.

Claudication Weakness and cramplike pain in the legs; inability to walk well.

Clearance Removal from the blood by an excretory organ of a particular substance, such as removal of urea, inulin, creatinine, and other materials by the kidney.

Clearance test Test for kidney function. It measures the excretory efficiency of the kidney to "clear" blood of a substance over a given period of time. It may also be used as a test for liver function to determine the ability of the liver to remove a substance from the blood.

Clearing factor A lipoprotein lipase present in various tissues, notably the heart, lungs, and adipose tissue. It appears in the plasma following a meal and "clears" the blood of its turbid and milky appearance by hydrolyzing the triglycerides present in the chylomicrons and in lipoproteins. It also mobilizes fatty acids from the fat depots. This enzyme is enhanced by *heparin* and activated by calcium and magnesium ions.

Cleft palate Congenital deformity characterized by incomplete closure of the lateral halves of the palate or roof of the mouth. This presents feeding difficulties as food passes through the roof of the mouth into the nasal cavity. See Dietary management of selected disorders, Appendix O.

Clinistix Enzyme-impregnated paper strip employed in the detection of sugar in the urine. The change in color on the strip is compared with a color guide, which gives a quantitative approximation of sugar concentration in the urine.

Clinitest Simple colorimetric method used in the quantitative estimation of sugar in the urine. It is a reagent tablet employing the principle of copper reduction without the application of heat. The test tablet is placed in a test tube to which 5 drops of urine and 10 drops of water are added. After 15 seconds, the contents are shaken and the color of the solution is compared with a color guide.

Clofibrate Drug used in lowering serum cholesterol and triglyceride levels.

Clonus Involuntary muscular contractions characterized by alternate rigidity and relaxation.

Clostridium Genus of anaerobic spore-forming rod-shaped bacterium that includes *Clostridium perfringens,* which causes gangrene, and *Clostridium botulinum,* which causes a fatal type of food poisoning. See *Botulism.*

Clot Semisolid coagulum of blood or lymph. See *Blood clotting.*

Clotting time The time it takes for blood to clot or coagulate. Normally it is $4\frac{1}{2}$ minutes.

Clysis Cleansing of a cavity by means of an enema.

CMI Abbreviation for *carbohydrate metabolic index.*

CMP Abbreviation for *cytidine monophosphate.* See *Cytidine phosphates.*

Co I, Co II, Co III Abbreviations for *coenzyme I, coenzyme II,* and *coenzyme III,* respectively.

CoA Abbreviation for *coenzyme A.*

Coagulation 1. Curdling or clotting; formation of a clot or coagulum, as in blood or milk. 2. In colloid chemistry the solidification of a sol into a gelatinous mass. Coagulation is usually an irreversible process.

Cobalamin Collective term given to the many forms in which vitamin B_{12} may appear in animal tissues, all of which contain cobalt as an integral part of the molecule. The members of the vitamin B_{12} group are identified by their prefixes. Hydroxo-, cyano-, and nitritocobalamin are among the forms known to exhibit vitamin activity; cyanocobalamin is the most active of the three. See *Vitamin B_{12}.*

Cobalt An essential trace mineral normally present in animal tissues as an integral part of vitamin B_{12}. The need for cobalt other than its role in the synthesis of vitamin B_{12} is not known. It seems that only ruminants are able to utilize cobalt in its inorganic form. It is present in large quantities in plants, especially green leafy vegetables, and occurs in animal tissues as cobalamin. Primary dietary deficiency is unlikely to happen unless animal products are not consumed. For further details, see Summary of minerals, Appendix H.

Cobamide Generic term given to vitamin B_{12}-containing coenzymes. Three forms have been identified and designated as 5,6-dimethylbenzimidazolylcobamide, benzimidazolylcobamide, and adenylcobamide. These three forms do not contain the cyano group attached to cobalt, as does cyanocobalamin. There is instead an adenine nucleoside linked to cobalt by a carbon-to-carbon bond.

Cocarboxylase Thiamin pyrophosphate (TPP) or diphosphothiamin (DPT), the thiamin-containing coenzyme that is a cofactor in the decarboxylation of pyruvic acid to acetate and the conversion of pyruvic acid to acetoin. It is also involved in the transketolase reaction and in the oxidation of pyruvic acid to acetyl coenzyme A.

Codecarboxylase Pyridoxal phosphate, the prosthetic group of enzymes that catalyzes the decarboxylation of amino acids.

Codehydrogenase I Diphosphopyridine nucleotide (DPN). See *Coenzyme I* under *Coenzymes I and II*.

Codehydrogenase II Triphosphopyridine nucleotide (TPN). See *Coenzyme II* under *Coenzymes I and II*.

Codelid An *elemental diet* preparation containing chemically defined amino acids, sucrose, vitamins, and minerals. It is fat-free and low in residue. (Schwarz/Mann.) See Proprietary foods: composition, features, and uses, Appendix P-1.

Codex Alimentarius Commission Committee created by FAO and WHO to develop international food standards on a worldwide, regional, or group-of-countries basis and to publish these standards in a food code called *Codex Alimentarius*. These food standards aim at protecting consumers' health and ensuring fair practices in the food trade. Also included are provisions in food hygiene, food additives, pesticide residues, contaminants, labeling and presentation, methods of analysis, and sampling.

Cod liver oil Oil obtained from the liver of the fish *Gadus morrhua*. It contains no less than 600 IU of vitamin A and 85 IU of vitamin D/gm. Cod liver oil is used in the treatment of diseases of bone and in vitamin A and D deficiencies.

Codon Sequence of three adjacent nucleotides that code a single amino acid.

Coefficient of digestibility Percentage portion of the ingested food constituent retained in the body and not excreted in the feces. The *average* coefficients of digestibility of foods are 98% for carbohydrate, 95% for fat, and 92% for protein. The *actual* coefficients of digestibility of specific foodstuffs vary considerably.

Coenzyme An organic dialyzable and heat-stable enzyme cofactor whose presence is required for the activity of many enzymes. Coenzymes usually contain vitamins as part of their structure, and they function as acceptors of electrons and functional groups. See *Enzyme; Cofactor;* and Vitamins as coenzymes, Appendix I-2.

Coenzymes I and II Hydrogen and electron transfer agents known to be a complex of nicotinamide, D-ribose, phosphoric acid, and adenine. They play a vital role in metabolism and participate in a wide variety of biologic oxidations. Their two major functions are the removal of hydrogen from certain substrates in cooperation with dehydrogenases and the transfer of hydrogen (or electrons) to another coenzyme in the hydrogen transport series.

Coenzyme I (Co I) Nicotinamide adenine dinucleotide (NAD); also called diphosphopyridine nucleotide (DPN); a complex of nicotinamide, two molecules each of D-ribose and phosphoric acid, and one molecule of adenine; formerly called codehydrogenase and cozymase.

Coenzyme II (Co II) Nicotinamide adenine dinucleotide phosphate (NADP); also called triphosphopyridine nucleotide (TPN); a complex of nicotinamide, adenine, two molecules of D-ribose, and three molecules of phosphoric acid;

formerly called Warburg and Christian's enzyme.

Coenzyme III (Co III) Cysteine sulfinic acid dehydrogenase, an enzyme that catalyzes the oxidation of cysteine sulfinic acid to cysteic acid. This dehydrogenase has been named coenzyme III because it requires as coenzyme a pyridine nucleotide similar in structure to *coenzymes I and II*. It is found in microorganisms and animal tissues, particularly in the liver, kidneys, and heart.

Coenzyme A (CoA) Pantothenic acid joined to adenosine phosphate by a pyrophosphate bridge and to beta-mercaptoethylamine by a peptide bridge. It functions in acetylation and acylation reactions, oxidation of keto acids and fatty acids, formation of acetylcholine, and synthesis of triglycerides, phospholipids, steroids, and porphyrins.

Coenzyme Q (CoQ) A lipidlike substance similar to vitamin K in its chemical make-up that belongs to a group of compounds known as *ubiquinones*. It is found in practically all living cells and appears to be concentrated in the mitochondria. It is believed to participate in the *redox system* for the release of energy.

Coenzyme R Factor necessary for the growth and respiration of the legume nodule bacteria *Rhizobium;* it has been identified as *biotin.*

Cofactor General term given to the nonprotein fraction of an enzyme necessary for its full activation. Cofactors are divided loosely into three groups: *prosthetic group,* which is firmly attached to the protein portion of the enzyme; *coenzyme,* which is easily dissociated from the protein enzyme; and *metal activators,* which are mono- and divalent cations such as K, Mn, Mg, Ca, and Zn and which may be either firmly or loosely bound to an enzyme protein. See also *Enzyme.*

Colchicine Alkaloid from the root of a lily plant, *Colchicum autumnale,* that is of value in the treatment of gout. However, it appears to induce reversible vitamin B_{12}

malabsorption by altering the function of the ileal mucosa.

Colic 1. Pertaining to the colon. 2. Abdominal pain, a symptom of various conditions.

Colitis Acute or chronic inflammation of the colon or large bowel due to one or more causes. *Mucous colitis* is characterized by abdominal distress, constipation, or diarrhea and the passage of mucous or membranous masses in the stools. *Spastic colitis,* also called irritable colon or unstable colon, is associated with increased tonus or abnormal activity of the colon. *Ulcerative colitis* is a chronic condition characterized by an ulceration of the mucosa and passage of pus and blood in the stools.

Collagen An albuminoid; the insoluble protein of connective tissue, bones, tendons, and skin. It is resistant to animal digestive enzymes but hydrolyzed to soluble gelatin by boiling in water, dilute acids, or alkalies. Collagen constitutes one third of the body proteins and possesses remarkable qualities. It has the "tensile strength of light steel wire, toughness of leather, tenacity of glue and viscosity of gelatin."

Colloids A two-phased system; a state of subdivision of matter in which the individual particles are of submicroscopic size (1 mμ to 0.1μ in diameter), do not dissolve but are distributed uniformly in the second phase, and yet will not settle out of the system. Such particles are referred to as the *dispersed phase;* the second phase is called the *dispersion medium.* The most common types of colloidal systems are *aerosol, emulsion, gel,* and *sol.*

Colon Part of the large intestine that extends from the cecum to the rectum.

Ascending c Part of the colon on the right side, going upward from the cecum.

Descending c Part of the colon on the left side between the transverse colon and the sigmoid colon.

Sigmoid c Part of the colon between the descending colon and the rectum.

Transverse c Part of the colon that runs transversely across the upper part of the abdomen from right to left.

Color blindness Inability to perceive one or more colors.

Colorimeter Instrument for measuring intensity of color in compounds. It is used in food laboratories for determination of vitamins and in hospital laboratories for blood and urine analysis.

Colorimetry Quantitative determination of the concentration of the constituents of a solution that possess inherent colors or that may be made to react stoichiometrically with suitable reagents to produce colored compounds. Colorimetric analysis is fast, simple, convenient, and sensitive, although it is less accurate than the gravimetric and volumetric methods of analysis.

Color index Expression of the amount of hemoglobin contained in red blood cells relative to normal values.

Colostomy Formation of an artificial outlet from the colon through the walls of the abdomen. The need arises when part of the colon becomes obstructed or has to be removed because of a diseased condition.

Colostrum First milk secreted by the mammary gland a few days after parturition. Compared to later milk secretion, it is higher in protein content and is chiefly immune globulins that contain antibodies responsible for the immunity of the newborn. Colostrum is also higher in beta-carotene, riboflavin, and niacinamide content but has less fat and carbohydrate.

Coma State of unconsciousness from which a patient cannot be aroused. It may follow brain injury, trauma, or hemorrhage; poisoning with narcotics or alcohol; poisons developed in the body by disease, as in uremia and ammonia intoxication; or disturbances of the acid-base balance, as in diabetic acidosis.

Diabetic c Serious complication of diabetes mellitus in which unconsciousness is an essential feature. It is often due to infection, too little intake of insulin, or too much eating. Preceding the comatose state, symptoms such as intense thirst, nausea and vomiting, dim vision, labored breath-ing, and "sweet" or acetone breath appear. See also Dietary management of selected disorders, Appendix O.

Hepatic c State of unconsciousness seen in patients with advanced liver disease due to ammonia intoxication. The precomatose state is characterized by disorientation, drowsiness, mental confusion, and flapping tremors of the distended arms. The condition culminates in deep stupor, unconsciousness, and the characteristic fecal odor of breath (fetor hepaticus). See Dietary management of selected disorders, Appendix O.

Commodity Distribution Program Program of the federal government that supplies foods purchased under the agricultural support program to low-income people. This program is being replaced by the *Food Stamp Program.*

Compleat B A ready-to-use commercial blenderized tube feeding formula containing meat, vegetables, fruit, and milk, with added vitamins and minerals. (Doyle.) See Proprietary foods: composition, features, and uses, Appendix P-1.

Complement A nonspecific substance composed of mixed globulins normally present in the serum. It can bind antigen and antibody in such a way that destruction of the antigen is facilitated.

Complemental air Also called inspiratory reserve volume; the volume of air that can be inspired by the deepest possible inspiration after an ordinary inspiration.

Complemental feeding See *Infant feeding.*

Complete protein See *Protein quality.*

Compound A 11-Dehydrocorticosterone.

Compound B Corticosterone.

Compound E Cortisone (16-hydroxy-11-dehydrocorticosterone).

Compound F Hydrocortisone (17-hydroxycorticosterone).

Computer Device that receives, processes, and presents information. It has four distinct parts: input equipment to enter data and instructions into the system, storage unit to store data until called for or needed, control unit to interpret the stored instructions, and output equipment to release the processed data from the system. Access to the computer is normally made through *data terminals*. Computers have found wide application in nutrition and food research, especially in nutrient analysis, epidemiologic and dietary studies, menu planning, and food cost accounting.

Conarachin A simple protein of the globulin type found in peanuts.

Conception Fertilization of the ovum by a spermatozoon.

Condensation Type of chemical reaction involving a combination between molecules or between parts of the same molecule.

Configuration In chemistry, the arrangement in space of the atoms of a molecule.

Congenital Existing at birth. *Congenital anomaly* is any abnormality or malformation in the body that develops during pregnancy; often called birth defect. It may be inherited or produced by harmful external factors such as the drug thalidomide.

Conjugated protein Protein combined with a non-amino acid group, generally called a prosthetic group. See Classification of proteins, Appendix C-2.

Conjunctiva Mucous membrane that covers the eyeball and lines the eyelids. Inflammation of the conjunctiva (conjunctivitis) may be due to allergy, infection, chemical irritants, or foreign bodies.

Conjunctival xerosis Condition characterized by dryness, thickening, pigmentation, lack of lustre, and diminished transparency of the conjunctiva of the exposed part of the eyeball. It is due to keratinization of the epithelial cells of the conjunctiva, and is seen in *vitamin A* deficiency.

Connective tissue General term for all the tissues that bind together and support the various structures of the body. It is present in tendons, ligaments, bone matrix, areolar tissue, adipose tissue, and supporting tissues of all organs. The three main types of connective tissue fibers are *collagenous* or white fibers found in regions of the body where strong support is needed; *elastic* or yellow fibers found in the walls of blood vessels and in the lungs and bronchi where its stretching properties are of special value; and *reticular* fibers, which constitute the framework of blood-forming lymphoid tissues such as the spleen, lymph nodes, and bone marrow.

Conservation of energy Energy cannot be created or destroyed, although it can be changed from one form to another. Thus the sum of all forms of energy remains constant. For example, the amount of heat (or energy) obtained from food is equal to the amount of energy expended in the forms of heat, work done, and energy in waste products (assuming that there is no gain or loss of weight). Energy intake greater or less than its expenditure would result, respectively, in storage or utilization of potential energy in the form of depot fat.

Constipation Infrequent or difficult bowel movement; retention of the feces in the colon beyond the normal length of emptying time. Chronic or habitual constipation often causes headache, feeling of malaise, loss of power to concentrate, foul breath, and dullness of special senses. See Dietary management of selected disorders, Appendix O.

Atonic c Sometimes called "lazy bowel" constipation because of lack of tonus of the colon with enlargement of a part or the whole colon. The urge to defecate is lacking and the feces are large and hard. Common causes include faulty diet (one low in fiber or insufficient in fluids), lack of exercise or activity, change of environment, and excessive use of laxatives.

Spastic c Constipation due to increased tonicity of the colon, resulting in spasmodic constriction and narrowing of parts of the colon. It is characterized by small, ribbonlike stools. Common causes are nervous disturbance, obstruction or stasis in the colon, and anxiety or worry.

Controlyte A high calorie, protein-free, low

electrolyte dietary supplement for protein-restricted diets. It is a hydrolysate of cornstarch and vegetable oil; 1 tablespoon of powder gives approximately 50 calories. It may be added to a variety of foods or mixed with water and served as a beverage. (Doyle.) See Proprietary foods: composition, features, and uses, Appendix P-1.

Convenience foods Those foods offered for sale as ready to eat or partially prepared or cooked.

Convertin A relatively stable substance in the blood that is essential for the optimal conversion of prothrombin to thrombin by thromboplastin. It exists in the inactive form (proconvertin), which, in the presence of calcium ions, interacts with thromboplastin to form convertin.

Convulsion A violent involuntary contraction of the voluntary muscles, which may be either tonic (without relaxation) or clonic (with alternate contraction and relaxation). There may or may not be loss of consciousness. Convulsions are due to central nervous system damage, as seen in some forms of epilepsy, toxic nephritis, insulin shock, and pyridoxine deficiency in infants.

Copper An essential trace mineral found in all tissues in the body. It is necessary for normal hemoglobin synthesis, elastin synthesis, iron utilization, and metabolism of fatty acids, ascorbic acid, and tyrosine. There has been no evidence that specific dietary deficiency of copper occurs in man. Copper is widely distributed in foods; richest sources are liver, kidneys, heart, shellfish, nuts, and dried legumes. For further details, see Summary of minerals, Appendix H.

Coprophagy Eating of feces. Animals that eat their own feces make use of certain vitamins synthesized by intestinal bacteria. This may present a problem in experimental studies with animals.

Coprosterol Sterol found in the feces produced by bacterial reduction of cholesterol in the lower intestine.

CoQ Abbreviation for *coenzyme Q.*

Cori cycle Series of reactions that make possible the conversion of muscle glycogen to blood glucose. Muscle glycogen cannot contribute directly to blood glucose because of lack of glucose-6-phosphatase, which is present only in the liver. In the absence of oxygen, lactic acid formed in the muscles diffuses into the blood and is taken up by the liver, which is able to convert lactic acid to glucose and, eventually, liver glycogen.

Cornea A transparent, colorless, nonvascular, connective tissue structure on the anterior portion of the eyeball. It receives nourishment from lymph vessels at its margin and is surrounded by a rich plexus of pain fibers.

Corneal vascularization Formation of fine capillary blood vessels on the periphery of the cornea due to congestion of the normal limbal plexus. It may be nonspecific and occur in any inflammatory or irritating process affecting the cornea. It is also seen in *riboflavin deficiency.*

Corneal xerosis Hazy, milky, or opaque appearance of the cornea, usually most marked in the lower central area. It is due in part to cellular infiltration of the corneal stroma; it is seen in *vitamin A deficiency.*

Corn-soy-milk (CSM) A high protein food supplement consisting of partially gelatinized cornmeal, toasted soy flour, and nonfat dry milk fortified with vitamins and minerals. It is used primarily in developing countries as a food supplement for preschool children. See Protein food mixtures, Appendix P-2.

Coronary heart disease (CHD) Condition characterized by inadequate coronary circulation because of narrowing of the lumen or complete occlusion of the coronary arteries due to atherosclerosis, thrombus formation, or embolism. As a consequence, the heart is deprived of its oxygen and nutrient supply. Epidemiologic and clinical investigations have identified several risk factors associated with susceptibility to coronary heart disease. These include high blood pressure, elevation in plasma lipids, especially cholesterol, obesity, physical inactivity, and heavy cigarette smoking. Hardness of water and iodine and sugar intake have also been implicated, although the exact relationship with the disease has not been exactly defined.

Corticosteroid Term applied to the steroid hormones secreted by the adrenal cortex and other natural or synthetic compounds having the same activity as the *adrenocortical hormones.*

Corticosterone Steroid hormone found in the adrenal cortex. It influences carbohydrate metabolism and electrolyte balance.

Corticotropin Another name for *adrenocorticotropic hormone.*

Cortin Original name given to the adrenal cortex hormones, now recognized to consist of several hormones.

Cortisol 17-Hydroxycorticosterone, the major adrenal cortical steroid influencing carbohydrate metabolism. It increases the release of glucose from the liver, stimulates gluconeogenesis from amino acids, and decreases the peripheral utilization of glucose. Cortisol is released into the blood and transported to the tissues in combination with a globulin as transcortin.

Cortisone 17-Dehydro-17-alpha-hydroxycorticosterone, a constituent of adrenal cortical extract; it is manufactured commercially for treatment of adrenal insufficiency and several acute diseases; it gives the body resistance to various forms of stresses; formerly called compound E.

Coumarin A fragrant neutral principle obtained from the Tonka bean and made synthetically from salicylic aldehyde; used to disguise unpleasant odors. Coumarin is an anticoagulant and has a hypoprothrombinemic effect, especially when the dietary intake of vitamin K is inadequate.

Coupling reaction Coupling mechanism is best explained as the transfer of hydrogens (or electrons) along the respiratory chain when adenosine diphosphate (ADP) and inorganic phosphate (P_i) are simultaneously converted into adenosine triphosphate (ATP) within the mitochondria. In other words, oxygen cannot be utilized unless ADP and P_i are available, which in turn depend on the rate at which ATP is split in the performance of work. Thus hydrogen is transported through the electron transport chain by coupling and uncoupling with ATP. See also *Phosphorylation.*

Cozymase Nicotinamide adenine dinucleotide (NAD) or diphosphopyridine nucleotide (DPN). See *Coenzyme I* under *Coenzymes I and II.*

Creatine Methyl guanidine derivative of acetic acid. As creatine phosphate, it acts as a source of *high-energy phosphate* and plays an essential part in the release of energy in muscular contraction. It is present in the muscle, brain, and blood; trace amounts are also normally present in the urine. It is excreted in abnormally large amounts in conditions accompanied by failure to burn carbohydrate (as in starvation, diabetes mellitus, and severe liver disease), in diseases of muscles (as in myasthenia gravis and muscular dystrophy), and in conditions accompanied by excessive tissue breakdown (as in fevers and wasting diseases).

Creatine index Measure of the ability of the body to retain ingested creatine as determined under standard conditions. The percentage retained is high in hypothyroidism and low in hyperthyroidism and other conditions accompanied by muscle wasting.

Creatinine Anhydride of creatine, formed largely in the muscles by irreversible and nonenzymatic removal of water from creatine phosphate. Free creatinine occurs in both blood and urine. The amount excreted in the urine is an index of muscle mass and may be used as a measure of basal heat production.

Creatinine clearance test Test for renal function based on the rate at which ingested creatinine is filtered through the glomeruli.

Creatinine coefficient Amount of urinary creatinine excreted in 24 hours/kg body weight. When expressed in terms of body size, the creatinine excretion of different individuals of the same age and sex is constant from day to day. The creatinine coefficient may thus be regarded as an index of muscle mass.

Cremation Burning of dead bodies.

Crenation Notched appearance of the borders of erythrocytes as a result of shriveling. This occurs when erythrocytes are placed in hypertonic solution or when they are exposed to the air.

Cretinism Chronic condition occurring in fetal life or early infancy due to deficient thyroid activity. It is characterized by arrested physical and mental development, dry skin, chubby hands, large protruding tongue and abdomen, and low basal metabolic rate. See also *Myxedema*.

Crocetin One of the *carotenoids;* partly responsible for the deep orange-yellow color of saffron.

Crude birth rate Number of live births reported in the calendar year per 1000 enumerated or estimated population at the middle of the year.

Crude death rate Number of deaths reported in the calendar year per 1000 enumerated or estimated population at the middle of the year.

Crude fat The fat, lipids, and other fat-soluble materials in food that are extractable by fat solvents, such as petroleum ether, ethyl ether, chloroform, or benzene. In the *proximate analysis* of foods this is sometimes referred to as ether extract or ether soluble fraction.

Crude fiber The ash-free insoluble residue left after boiling a food sample first with dilute acid and then with dilute alkali to simulate gastric and intestinal digestion. It is commonly called indigestible carbohydrate and consists of varying amounts of cellulose, hemicellulose, lignin, pectic substances, gums, and mucins. These compounds, particularly cellulose and hemi-cellulose, require enzymes of certain microorganisms that thrive in mammals, especially those having a rumen or large cecum. End products of fiber digestion are lower fatty acids (acetic, propionic, and butyric acid) and gases (carbon dioxide and methane). When digested, the energy obtained per gram of crude fiber is about the same as digested starch or sugar. Depending on the intestinal microflora, crude fiber digestion in man could be of sufficient magnitude (25% to 62% digestible) as to merit consideration in estimating net energy value of foods.

Crude protein Food nitrogen content, as derived from protein and nonprotein nitrogenous materials. Crude protein is obtained by multiplying the nitrogen content of foods (as determined by the Kjeldahl process) by the factor 6.25. See *Kjeldahl method.*

Cryogenics Science that deals with production of very low temperatures and their effect on matter. Very low temperature storage greatly reduces biologic activity, making preservation of life possible for an indefinite period. Practical applications for storage of living cells and tissues (cryopreservation) are seen in biologic research, blood banks, sperm banks for artificial insemination, and food preservation. Low temperatures can also be used for selective destruction of tissues (cryosurgery), or applied as a therapeutic agent (cryotherapy).

Cryptoxanthin A yellow pigment belonging to the *carotenoid* group that can be converted into *vitamin A* in the body. It is one of the chief pigments in yellow corn, paprika, and oranges.

CSM Abbreviation for *corn-soy-milk.*

CTC Abbreviation for *chlortetracycline.*

CTP Abbreviation for *cytidine triphosphate.* See *Cytidine phosphates.*

Culture Growth or propagation of microorganisms in a controlled or special media. It may be a culture of microorganisms (e.g., bacterial culture) or one of animal or plant cells (e.g., tissue culture). Cultures require a suitable culture medium and controlled environmental temperature.

Curie Unit used in measuring radioactivity. One curie is equivalent to the number of atomic disintegrations occurring per second in a gram of pure radium (equals 37 billion disintegrations per second).

Curled toe paralysis Condition seen in chickens as a result of *riboflavin deficiency*. The chickens walk on their hocks with their toes curled inward. The legs eventually become paralyzed.

Cushing's syndrome Condition due to hypersecretion of the adrenocortical hormones because of hyperplasia or tumor of the adrenal cortex, basophilic adenoma of the pituitary gland, or prolonged use of large doses of adrenocorticotropic hormone (ACTH). The chief features of the syndrome include obesity of the trunk, face, and buttocks, purplish striae over the abdomen, pigmentation of the skin, hypertension, hyperglycemia, excessive growth of hair, and loss of sexual function.

CVD Abbreviation for *cardiovascular disease*.

Cyanocobalamin A *cobalamin* with a cyanide group; the designated term for alpha-5,6-dimethylbenzimidazolylcobamide cyanide, more commonly known as *vitamin B₁₂*.

Cyanogen Compound of two carbon and two nitrogen atoms $(CN)_2$. Many plant foodstuffs contain cyanogenetic glucosides or cyanide in the form of nitrile. Sources of these glucosides habitually consumed by man include cassava, sweet potato, sorghum, millet, lima bean, kidney bean, bamboo shoots, and the seeds of apples, almonds, pears, cherries, plums, and apricots. Fortunately poisoning is rarely produced because cyanogens are present in small amounts or in parts of the food that are not normally eaten. A nonfatal dose may produce headache, sensation of tightness in the throat and chest, palpitation, and muscle weakness. Severe poisoning results in mental confusion and stupor, cyanosis, twitching, and convulsions with terminal coma.

Cyanosis Bluish appearance of the skin due to insufficient oxygenation of the blood.

Cycasin Plant toxin occurring in the *Cycas* family, which is widely distributed in tropical and subtropical areas. It is a potent carcinogen and produces malignant liver and kidney tumors in animals. The cycas plant is used as a source of starch for thickening and bread making. Soaking and washing the cycas kernels in water will remove the toxic principle.

Cyclamate Sodium or calcium salt of cyclohexylsulfamic acid; a nonnutritive or artificial sweetener about 30 to 60 times sweeter than sucrose. The use of cyclamates in beverages and food products has been prohibited because of findings that they form toxic compounds and that high intakes produce cancer in rats and genetic damage in chicken embryos. Cyclamate was transferred from the *GRAS* category as a food additive to drug status to permit its use under medical supervision. See *GRAS list*.

Cyclic AMP (cAMP) Abbreviation for *adenosine-3',5'-monophosphate*. This compound mediates the effects of hormones and thus may be a "second messenger." It plays a role in many metabolic reactions. See *Adenosine phosphates*.

Cyst A sac, especially one containing a liquid or semisolid.

Cystathionine An intermediate product in the conversion of methionine to cysteine.

Cystathioninuria Inborn error of metabolism characterized by mental retardation and elevated cystathionine in blood and urine. It is probably a defect in the methionine-cysteine pathway. In some instances the biochemical abnormality can be corrected by administration of pyridoxine.

Cysteine Alpha-amino-beta-mercaptopropionic acid, a sulfur-containing amino acid formed by the reduction of cystine.

Cystic fibrosis Fatal disease occurring in young children characterized by generalized dysfunction of the exocrine glands involving the pancreas, respiratory system, salivary glands, gastrointestinal tract, biliary system, and paranasal glands. The sweat contains large amounts of sodium chloride and, to a lesser extent, potassium. Abnormal mucus secretion results in obstruction of mucus-producing cells or organ passages. Lack of pancreatic enzymes interferes with the utilization of protein, fat, and carbohydrate. Vitamin deficiencies occur because of digestive defects and death usually results from malnutrition or bronchopneumonia. An integrated treatment includes pancreatic enzyme replacement, therapy for the digestive defect, and dietary management. See Dietary management of selected disorders, Appendix O.

Cystine A sulfur-containing nonessential amino acid found in large amounts in *keratins*. It is relatively insoluble at the pH of normal urine and can crystallize or precipitate to form cystine stones.

Cystinosis A rare hereditary disease characterized by accumulation of cystine crystals in bone marrow, cornea, and internal organs. Cystine level in the plasma is normal, but free cystine concentration in leukocytes is about 80 times greater than normal. The primary defect is believed to be due to an abnormal subcellular compartmentalization of cystine.

Cystinuria Inborn error of metabolism characterized by high urinary excretion of cystine crystals. The condition is due to a defect in the renal tubular reabsorption of amino acids, especially cystine, and basic amino acids such as lysine, arginine, and ornithine. Cystine, being the least soluble, tends to precipitate out of the urine and form kidney and bladder stones. Increasing the water intake to dilute the urine is desirable. See also Dietary management of selected disorders, Appendix O.

Cystogram Radiograph of the urinary bladder.

Cystolithiasis Formation of stones or calculi in the urinary bladder.

Cystolithotomy Surgical removal of calculus from the bladder.

Cytidine A pyrimidine nucleoside composed of cytosine and D-ribose.

Cytidine phosphates Mono-, di-, and triphosphoric esters of cytidine, as cytidine monophosphate (CMP), cytidine diphosphate (CDP), and cytidine triphosphate (CTP). As cytidine phosphate derivatives, they are involved in the biosynthesis of lecithin and cephalins.

Cytochrome oxidase An iron-containing oxidase that accepts electrons from the other cytochromes and passes them on to oxygen, which is the ultimate hydrogen acceptor. Of all the cytochromes, it is the terminal catalyst in the sense that it effects the direct union of oxygen with the electrons derived from substrates.

Cytochromes Group of oxidation-reduction enzymes that are primarily concerned with the transfer of electrons from flavoproteins and other substrates to oxygen or other electron acceptors.

Cytology Science that deals with the structure, behavior, growth, reproduction, chemistry, and function of cells.

Cytoplasm Viscous, fluidlike mass outside of the nucleus that contains various specialized structures called *organelles*. It contains water, nucleic acid, enzymes, proteins, and various chemicals involved in cell functions.

Cytosine 2-Oxy-4-aminopyrimidine, a *pyrimidine* found in nucleic acids.

D

Dairy food substitutes Foods that resemble or imitate dairy food products but are different in composition and nutrient content. Examples are coffee whiteners (imitation cream) and mellorine (imitation ice cream).

Dalton's law Total pressure exerted by a mixture of gases is equal to the sum of the partial pressures of the various gases.

Dark adaptation Speed with which the eye adjusts to a change in intensity of light. This depends on the amount of vitamin A in the body. In man, maximal dark adaptation of the rods requires about 25 minutes; it is longer in vitamin A deficiency.

Data communication A rapid way of transmitting information that can be directly used by *computers*. Data communication is also used to report conditions happening in remote places. A typical use in medicine is the transmission of electrocardiogram tracings from a small hospital or from a patient's home to the office of a cardiologist so that a quick diagnosis can be made.

Data processing system Procedure that describes the orderly sequence of operations to be followed in processing data information.

Data terminal Device for transmitting computer data. It may be in the form of punched cards, punched paper tape, magnetic tape, or other physical media.

DBI Trade name for phenformin, an oral hypoglycemic agent used in adult-onset diabetes and as a supplement to insulin in certain young diabetics. See *Oral hypoglycemic agents*.

DBW Abbreviation for *desirable body weight*. See *Weight*.

Deamination Removal of an alpha amino group from an amino acid. The reaction is catalyzed by the enzyme *deaminase;* it occurs chiefly in the liver and possibly in the kidneys and other organs.

Debranching enzyme Amylo-1,6-glucosidase, an enzyme that removes the branching points in glycogen. In the breakdown of glycogen to glucose-1-phosphate, phosphorylase acts only on the 1,4 linkages and ceases as points of branching are approached. The 1,6 branch linkages are removed hydrolytically by the action of this enzyme. See also *Branching enzyme*.

Decalcification Demineralization; the loss of calcium salts from bones and teeth.

Decarboxylation Removal of the carboxyl group (carbon dioxide) from a molecule by the enzyme *decarboxylase*.

Decompensation Failure or inability of the heart to maintain adequate circulation. The condition is characterized by dyspnea, cyanosis, edema, and venous engorgement.

Decubitus ulcer A pressure sore caused by prolonged confinement and immobility in bed.

Defecation Evacuation or excretion of fecal matter through the anus. Fecal contents are variable and include undigested and unabsorbed food residues, substances excreted from the body into the digestive tract, living and dead microorganisms that normally inhabit the alimentary tract, and small amounts of water. Normally the fecal material is liquid on entry into the colon. It loses water to become a semisolid mass by the time it reaches the rectum.

Deficiency disease Condition arising from the deficiency or lack of one or more of the essential nutrients because of *primary* or dietary inadequacy or as a result of *secondary* or conditioned inadequacy. The condition may be conceived as a progressive and continuous process that, if uncorrected, eventually leads to depletion of body nutrient reserves. Biochemical changes or "lesions" occur in selected tissues or in the body at large; these eventually result in functional changes such as loss of appetite, easy fatigability, and gastrointestinal disturbances. As the nutritional deficiency continues, anatomic lesions develop and gross clinical signs and symptoms like glossitis, cheilosis, and dermatitis become manifest. In summary, the development of a deficiency disease may be envisioned to occur in five stages, i.e., nutritional inadequacy, tissue depletion, biochemical changes, functional changes, and anatomic lesions. For manifestations of mineral and vitamin deficiencies, see Summary of minerals and Summary of vitamins, Appendices H and I-1. See also Methods of research in nutrition: clinical tests, Appendix M-3.

Primary Also called dietary deficiency disease; a condition due to the failure to ingest an essential nutritional factor in amounts sufficient to meet existing requirements of the body. This may in turn be due to poor food habits, poverty, ignorance, lack of food, or excess consumption of highly refined foods.

Secondary Also called conditioned deficiency disease; due to failure to absorb or utilize an essential nutrient because of environmental condition or bodily state and not because of dietary lack or failure of ingestion. These conditioning factors may be grouped into six categories, i.e., interference with ingestion, interference with absorption, interference with utilization,

increased nutrient requirement, increased nutrient destruction, and increased nutrient excretion.

Dehydrase Enzyme that catalyzes the removal of water from a substrate.

Dehydration 1. Drying; removal of water from food, tissue, or substrate. 2. Condition resulting from excessive loss of fluids from the body.

Dehydroascorbic acid Oxidized form of *vitamin C;* the reduced form is ascorbic acid. These two compounds are readily and reversibly oxidized and reduced. Both are biologically active, although dehydroascorbic acid is somewhat less stable than ascorbic acid.

7-Dehydrocholesterol See *Vitamin D.*

Dehydrogenase Enzyme that catalyzes the transfer of hydrogen from a substrate to a carrier. There is a specific dehydrogenase for each substrate. The aerobic dehydrogenase transfers hydrogen directly to oxygen, resulting in the formation of hydrogen peroxide. The anaerobic dehydrogenase, on the other hand, requires a hydrogen acceptor or carrier, forming water as the final product.

Dehydrogenation Removal of hydrogen by reaction with a hydrogen acceptor. The oxidation of organic compounds is synonymous with dehydrogenation.

Dehydroretinol New term for vitamin A_2 or 3-dehydroretinol. See *Vitamin A.*

Delaney clause The anticancer clause in the Federal Drug and Cosmetic Act that requires the removal of any food additive shown to be capable of inducing cancer in experimental animals.

Delirium tremens Kind of mental disturbance associated with chronic alcoholism; usually accompanied by hallucination, delirium, trembling, disorientation, loss of appetite, and nausea.

Demographics Characteristics of human population, such as size, distribution, and vital statistics.

Demulcent A substance that is soothing and allays irritation.

Denaturation Any alteration in the structure

of a *native protein,* giving rise to definite changes in chemical, physical, or biologic properties such as decrease in solubility at the isoelectric point, loss of biologic specificity, loss of ability to crystallize, increase in viscosity and digestibility, and changes in molecular shape. Denaturation may be brought about by heating, freezing, irradiation, pressure, and treatment with organic solvents.

Dendrite A branched protoplasmic extension from a nerve cell that conducts impulses toward the cell body.

Density Mass of a substance divided by its volume $(D = W/V)$.

Dental caries Teeth decay; demineralization of the inorganic portion and dissolution of the organic substance of the teeth. Three factors are involved in the development of dental caries: host and teeth, microflora, and substrate in the mouth. Dental caries will not develop if the teeth are caries resistant and the mouth is kept clean and free of food particles that will sustain the growth of cariogenic bacteria. Evidence indicates that sucrose, especially if taken between meals, is the chief dietary component promoting dental caries. The production of acid from the bacterial fermentation of carbohydrates is the immediate cause of the breaking down of the enamel and dentin. Fluorine and other nutrients in foods can also accelerate or reduce the development of dental caries. The following are recommended dietary measures to prevent tooth decay: (a) fluoridation of drinking water where the supply is deficient in natural fluorine, (b) restricted consumption of sticky and sugary confections, and (c) avoidance of between-meal consumption of sweets.

Dentin Also called dentine; the chief substance of calcified tissue that surrounds the tooth pulp and root canals. It is covered by the *enamel* on the crown or exposed part of the tooth and by the *cementum* over the roots implanted in the jaw. Dentin resembles bone but is harder and denser.

Dentition Teething; eruption of the teeth. See *Nutrition, dental health.*

Deoxy- Prefix signifying loss of oxygen from a compound.

Deoxycorticosterone (DOC) Also called desoxycorticosterone; a hormone produced by the adrenal cortex. It is corticosterone without the oxygen atom at carbon atom 11. Except for aldosterone, it has a greater electrolyte-regulating effect than the other corticoids. It is prepared synthetically as the acetate (Doca) and is useful in the treatment of Addison's disease.

Deoxycorticosterone acetate (DOCA) Acetic acid ester of deoxycorticosterone. It is the active principle in the commercial preparation of Doca.

Deoxypyridoxine Structural analog and antagonist of *pyridoxine.* It is used in the experimental induction of pyridoxine deficiency in animals as well as human adults.

Deoxyribonucleic acid (DNA) Also called deoxyribose nucleic acid; the main carrier of genetic information necessary for the synthesis of specific proteins. It is found in the nuclei of cells as part of the chromosome structure and consists of phosphoric acid, purines (adenine and guanine), pyrimidines (cytosine and thymine), and the sugar deoxyribose. The DNA structure is envisioned as a double helix in which the purine and pyrimidine bases are inside the helix, with the sugar and phosphate backbone outside the helix. The chains are held together by hydrogen bonding.

Depot fat Stored body fat. See *Adipose tissue.*

Depressor nerve An *afferent* nerve that promotes a fall in blood pressure by slowing the heart or by vasodilatation.

Dermatitis Inflammation of the skin. There are many forms and causes, e.g., prolonged exposure to the sun's rays, allergy, and infection. Dermatitis is also seen in association with deficiency states due to lack of biotin, niacin, vitamin B_6, and essential fatty acids.

Dermatology Science that deals with the structure, function, and diseases of the skin. See *Nutrition, dermatology.*

Dermis True skin. It is highly vascular and supplied with sensitive nerve endings. See *Skin.*

Desiccator A closed container that contains a hygroscopic agent such as calcium chloride to keep materials inside it dry and free from moisture.

Desmoglycogen Form of glycogen in tissue; bound to protein, particularly myosin.

Desmosterol The immediate precursor of cholesterol in its biosynthetic pathway.

Desoxy- Prefix signifying loss of oxygen from a compound. The preferred form is *deoxy-*. For words beginning as desoxy-, see those beginning as deoxy-.

Detoxication Also called detoxification; the chemical changes in the body that serve to convert toxic substances into forms that are less toxic and more readily excretable. The detoxication mechanism involves oxidation, reduction, hydrolysis, or conjugation with a compound occurring normally in the body, such as glycine, cysteine, and glutamine. Toxic products in the body are either metabolic in origin, ingested, or produced by bacteria in the large intestines.

Deuterium Heavy hydrogen; the *isotope* of hydrogen with an atomic weight of 2. It is used in tracer studies and body water determinations.

Dextran Polysaccharide of glucose produced by the action of microorganisms on sugar. It is used in gel filtration chromatography and as a substitute for blood plasma in the treatment of severe burns and hemorrhagic shock.

Dextrimaltose Preparation of dextrin and maltose; used as a carbohydrate modifier in infant milk formulas.

Dextrin Polymer of D-glucose that is intermediate in complexity between starch and maltose. It is formed by partial hydrolysis of starch during digestion or by the action of dry heat on starch and is used as an emulsifying, sizing, and thickening agent.

Dextrorotatory Having the ability to rotate a plane of polarized light to the right; designated by a plus (+) sign. See *Optical activity.*

Dextrose Also called glucose. See *Glucose.*

Diabetes Condition characterized by excessive thirst and excessive urination. If used unqualified, the term refers to *diabetes mellitus.*

D alloxan Hyperglycemia (high blood sugar) following the experimental administration of *alloxan* in animals. Symptoms produced are similar to those seen in human diabetes mellitus.

D insipidus Condition characterized by the excretion of large quantities of urine of low specific gravity, excessive thirst, and dehydration. It is due to a disorder of the hypothalamus or the pituitary gland.

D, juvenile Infantile or childhood diabetes mellitus. Diabetes in children is likely to be more severe than in adults. The onset is quite sudden and the majority of children are underweight when the disease is first recognized. The condition is generally unstable and difficult to regulate, and the patients are insulin dependent (i.e., they need insulin to be metabolically balanced) and insulin sensitive (i.e., a small change of insulin dosage may cause large changes in the concentration of blood sugar).

D, lipoatrophic Syndrome characterized by insulin-resistant diabetes, less of a tendency to develop ketosis on omission of exogenous insulin, complete absence of subcutaneous intra-abdominal and peripheral fat, hepatosplenomegaly, hyperlipemia, and marked elevation of basal metabolic rate without other evidence of hyperthyroidism.

D mellitus Metabolic disorder characterized by varying degrees of impairment in the body's ability to utilize carbohydrate. For some individuals, diabetes presents no symptoms unless detected clinically. When symptoms are present, the most characteristic are increased appetite or polyphagia, excessive urination or polyuria, increased thirst or polydipsia, weakness, and loss of weight. Visual disturbances and pruritus vulva are also seen. The etiologic development of the disorder is not clear, but it seems that the entire endocrine system is involved, particularly the pancreas as well as the anterior pituitary, adrenal cortex, and thyroid. An imbalance in one or several of these endocrine glands may be implicated in diabetes. Heredity seems to be a significant factor; a familial tendency to diabetes exists, although the precise genetic factor and the mode of inheritance are not known. For many years it was thought that diabetes was simply caused by diminished secretion of insulin by the beta cells of the islet of Langerhans in the pancreas. Recent observations show that in some diabetics, the blood level of insulin or insulin-like activity is normal or even slightly increased. Two explanations have been offered: that insulin may be present in bound form and not available to the tissues, or that there may be an antagonist that interferes with the action of insulin or counteracts its effect in the tissues. The better known insulin antagonists are the *glucocorticoids, thyroxine, glucagon, insulinase,* and *synalbumin.* Other possible causes of diabetes include the development of *autoimmunity,* deficiency in minerals (such as chromium, potassium, and probably zinc), dietary factors (particularly a diet rich in soluble carbohydrate), and a genetic defect in the polypeptide synthesis of insulin. See *Diet, diabetic* and Dietary management of selected disorders, Appendix O.

D, renal Form of diabetes due to low renal threshold for glucose, resulting in excretion of glucose in the urine even with a normal blood sugar level. See also *Phlorizin.*

Diabetogenic hormone Factor in the anterior pituitary gland capable of raising the blood sugar level. Whether or not this factor in the pituitary gland exists as a separate substance is not known. Several pituitary hormones such as growth hormone, ACTH, and TSH have diabetogenic properties and can cause hyperglycemia when secreted in large amounts.

Diabinese Trade name for chlorpropamide, an *oral hypoglycemic agent.*

Diacetyl A butter flavor component produced during ripening of butter by microbial action. It is produced artificially and used commercially to give the "butter" flavor to margarine.

Dialysis Separation of substances in solution by selective diffusion through a semipermeable membrane. Substances smaller than the pores of the membrane pass through, leaving the larger molecules behind. Some membranes suitable for dialysis are collodion, dialyzing cellophane, animal parchment, vegetable parchment, and fish bladders. See also *Hemodialysis.*

Diaphysis Shaft of a long bone, as the arm bone, shin bone, or thigh bone.

Diarrhea Condition characterized by frequent passage of loose, watery, and unformed stools. It may be functional or organic in nature and may be due to a number of causes, e.g., intestinal infection, ingestion of poison, overeating, nervous disorder, endocrine disturbance, and food malabsorption and sensitivity. Diarrhea may also be associated with nutritional disorders such as pellagra. See Dietary management of selected disorders, Appendix O.

Diastole Period of dilatation of the heart. See *Blood pressure.*

Diathesis Condition or constitution of the body or a combination of attributes in one individual that makes him more susceptible to disease.

Dicumarol Trade name of bishydroxycoumarin; an anticoagulant present in spoiled sweet clover that is structurally similar to vitamin K. It counteracts the formation of clotting factors, notably prothrombin, whose production requires the presence of vitamin K. Dicumarol and its various derivatives are prepared synthetically and used in the treatment of thrombosis.

Diet 1. The usual food and drink regularly consumed. 2. To take food according to a regimen. 3. Food prescribed, regulated, or restricted as to kind and amount for therapeutic or other purposes.

Diet, adequate Diet that meets all the nutritional needs of an individual. A dietary pattern based on the *basic four food groups* is a practical way of planning for dietary adequacy to meet the *recommended dietary allowances* for specific nutrients.

Diet, Alvarez A "smooth" diet consisting of three full meals with between-meal feedings of 6 ounces of milk-egg mixture (2 eggs/quart milk) every 2 hours and after supper until two or three o'clock the following morning. This diet was prescribed by Alvarez for convalescing peptic ulcer patients. Foods included in the diet are orange juice, coffee and tea in moderation, cocoa or chocolate, white bread or toast, cream soups, smooth mush (such as farina, cream of wheat, strained rolled oats, rice, and potatoes), purees of peas, beans, or lentils, small portions of meat, fish, and chicken, plain puddings, custards, ice cream, cake and gelatin, and ripe banana and stewed fruits.

Diet, Andresen Diet prescribed for bleeding peptic ulcers and following gastric surgery. It consists of a 6-ounce mixture of milk, cream, gelatin, and dextrose given every 2 hours. On the fifth or sixth day, soft cooked egg or 3 ounces of cereal, custard, plain gelatin, or ice cream is added to three or four of the feedings during the day. Other bland and low fiber foods are gradually added to the diet until the patient is receiving stage II of the *progressive bland diet.*

Diet, ash The mineral elements in foods (ash) form a residue that is excreted in the urine. Ash diets are classified as acid-ash, alkaline- or basic-ash, and neutral-ash, depending on the effect that the predominant mineral elements have on the pH of the urine. The acid-forming elements in foods such as sulfur, phosphorus, and chloride decrease the pH of the urine. On the other hand, the alkaline-forming elements in foods such as sodium, potassium,

magnesium, and calcium bring about a pH increase in the urine. Foods that have no effect on urine pH are neutral-ash foods. Thus by changing the composition of the diet the urine may be made either acidic or alkaline. In general, cereals and protein-rich foods have a predominance of the acid-forming elements. Fruits, vegetables, and milk contain mostly alkaline-forming elements. Fats, oils, and sugars give a neutral ash.

Acid-ash d Diet emphasizing the use of large amounts of acid-forming foods such as meat, fish, eggs, and cereals while restricting the intake of alkaline-forming foods such as fruits, vegetables, and milk. The diet is prescribed for kidney stones consisting of calcium and magnesium phosphates, carbonates, and oxalates. It is believed that acidifying the urine will keep these stones in solution. When properly planned, the diet is nutritionally adequate.

Alkaline-ash d Diet emphasizing the intake of large amounts of alkaline-forming foods such as fruits, vegetables, and milk while limiting the intake of acid-forming foods such as meat, fish, eggs, and cereals. The diet is prescribed for uric acid and cystine stones in the kidneys. A change in the urine toward the basic side is believed to be beneficial in keeping these stones in solution. The diet is nutritionally adequate if foods are chosen properly.

Diet, balanced Diet containing all the required nutrients in *proper proportion* with respect to one another for optimum nutrition. A more appropriate term to use is *adequate diet,* since a diet that is quantitatively "balanced" for "optimum" nutrition is rather difficult to attain.

Diet, basic-ash See *Alkaline-ash diet* under *Diet, ash.*

Diet, bland Diet consisting of bland and mild-flavored foods. In the past, "bland" foods have been defined as those that are soft or smooth in consistency, not mechanically or chemically irritating to the stomach, and not stimulating excessive flow of gastric juice. Excluded from the diet are foods that are fibrous, hard, and harsh; strong-flavored vegetables such as cabbage, broccoli, cauliflower, and turnips; nonprotein nitrogenous meat extractives; and flavoring substances such as spices, herbs, and condiments. There is no evidence that such foods irritate the gastric mucosa. Except for alcohol and spices such as black pepper, chili powder, cayenne pepper, curry, and possibly nutmeg, other foods do not seem to cause gastric irritation. Present diet therapy emphasizes small frequent feedings and puts fewer restrictions on the type of food allowed. Individualization is the rule, and only those foods known to be disagreeable to the patient are omitted from the diet. The bland diet is indicated for patients with gastric and duodenal ulcers, hiatus hernia, and esophagitis with reflux of gastric secretion. See also *Diet, progressive bland.*

Diet, Boas test Test meal consisting of a pint of thin oatmeal gruel given on an empty stomach prior to gastric analysis to stimulate the secretion of gastric juices.

Diet, Borst Protein-free diet advocated by Borst in cases of uremia and acute renal failure. It consists of ¾ cup sugar and ¾ cup butter given in the form of frozen butter balls or in the form of butter soup mixed in 2 cups water and thickened with 2 tablespoons flour. The whole mixture, given in six equal feedings, contains approximately 1800 calories, 150 gm carbohydrate, 135 gm fat, and 1400 mg sodium. The diet is adequate in vitamin A but is lacking in calcium, iron, ascorbic acid, and the B complex vitamins. For variation, the butter-sugar mixture may be flavored with coffee, tea, or vanilla.

Diet, brat Diet consisting of banana, rice, apple, and tea; prescribed for diarrhea, especially in infants and children.

Diet, Bull Protein-free diet similar to Borst diet, except that peanut oil is used instead of butter. See *Diet, Borst.*

Diet, butter-sugar See *Diet, Borst.*

Diet, Caesar's Diet of milk and barley water formerly used in the early stages of gout.

Diet, calcium-phosphorus–restricted Diet prescribed in the treatment of calcium phosphate stones. It restricts the intake of calcium and phosphorus to minimal levels while maintaining nutritional adequacy. Foods high in these minerals (such as milk and milk products, whole grain cereals, organ meats, sardines, leafy greens, legumes, nuts, and cocoa) are either restricted or omitted from the diet, depending on the level of intake prescribed by the physician. A strict to moderate restriction ranges from 200 to 400 mg calcium and 700 to 1000 mg phosphorus.

Diet, calcium test Calculated diet used in the study of calcium metabolism under conditions of minimum intake. The diet contains approximately 170 mg calcium and 600 mg phosphorus. A weighed diet plan is made and used during the entire test period, which usually lasts for 1 week.

Diet, calorie modified Diet in which the total intake of calories is either increased or decreased from the normal intake to allow for a gain or loss in body weight.

Low calorie d Diet planned to permit loss of weight while maintaining health. A reduction of 500 calories/day, while keeping activity constant, should bring about a loss in body weight of about 1 pound/week. It is best to arrive at a caloric allowance that is tolerable to the patient. A weekly weight loss of 1 to 2 pounds is considered satisfactory. Weight loss of more than 2 pounds/week is not advisable unless under the close supervision of a physician. Care should be observed in planning the diet; caloric levels below 1200 are marginal in nutrient content and may necessitate vitamin supplementation. A liberal protein intake is essential for its satiety value and to prevent negative nitrogen balance; carbohydrate and fat are restricted to the caloric level desired. Foods to avoid include sauces, gravies, nuts, sweets, desserts, and fried foods.

High calorie d Diet with a prescribed caloric intake above normal to meet increased energy requirements and to provide weight gain. It is indicated in febrile conditions, hyperthyroidism, athetosis, undernutrition, and other conditions that have resulted in loss of weight. The caloric increase may vary from 30% to 100% above the usual intake. It is best to individualize the diet. Observations with patients of different sexes and ages show that men seem to prefer the additional calories through extra portions of the usual foods served at meals, children and adolescents prefer between-meal nourishment, and women seem to favor more concentrated foods.

Diet, Cantani's An exclusive meat diet formerly used for diabetes.

Diet, carbohydrate modified Diet that provides a specified level of carbohydrate or is restricted in the amount of a particular type of carbohydrate such as glucose, sucrose, fructose, galactose, or lactose.

High carbohydrate d Diet high in available carbohydrate to allow for glycogen formation, to ensure sufficient calories to meet needs, to spare protein, and to minimize tissue catabolism. It is indicated in liver diseases, Addison's disease, fasting hypoglycemia, acute glomerulonephritis, uremia, pernicious vomiting, and toxemias of pregnancy. The diet is modified in consistency or other nutrient content to suit specific disease conditions. Emphasis is placed on easily available carbohydrates such as sugar, syrups, jellies, and jams.

Restricted carbohydrate d Diet limited in carbohydrate content to reduce available glucose when carbohydrate metabolism is impaired, as in spontaneous hypoglycemia. It is also indicated for dumping syndrome, epilepsy, and obesity. Restrictions in specific types of carbohydrates such as sucrose, lactose, maltose, and galactose are also indicated in cases of carbohydrate intolerance to these sugars. See *Diet, galactose-free; Diet, lactose-free; Diet, maltose-free;* and *Diet, sucrose-restricted.*

Diet, chemically defined See *Diet, elemental.*

Diet, Chittenden's Diet that limits the intake of protein to 45 to 55 gm/day. The diet is based on the rationale that a low protein intake is more beneficial to health than higher intakes.

Diet, cholesterol-restricted Diet in which the intake of dietary cholesterol is restricted to a prescribed level. It is indicated for hypercholesterolemia, atherosclerosis, and gallbladder stones with cholesterol esters. Individuals who eat one or more eggs a day and use organ meats at regular intervals ingest 1000 mg cholesterol/day or more. Omission of eggs and organ meats will bring down the intake of cholesterol to 300 mg/day. This amount can be further reduced if butter is not used and skim milk is substituted for whole milk.

Diet, cholesterol-restricted, fat-controlled Diet designed to lower blood cholesterol level by restricting the intake of foods high in cholesterol and saturated fats and by increasing the use of vegetable oils and special margarines high in polyunsaturates. This may be accomplished by limiting the intake of meat, fish, and poultry to two average servings per day (3 to 4 ounces/serving); restricting the intake of egg (i.e., egg yolk) to three per week; limiting the intake of cheese, shellfish, and organ meats (liver, kidney, sweetbreads, and heart) to a 2-ounce portion as a substitute for an egg; restricting the intake of saturated fats by trimming visible fat and using only lean cuts of meat; using only liquid vegetable oils and margarines made from oils rich in polyunsaturates such as corn, cottonseed, soybean, and safflower oil; avoiding commercially prepared and packaged foods containing whole egg, whole milk, and saturated fats; and eliminating cholesterol-rich foods such as fish roe, caviar, and brain. This dietary regimen restricts the intake of cholesterol to about half the normal intake of cholesterol in the average American diet (approximately 300 to 350 mg/day). A further reduction in cholesterol would necessitate total omission of eggs from the diet. In order to have a high polyunsaturated/saturated fat ratio, at least 1 teaspoon vegetable oil or margarine high in polyunsaturates is needed per ounce of cooked meat. For the overweight person, weight reduction is desirable as this has the effect of lowering blood cholesterol.

Diet, Coleman-Shaffer Diet formerly used for typhoid fever; composed of eggs, cream, cocoa, milk, sugar, bread, and butter and given in small frequent feedings.

Diet, copper-restricted Diet calculated not to exceed 1 mg of copper/day; normal copper intake is about 2.5 mg daily. The diet is prescribed for the treatment of Wilson's disease, which is characterized by low plasma copper level but high copper storage in the liver and nervous tissue. Food sources rich in copper are eliminated from the diet; these include liver and organ meats, nuts, dried fruits, peas and lentils, whole-grain cereals, shrimp, shellfish, oysters, mushrooms, molasses, spinach, and other leafy greens. Only chemically pure salt can be used, as table salt has varying and significant amounts of copper.

Diet, Cutler-Power-Wilder test Calculated low sodium, high potassium test diet for diagnosis of adrenocortical insufficiency. The standard test diet is weighed and given for 2½ days. Under the conditions of the test, a urinary chloride concentration above 225 mg% indicates poor function of the adrenal cortex; a chloride concentration of 125 mg% or less indicates normal function. The test is of limited value when glomerulonephritis or uncontrolled diabetes is present.

Diet, desensitizing Diet aimed at decreasing the sensitivity of a person to a given food allergen. The food allergen is first excluded from the diet for an indefinite period. Then the offending food is gradually added to the diet in small amounts until an average portion is tolerated by the individual.

Diet, dental soft See *Diet, mechanical soft.*

Diet, diabetic The diabetic diet follows the pattern of a normal diet for maintenance of good health and normal activity. It is no longer necessary to require a diabetic (with no complications) to follow detailed dietary regulations and precise food measurements and meal patterns. Except for simple sugars that are rapidly absorbed and can produce hyperglycemic peaks, a diabetic can have more freedom in his choice of foods. However, individualization is the rule; the dietary requirements of diabetics differ with the severity of the disease, the type and extent of insulin therapy received, and the amount of activity performed. The most important consideration is adjustment of total caloric intake to attain and maintain desirable body weight. Also important are the proper spacing and regularity of meals, particularly among those receiving insulin therapy, to avoid intermittent hypoglycemia.

Diet, elemental Also called chemically defined diet; a mixture of basic nutrients of known quantitative composition. It consists of either hydrolyzed protein or synthetic L-amino acids, simple sugars, and all other nutrients presently known to be required for human nutrition. This diet was originally designed for space travel. The mixture requires very little digestion; it is almost completely absorbed by the upper small bowel and is very low in residue. Elemental diets are now used in malabsorption, short bowel syndromes, and severe nutritional problems involving the gastrointestinal tract.

Diet, elimination A normal diet that excludes the intake of a specific food or food group known to produce allergic manifestations. Attention should be given to commercially processed or packaged foods that may contain the offending substance in disguised form. The patient should be taught to read the list of ingredients on all labels and packages.

Diet, elimination test A series of allergy test diets beginning with a basic diet that consists of a few carefully selected foods least likely to cause allergic reactions. If the patient remains asymptomatic on the basic diet for 2 weeks, other foods are gradually added at 4-day intervals. Milk, eggs, and wheat are added last because these items are the most notorious food allergens. If relief of symptoms is not obtained even on the basic diet, it is probable that an agent other than food is the offending allergen. The most widely used test diet is the one designed by Rowe. See *Diet, Rowe's elimination.*

Diet, Ewald test Test meal given on an empty stomach prior to gastric analysis. It consists of 1½ glasses (300 to 400 ml) water or weak tea without cream or sugar and 2 slices of white bread or toast. The stomach content is extracted 45 minutes after the meal for examination of free hydrochloric acid and total acidity.

Diet, faddist A craze diet based on the purported "magic quality" in some peculiar kind of food to treat or cure conditions. Common fad diets are the *Zen macrobiotic diet,* molasses diet, fruit diet, and various formula diets that have caught the fancy of overweight persons.

Diet, fat modified Diet that prescribes a specified level of fat in the diet, fatty acids ratio, or percentage of calories from fat. Modifications in the fat content of the diet are necessary in weight reduction, diseases of the gallbladder, pancreas, and cardiovascular system, and disturbances in fat absorption in association with such diseases as sprue, cystic fibrosis, and pancreatitis.

Fat-controlled d Also called proportioned fat diet; one in which both the *amount* and *kind* of fat are regulated. The diet is generally planned to provide 30% of the calories from fat. The total amount of fat is then "controlled" or proportioned into two categories: basic or unavoidable fat of meats and other foods, and saturated, monounsaturated, and polyunsaturated fatty acid portion. The objective of the diet is to increase the intake of polyunsaturated fatty acids and reduce the intake of saturated fatty acids to bring about a decrease in serum cholesterol and triglycerides. Polyunsaturated fatty acids are supplied by such oils as corn, soybean, cottonseed, and safflower. Saturated fatty acids are high in animal products, palm oil, and hydrogenated oil products. A high polyunsaturated/saturated fat (P/S) ratio may be attained by trimming visible fats from meats, using lean meats, fish, and poultry without the skin, substituting skim milk for whole milk, and using oils rich in polyunsaturates in food preparation. An allowance of 1 tablespoon vegetable oil rich in polyunsaturates per average serving of meat is generally considered sufficient to give the desired P/S ratio.

Liberal fat d A liberal fat allowance is about 40% of caloric intake or approximately 100 to 130 gm of fat/day. A liberal fat intake often accompanies a high protein, high calorie diet prescription for certain conditions that do not require any restriction in the fat content of the diet, such as in undernutrition, burns, nephrosis, and ulcerative colitis. A high fat intake is indicated in conditions that restrict the intakes of carbohydrate and/or protein, as in dumping syndrome, functional hyperinsulinism, and uremia. In such cases it is best to supply fat in the form of butter, margarine, cream, salad dressing, and vegetable oils.

Low fat d Reduction in the fat content of the diet to from 10% to 15% of caloric intake or approximately 20 to 40 gm of fat/day is indicated during acute attacks of pancreatitis and cholecystitis. This amount of fat is essentially supplied by 5 to 8 ounces of lean meat, fish, or poultry. Any fat restriction lower than 20 gm/day will impose further limitation in the selection and intake of animal protein foods; the intake of the B complex vitamins will also be limited. All foods rich in fat are not allowed. Visible fats of meat are trimmed and foods are prepared simply by broiling, roasting, baking, or boiling. The use of sugar, sweets, fruits, cereals, and starchy vegetables will increase caloric intake, and protein may be increased through the use of skim milk, egg white, and gelatin.

MCT fat d Diet in which MCT oil is used in place of ordinary cooking fats and oils. MCT is a unique oil containing triglycerides of medium-chain fatty acids, which are more easily hydrolyzed and absorbed than the long-chain triglycerides present in conventional dietary fats. The diet is indicated for conditions wherein ordinary dietary fats are poorly digested and absorbed, as in pancreatitis, cystic fibrosis, chyluria, sprue, intestinal resection, pancreatic insufficiency, deficient bile secretion, and biliary obstruction. Three to four tablespoons MCT oil (about 40 to 55 gm fat) or an amount recommended by the physician may be used in cooking, in salad dressings, sauces, or marinades for meats and vegetables, or simply mixed with fruit juices. The oil is colorless, odorless, and tasteless and mixes well with liquids.

Moderate fat d Diet with a fat allowance of from 20% to 30% of caloric intake or about 50 to 70 gm of fat/day. A moderate fat intake is indicated in hepatitis, cirrhosis of the liver, and chronic gallbladder and pancreatic diseases. It is also recommended in weight reduction to lend palatability and satiety value to the diet. Fried foods, nuts, sauces, gravies, and other fatty foods should be avoided. It is best to get the fat allowance from lean meats, eggs, milk, butter, and other highly emulsified fats. Whenever necessary, additional calories may be supplied by sugar, sweets, and other carbohydrate-rich foods.

Very high fat d One in which fat is approximately 80% or more of caloric intake. Carbohydrate intake is severely restricted to not more than 30 gm/day, and protein allowance is slightly below normal levels. The aim of the diet is to maintain a keto-genic/antiketogenic ratio that will produce a state of ketosis. See *Diet, ketogenic*.

Diet, fat test Two test diets are used in the diagnosis of gallbladder disease and the determination of fat absorption.

Fat-free test d A test meal given the night before a gallbladder radiologic examination. The meal may consist of fat-free broth or consommé, fruits, plain gelatin, skim milk, and black coffee or tea. Nothing is given orally after midnight, and breakfast is withheld until after the x-ray examination is made. In some cases the x-ray examination is repeated after a *fatty meal*, which may consist of two fried eggs, buttered toast, whole milk, and coffee with cream.

High fat test d Calculated 100 gm fat test diet used to diagnose steatorrhea or azotorrhea. It is usually given for 3 days unless otherwise indicated. The fat allowance should come mainly from eggs, meats, whole milk, and highly emulsified fats such as butter and cream. It is important to choose foods that are simply prepared to facilitate fat intake calculation.

Diet, fiber modified Diet in which the amount of fiber or indigestible portion of food is modified higher or lower than the normal intake of about 4 gm daily. Fiber in plant foods is chiefly associated with the skins and seeds of fruits and vegetables, whole-grain cereals, nuts, and legumes. Fiber in meat is associated with the gristle or tough yellow connective tissue that is not changed by moist heat to gelatin during cooking.

High fiber d Also called high roughage diet; a normal diet with an additional two to three servings of foods high in roughage or indigestible carbohydrate. Excellent sources of fiber are whole grain cereals and unrefined breads, long-fibered vegetables, raw fruits, and legumes. The diet is prescribed in atonic constipation to stimulate peristalsis in the sluggish colon.

Low fiber d Diet that contains a minimal amount of indigestible carbohydrate and tough connective tissue. It is indicated in narrowing or stenosis of the intestines and in cancer of the bowel. The fiber content of the diet may be reduced by removing gristle and tough connective tissue in meats, removing seeds and skins of fruits and vegetables, omitting long-fibered foods or chopping or mincing these to cut down fibers, cooking foods to soften fibers, and using refined cereals and breads.

Diet, fluid See *Diet, liquid.*

Diet, formula A commercial preparation with balanced nutrient content to satisfy dietary needs in specific disorders. It comes in liquid or dry form. Examples are commercially prepared tube feedings and preparations designed for weight reduction such as Metrecal.

Diet, fructose-restricted Diet that restricts the intake of fructose from fruits and foods high in sucrose content (sucrose yields on hydrolysis glucose and fructose). These include table sugar, syrups, sweets, and processed foods with added sugar. Milk, meat, fish, poultry, and cereals can be given in normal amounts. Vegetables are allowed, except for sugar beets, green peas, and sweet potatoes.

Diet, full hospital Also called regular, general, or house diet. See *Diet, regular.*

Diet, galactose-free Diet eliminating foods containing galactose and lactose for the treatment of galactosemia. The chief dietary modification involves the elimination of milk and milk products, galactose-storing organ meats such as liver, pancreas, and brain, and vegetables such as beets, peas, soybeans, and lima beans because they have galactose-containing oligosaccharides in the form of raffinose and stachyose. Hidden sources of galactose and lactose in commercially prepared and packaged products can be detected by carefully reading package labels. Those with added milk, lactose, casein, whey, dry milk solids, or curds should be avoided. For infants a protein hydrolysate (such as Nutramigen) or a meat base formula may be

used in place of milk. The use of soya milk preparations like Soyalac and Sobee has been the subject of controversy. While there is no evidence that raffinose and stachyose in soybeans are hydrolyzed in the digestive tract, it may be wise not to use soya milk for infants until it is established that galactose is not liberated during digestion.

Diet, general Also called regular hospital diet. See *Diet, regular.*

Diet, Gerson-Hermannsdorfer Diet formerly prescribed for tuberculosis. It is high in fat, vitamins, and minerals, but somewhat limited in protein, carbohydrate, and salt.

Diet, Giordano-Giovannetti Highly restricted, selected protein diet prescribed for patients in acute kidney failure. The diet contains about 20 gm protein of the highest biologic value and 2000 to 3000 calories for daily maintenance in the form of carbohydrates and fats. This amount of protein will supply a minimal amount of the essential amino acids needed for maintenance of nitrogen balance; no provision is made for the nonessential amino acids in order to force the patient to utilize his elevated blood urea nitrogen supply in the synthesis of these amino acids. This serves to decrease the patient's blood urea level. The American adaptation of the original Giovannetti diet consists of a daily intake of 1 egg and ¾ cup of milk to supply the minimum requirements for essential amino acids. The remainder of the protein comes from low protein fruits, vegetables, and cereals. Additional calories are provided by sugars, fats, and special wheat starch products.

Diet, gliadin-free Diet eliminating wheat, oat, rye, barley, buckwheat, and products containing these cereal grains. The diet is used in the treatment of gluten-induced enteropathy. In place of the excluded cereals, rice, corn, potato, soybeans, the products of these, and gluten-free wheat starch may be used as desired. Milk, meat, fish, poultry, eggs, fruits, vegetables, fats, and sweets are allowed freely. It is important to read labels carefully, as many processed foods contain the restricted cereals in disguised form. Examples of such foods are malted milk, Ovaltine, beer, instant coffee, cold cuts, and sausages with wheat binders.

Diet, glucose-restricted Diet prescribed in rare cases of glucose intolerance. This diet is difficult to plan as glucose is present, either as free glucose or as a disaccharide component in milk, fruits, vegetables, and cereals. Newly born infants require the use of a special proprietary formula based on calcium caseinate, fructose, and corn oil with added vitamins and minerals. This regimen is usually followed until 6 months of age. Semisolid foods low in starch content are gradually introduced by the seventh month. At the age of 1 year the infant should be taking egg, fish, meat, and restricted amounts of fruits and vegetables. Milk and starchy foods are not introduced until about 2 to 3 years of age.

Diet, gluten-free Diet eliminating the use of cereals high in gluten content such as wheat, rye, oat, and barley. The current accepted terminology is *gliadin-free diet.*

Diet, Guelpa One of the early diets prescribed for diabetes. It starts with 3 days of fasting with purgation followed by a day's diet of milk, then vegetables, and gradual resumption of a normal diet.

Diet, high altitude High carbohydrate (68%), low fat (20%) liquid diet recommended prior to rapid ascent to high altitudes. This diet has been found beneficial in reducing the clinical symptoms observed at high altitudes. Major mountain sickness symptoms manifest their maximal severity within 4 to 12 hours after a liquid meal, in contrast to 36 hours after ingestion of a normal diet.

Diet, hospital One used for hospital patients. The routine hospital diets are the *regular, soft,* and *liquid* diets. These may be modified to suit individual requirements for certain therapeutic purposes. See *Diet, modified.*

Diet, house See *Diet, regular.*

Diet, hydroxyproline test Test diet eliminating meat and meat products, fish, gelatin, ice cream, marshmallows, salad dressings, and puddings during the test period for urinary excretion of hydroxyproline to study bone collagen turnover in hyperparathyroidism and Paget's disease.

Diet, Jarotsky Diet formerly prescribed for gastric ulcer patients consisting of egg white and olive oil given separately several hours apart.

Diet, Karell Low calorie milk diet prescribed in the initial stages of congestive heart failure and myocardial infarction. It consists of 800 ml of milk given in four feedings of 200 ml each (6½ ounces) at 4-hour intervals. No other food and little additional fluid is given. After 3 to 4 days, the amount of milk is increased to 1000 ml and other simple foods such as soft cooked egg, toast, cereal gruel, gelatin, custard, and fruit and vegetable purees are gradually added.

Diet, Kempner Rice-fruit diet used in the treatment of hypertensive vascular disease and kidney disease. The diet consists of 300 gm raw rice, sugar, and liberal amounts of fresh, canned, or preserved fruits. Rice is cooked simply by boiling or steaming without added milk, fat, or salt. To increase calories, generous amounts of sugar may be added to cooked rice, fruit, or fruit juice. Fluids are limited to from 700 to 1000 ml of fruit juice; additional water is not allowed. The diet is low in protein, sodium, and fat and practically free of cholesterol.

Diet, ketogenic Calculated high fat, low carbohydrate diet prescribed in the treatment of epilepsy. The proportions of carbohydrate, protein, and fat are regulated so that the ketogenic/antiketogenic ratio equals 2 or more. Such a ratio will produce a state of ketosis, which is believed to be effective in controlling certain types of convulsive seizures. Concentrated fat sources such as butter, cream, bacon, mayonnaise, and salad dressing are taken in generous amounts. Foods high in carbohydrate such as breads, cereals, fruits, desserts, sweets, and beverages containing sugar are excluded from the diet. The diet is monotonous and unpalatable. A modified ketogenic diet using medium-chain triglycerides (MCT) in place of the usual dietary fats is more effective in inducing ketosis. It also allows more carbohydrate, making the diet more palatable.

Diet, Kolff Low protein diet prescribed during acute renal failure. It consists of a creamy emulsion of 150 gm butter, 150 gm sugar, and water to make 600 ml. It is thickened with flour and flavored with strong coffee extract. The mixture is given in six equal feedings a day. The entire recipe provides 2 gm protein and 1775 calories.

Diet, lactose-free Diet excluding lactose in the form of milk and milk products or any processed food with added lactose. It is indicated for galactosemia and lactose intolerance in infants, children, and adults. (Generally the infant and child with lactase deficiency require more strict control of lactose intake than the adult.) Care should be taken in the selection of foods. Lactose is often present in disguised form. Examples of foods that may have added lactose are canned and frozen fruits and vegetables, cordials and liqueurs, dietetic and diabetic preparations, dried soups, health and geriatric foods, instant coffee and instant mixes, meat products with milk binders, monosodium glutamate extenders, powdered soft drinks, salad dressings, and spice blends.

Diet, Lenhartz Diet prescribed for bleeding peptic ulcers. It is similar to the *Sippy diet* but contains more protein. Raw egg is occasionally substituted for milk.

Diet, light Diet that consists of foods that are easily digested and readily emptied from the stomach. It is often prescribed prior to surgery or gastric analysis; it is also indicated for patients, especially the older ones, who are quite sick and cannot tolerate rich and heavy foods. The diet is given in three small meals with between-meal feedings. Foods are prepared simply; fatty foods, rich pastries, concentrated desserts, and fibrous fruits and vegetables are not given.

Diet, liquid Diet consisting of a variety of foods that are liquid, can be liquefied, or can easily melt in the mouth or at body temperature.

Clear liquid d Diet of clear liquids that leave little or no residue. It is used in pre- and postoperative cases, food intolerance, acute infections, and acute inflammatory conditions of the gastrointestinal tract. The primary purpose of the diet is to relieve thirst and help maintain water balance. Plain tea, black coffee, fat-free broth, ginger ale, plain gelatin, and glucose solution are the usual liquids given. Other liquids such as Popsicle, fruit ices, fruit drinks, carbonated beverages, and clear fruit juices such as apple, grape, and cranberry are often allowed to contribute additional calories. The diet is nutritionally inadequate and must not be used for more than 2 days.

Cold liquid d Diet prescribed after tonsillectomy and other minor mouth or throat operations. Only cold liquids such as ginger ale, iced tea, plain gelatin, and bland juices are given to prevent bleeding.

Full liquid d Diet consisting of foods that are liquid or easily become liquid in the mouth or at body temperature. This diet bridges the gap between the clear liquid diet and the soft diet. It is used in acute conditions, for patients with fractured jaws, after oral and other types of surgery, and for patients too ill to eat solid foods. When properly planned, the diet can be made nutritionally adequate and can be used for relatively long periods of time. Six or more feedings per day are recommended. All liquids and foods that easily become liquid such as plain ice cream, plain gelatin, strained cream soups, strained cereal gruel, soft custard, and puddings are allowed in the diet.

Diet, macrobiotic See *Diet, Zen macrobiotic.*

Diet, maltose-free Diet prescribed for maltose intolerance that eliminates maltose or available maltose. Excluded from the diet are corn syrup, corn sugar, beets, malted cereals, and other malted products. Since maltose is an intermediate product of starch digestion, the intake of starchy foods such as wheat, rice, corn, potato, and sweet potato is limited.

Diet, MCT See under *Diet, fat modified.*

Diet, meat-free test Test diet for the diagnosis of occult blood in the feces. Meat, fish, poultry, and products made with meat, including gravies and soups, are not given for 3 days prior to the test.

Diet, mechanical soft Also called dental soft or geriatric soft diet; this diet is indicated for patients who have difficulty in chewing due to poor dental condition or lack of teeth or presence of sores and lesions in the mouth. It consists of foods that are soft in texture and easy to chew. Food is well cooked and, if necessary, chopped, diced, or minced. All beverages are allowed, although patients with lesions in the mouth may not be able to tolerate tart fruit juices.

Diet, Meulengracht A liberal dietary regimen for bleeding ulcer patients. It consists of an abundant amount of a "full puree" diet, which consists of milk, eggs, pureed fruits and vegetables, custard, ice cream, gelatin, plain pudding, crackers, bread, and butter. After 2 days, ground or minced broiled meats including liver and poultry and broiled, baked, or creamed fish are included, and the patient is encouraged to eat well. Foods not allowed in the diet include coffee, tea, cocoa, soft drinks, alcoholic beverages, spices, nuts, and pastries.

Diet, modified A normal diet altered to meet specific body requirements under different conditions of health or disease. The diet may be modified in consistency, content (calories, carbohydrate, protein, fat, or specific nutrient), flavor, methods of preparation or service, and frequency of feeding. A modified diet is described as *high* or *low* if it provides substantially more or less of the nutrient than is ordinarily required. The word *restricted* is used when the intake of a specific nutrient is severely limited in amounts. The word *free* is used when a particular nutrient is eliminated from the diet.

Diet, Moro-Heisler Diet of grated apple for diarrheal conditions in infants.

Diet, Mosenthal test Test diet for kidney function to determine the concentrating power of the kidney. It is a "meal" consisting of 1 pint of water, tea, or coffee given at each of the patient's three regular meals before the test and on the day of the test. No food or fluid is allowed between meals and until after 8 A.M. the following morning. See also *Mosenthal concentration test.*

Diet, motor test meal Test diet to determine the emptying time of the stomach. It consists of rice and raisins or berries with seeds, or a meat sandwich with 2 tablespoons of raisins, or a meal with stewed prunes given 12 hours before gastric analysis. The presence of fibers in the gastric contents indicates decreased stomach motility.

Diet, NASA See *Diet, chemically defined.*

Diet, Newburgh High fat diet prescribed for diabetics before the discovery of insulin.

Diet, normal Diet that supplies all the nutritional needs of a normal healthy individual with due consideration for his age, sex, activity, and physiologic needs. It contains enough calories for energy, adequate protein for growth and repair of tissues, and enough minerals and vitamins for the proper functioning of the body.

Diet, optimal The *best possible* diet that will supply all the essential nutrients at the *highest possible* level to achieve the *ulti-*

mate goal of nutritional intake. The optimal diet is difficult to define in precise quantitative terms, as the optimum intake for each nutrient has not yet been established.

Diet, oxalate-restricted Diet prescribed for urinary calcium oxalate stones. Foods high in oxalic acid such as spinach, chard, endive, beet greens, sweet potato, figs, plums, rhubarb, strawberries and other berries, almonds, cashew nuts, tea, and cocoa are eliminated from the diet.

Diet, phenylalanine-restricted Diet restricting the intake of phenylalanine to approximately 15 to 25 mg/kg body weight, depending on the age of the patient and his tolerance for the amino acid. Since natural protein foods contain about 5% phenylalanine, the diet is planned on the basis of a proprietary formula low in phenylalanine such as *Lofenalac*. As the child grows older, small amounts of low protein fruits and vegetables are gradually added to the diet.

Diet, phosphorus-restricted Diet restricting the phosphorus intake to the minimal level. The intake of foods rich in phosphorus is limited. These include milk and milk products, legumes, fish, meat, leafy greens, nuts, and whole-grain cereals. Calcium intake is also limited if the diet is prescribed for urinary calcium phosphate stones.

Diet, phytanic acid–restricted Special diet restricting the intake of phytanic acid and phytol to less than 21 and 1 mg, respectively. Eliminated are foods known to be rich sources of phytanic acid (primarily dairy products) and phytol (primarily green vegetables). The diet is indicated for Refsum's syndrome.

Diet, potassium-free Essentially a protein-free diet, since all foods except for sugar and fat naturally contain potassium. Only butter soup, butter balls, hard candies, and *Controlyte* powder in potassium-free beverages (such as ginger ale, root beer, and Kool-Aid) are allowed in the diet. Foods with negligible potassium content

such as Popsicle, ice sherbet, cranberry juice, and gelatin may be given to lend variety to the diet.

Diet, potassium-restricted Diet prescribed in hyperkalemia restricting potassium intake to 1500 to 2000 mg/day (37 to 50 mEq K), which is about half the average potassium content of a regular mixed diet. Since potassium is widely distributed in foods, its restriction also limits the intake of other essential nutrients, particularly protein and vitamin. Milk, meats, legumes, whole grains, leafy vegetables, and some fruits (bananas, prunes, melons, and citrus fruits) supply considerable amounts of potassium. Many other foods are supplementary sources. The diet thus requires careful planning and selection of foods.

Diet, progressive bland Dietary regimen prescribed for gastric and duodenal ulcers and other gastrointestinal disorders. It consists of five stages designed to provide gradual increases in amounts and selection of food. A patient may be placed on any stage or may start on the first stage and gradually progress to the succeeding stages, depending on his condition. Foods are prepared simply and moderately seasoned. Alcohol is not allowed in any of the five stages.

Stage I Hourly feeding of 2 to 3 ounces of whole or skim milk or a milk-cream mixture, alternating with antacids on the half hour.

Stage II Six ounces of whole or skim milk or a milk-cream mixture, given in seven to eight feedings at 2-hour intervals. Three small meals are given in place of the milk regimen. Food selection includes soft egg, refined cooked cereals, white bread and crackers, white potato without skin, strained cream soups, cottage cheese, plain pudding, gelatin, ice cream, and custard.

Stage III Three small meals of larger variety and volume (10 to 12 ounces/meal) are given with three small between-meal feedings. The diet includes tender meat, fish, and poultry; well-cooked or canned beets, carrots, winter squash, peas, spinach, green or wax beans; ripe banana; cooked or canned low fiber fruits; fruit juices and fruit whips; sponge and other plain cakes; and plain cookies.

Stages IV and V Three average-sized meals with three between-meal feedings. Gradually more foods are added as tolerated by the patient, including tomatoes, lettuce, and other tender greens. A cup of weak coffee or tea may be allowed during meals.

Diet, protein modified Diet that prescribes a specified level of protein or restricts the amount of a protein fraction or amino acid. An increase in protein intake is necessary in any of the following conditions: excessive metabolism of protein, as in fevers and hyperthyroidism; loss of protein from the body, as in severe burns and nephritis; failure of protein synthesis, as in liver disease; failure of protein absorption, as in sprue and celiac disease; and inadequate intake of protein, as in starvation and kwashiorkor. A reduction in protein intake is necessary whenever the body's ability to excrete waste products of protein metabolism is impaired, as in hepatic coma and acute glomerulonephritis. Restriction in a specific amino acid is called for in certain conditions, such as phenylketonuria and other inborn errors of amino acid metabolism. The suggested terminology for the different levels in protein content of the diet is listed below. See also *Diet, gliadin-free; Diet, phenyl-alanine-restricted;* and *Diet, taurine-restricted.*

High protein d An allowance of from 2.5 to 3.0 gm protein/kg body weight or approximately 120 to 150 gm protein/day. A high protein intake is indicated in pernicious anemia, liver cirrhosis, infectious hepatitis, ulcerative colitis, fractures, severe burns, and postoperative conditions to regenerate body tissues and cells. This allowance may be met by taking daily 2 eggs, 2 to 3 cups milk, and 10 to 12 ounces of meat, in addition to protein provided by breads, cereals, and vegetables. This high intake of protein is difficult to attain when the condition calls for restrictions in sodium and fat. A high intake of carbohydrate is essential because of its protein-sparing action, except in hyperinsulinism when carbohydrate level has to be drastically reduced.

High protein, low carbohydrate d Diet prescribed for patients who experience the *dumping syndrome* following gastric resection. Simple sugars, sweets, and concentrated desserts are limited, especially during meals; alcoholic drinks and sweet and carbonated beverages are not allowed. Fat intake should be relatively high to retard the passage of food in the stomach. Foods high in roughage are avoided; raw foods are taken as tolerated. The daily food allowance is divided into six small meals, with a maximum of 4 ounces (½ cup) fluid allowance during meals. Additional fluids may be taken between meals or 30 minutes before and after meals.

High protein, carbohydrate-restricted d Diet prescribed for spontaneous hypogly-

Suggested terminology	Allowance (gm/kg body weight)	Approximate level (gm/day)
Protein free	0	0-5
Minimal protein	0.2-0.3	20-25
Low protein	0.5-0.7	30-40
Normal protein	0.8-1.2	50-80
Liberal protein	1.5-2.0	90-110
High protein	2.5-3.0	120-150
Very high protein	3.0-4.0	150 or more

cemia and leucine-induced hypoglycemia. It contains about 2.5 gm protein/kg desirable body weight and an initial allowance of 150 gm carbohydrate. The protein in the diet should come chiefly from animal sources, although infants with leucine-induced hypoglycemia should not be given milk and eggs until tolerance to these foods has been established. Eliminated from the diet are sugars and other readily digested and absorbed carbohydrates; other carbohydrate-rich foods are limited. Carbohydrate is gradually increased, depending on the patient's tolerance. The daily food allowance is divided into four equal meals.

Liberal protein d An allowance of from 1.5 to 2.0 gm protein/kg body weight or about 90 to 110 gm protein/day. A liberal protein intake is indicated in chronic glomerulonephritis in the presence of albuminuria, in pulmonary tuberculosis to afford healing of tuberculous lesions, and in hyperthyroidism and fevers because of increased protein catabolism. About two thirds of the protein allowance should be provided by animal sources. Emphasis should be placed on eggs, milk, lean meats, and liver. Legumes and nuts also have a place in the diet. For maximum utilization of protein, the diet must also be high in calories, especially in readily available carbohydrates because of their protein-sparing action.

Low protein d A moderately restricted protein diet prescribed in chronic glomerulonephritis and as part of the progressive protein regimen in chronic uremia and hepatic coma. A protein allowance of 30 to 40 gm/day is based on a protein intake of 0.5 to 0.7 gm/kg body weight. The protein in the diet is supplied by 1 egg, ½ cup milk, 2 ounces meat, 3 slices bread or equivalent, fruits, and low protein vegetables. Additional calories are supplied by sugar and other sweets, fats, carbonated beverages, and baked products made from low protein wheat starches.

Minimal protein d An allowance of 0.2 to 0.3 gm protein/kg body weight or approximately 20 to 25 gm protein/day. It is prescribed for patients with chronic renal failure, acute glomerulonephritis and hepatic coma. The protein allowance is supplied by 1 egg, ½ cup of milk, 3 slices of bread or substitute, fruits and low protein vegetables such as cucumber, celery, squash, carrot, eggplant, radish, tomato, asparagus, cabbage, and lettuce. Extra calories are provided by liberal use of sugars, fat-rich foods, and protein-free starches. This dietary regimen will supply the essential amino acids for tissue synthesis; intake of nonessential amino acids is minimized. Because of their relatively greater content of nonessential amino acids in comparison with egg and milk proteins, meat, fish, and poultry are not recommended at this low level of protein intake.

Normal protein d The normal protein allowance for adults is from 0.8 to 1.2 gm/kg body weight, or about 50 to 80 gm protein/day. Higher protein allowances are required during pregnancy, lactation, and growth periods. These higher protein allowances, which may range from 1.5 to 3.0 gm/kg body weight, are also considered normal allowances. See Recommended Daily Dietary Allowances, Appendix A-1.

Protein-free d This diet permits no choice of food since even fruits and fruit juices contain small amounts of protein. A strict protein-free diet allows only sugar, fat, and carbonated beverages. These may be given in the form of commercial preparations such as *Controlyte* powder and *Lipomul-Oral* emulsion or as frozen butter-sugar balls or butter soup. Some physicians permit liberalization of the diet by allowing the inclusion of fruits and fruit juices. Several commercial mixes for low protein bread are available in the market. The protein-free diet is prescribed when the kidney is unable to remove nitrogenous waste products from the blood, as in acute anuria, or when the liver is unable to convert blood ammonia to urea, as in hepatic coma.

Very high protein d Diet allowing 3 to 4 gm protein/kg body weight. It is prescribed in nephrosis and celiac disease and for premature infants. Eggs, milk, cheese, meat, fish, and poultry are excellent protein sources of high biologic value. It is best to divide the protein allowance into three meals and three between-meal feedings. Skill in planning the menu is called for, especially when the diet has to be restricted in sodium, as in nephrosis, or fat, as in celiac disease.

Diet, provocative Allergy test diet containing the most allergenic foods such as milk, egg, and wheat unless the patient's previous history definitely contraindicates their use. If allergy is due to food, some manifestations will show up within a week; otherwise, allergy is due to a nonfood allergen.

Diet, pureed Also called blenderized diet; consists of a normal variety of foods that have been strained or put in a blender or osterizer and then combined with liquids to the consistency desired. It is indicated for patients who have difficulty in swallowing or who have had oral surgery.

Diet, purine-restricted Diet restricting the daily intake of purine to approximately 120 to 150 mg as compared to a normal intake of 600 to 1000 mg/day. The diet is prescribed for gout and is designed to lower the uric acid level in the blood. Chief food sources of purines such as glandular organs, anchovies, sardines, and meat extractives are eliminated from the diet. Fish and seafoods, meats, and poultry are restricted, depending on the patient's condition. These foods are not allowed during acute gouty attacks. A 2-ounce serving portion is permitted when the acute stage subsides, and 2 servings/day may be taken in chronic conditions. Foods that are essentially free of purines may be taken as desired. These include breads and cereals, cheese, egg, fats, sugars and sweets, milk and milk products, and vegetables (except peas, beans, lentils, cauliflower, mushrooms, and spinach). This diet is now seldom prescribed since the advent of drug therapy.

Diet, reducing Low calorie diet designed to reduce weight. The amount of caloric reduction from the normal intake varies and depends on the rate at which one expects to lose weight. Ideally this should be about 1 to 2 pounds/week, although a greater reduction in weight is necessary in extremely obese individuals. Reducing the number of calories from the normal intake by 3500/week or 500/day would, theoretically, reduce body weight by 1 pound/week. Several types of reducing regimens have been proposed, from starvation diets to nibbling and from formula diets to calculated food intake. A good reducing diet in order to be effective must be nutritionally adequate (except for calories), acceptable to the patient, compatible with the food pattern to which the patient is accustomed, economically feasible, palatable, offer variety, and give a sense of well-being.

Diet, regular Also called general, house, or full hospital diet; it is a normal diet planned to provide the recommended daily allowances for essential nutrients, but designed to meet caloric needs of a bedridden or ambulatory patient whose condition does not require any dietary modification for therapeutic purposes. It also serves as a basis for the modification of therapeutic diets in the hospital. While there is no restriction as to the amount and type of foods allowed, the diet calls for careful planning of menus, wise selection and proper preparation of foods, as well as attractive service so that it will appeal to patients with relatively poor appetites.

Diet, residue modified Diet that limits or eliminates the intake of foods that leave a high amount of residue in the colon. Foods with decreasing amounts of residue are carbohydrates with indigestible material, digestible carbohydrates, milk, fats, and protein.

Low residue d Diet often prescribed in the treatment of diarrhea and diseases involving the bowel, particularly in association with obstruction, distention, edema, and inflammation. A diet low in residue is desirable in these conditions where the presence of bulky fecal masses would strain the colon. Foods recommended are fish, tender cuts of meat, chicken, hard-cooked egg, liver, gelatin, refined cereals, and non-fibrous cooked or canned fruits and vegetables.

Minimal residue d Diet designed to leave the least amount of residue in the lower bowel after digestion and absorption has taken place proximally. The diet is indicated prior to and following intestinal surgery, particularly of the colon, and during radiation therapy of the pelvic area. It may also be used initially during the acute stage of diarrhea, ileitis, colitis, and diverticulitis. Eliminated are milk, tough cuts of meat, fish or poultry with skin, fibrous fruits and vegetables unless canned or cooked and strained, excessive fats, excessive sweets, spices, and condiments.

Diet, rice-fruit Diet consisting only of rice and fruit. See *Diet, Kempner.*

Diet, Riegel test Test meal consisting of 200 ml beef broth, 150 to 200 gm broiled beef, and 100 gm boiled potato given before gastric analysis for hypoacidity.

Diet, routine hospital Term referring to the *regular, soft,* and *liquid* diets commonly used in hospitals. They differ in the consistency and type of foods allowed.

Diet, Rowe's elimination Series of four test diets for the diagnosis of food allergy. Each of the first three diets contains a cereal or a starch, one or two meats, a group of fruits and vegetables, and condiments and seasonings. The fourth diet consists only of milk, tapioca, and sugar. The patient is placed on each diet for a period of 1 week unless relief of symptoms is obtained.

If the patient shows no improvement on any of the diets, the allergy is probably not caused by food.

Diet, Schemm Acid-ash, sodium-restricted diet prescribed in edema associated with heart and kidney disorders. Acidification of the urine is believed to incite the kidneys to eliminate sodium and water from the body.

Diet, Schmidt test Test diet for diarrhea to determine intestinal ability to digest protein, carbohydrate, and fat. It is a standard weighed diet given for 3 consecutive days. Included in the diet are easily digested foods such as milk, soft-cooked eggs, oatmeal gruel, boiled potato, scraped beef, toast, and butter.

Diet, Serotonin test Test diet eliminating bananas and vanilla 3 days prior to and during the urinary collection for the diagnosis of carcinoid tumor.

Diet, Sippy Diet prescribed for bleeding gastric and duodenal ulcers. It consists of hourly feedings of 3 ounces of equal parts of milk and cream or whole or skim milk from 6 or 7 A.M. to 9 or 10 P.M. and during the night if the patient awakens. Soft eggs and strained cereals not exceeding 3 ounces per feeding are added to the milk-cream mixture after 2 or 3 days. Bland and easily digested foods such as cream soups of various kinds, vegetable purees, and custards are included occasionally to lend variety to the diet. These additions are taken in place of or in addition to the milk-cream mixture; the total bulk at any one feeding does not exceed 6 ounces. An added feature of the regimen is the continuous neutralization of free hydrochloric acid with alkali taken between feedings.

Diet, sodium-restricted Diet in which the sodium content is limited to a specified level, which may range from mild restriction to severe restriction. Sodium restriction is used primarily for the elimination, control, and prevention of edema accompanying congestive heart failure, cirrhosis of the liver, nephritis, nephrosis, toxemias of pregnancy, and ACTH therapy. It is also beneficial in the treatment of some cases of hypertension. Retention of sodium in the body requires retention of water to keep the sodium concentration of the fluid constant. As a consequence, edema or swelling of tissues results. The average American diet contains approximately 3 to 6 gm sodium (about 7 to 15 gm salt, or NaCl)/day. Sodium in the diet comes from two sources: sodium *naturally* present in foods and sodium *added* during cooking and food processing. Foods differ widely in natural sodium content. In general, animal foods are relatively high in sodium; plant foods are generally low in sodium. Most of the sodium added to foods comes from table salt (or sodium chloride) and monosodium glutamate. The other forms of sodium commonly used in food processing are sodium bicarbonate, sodium citrate, sodium alginate, sodium benzoate, sodium hydroxide, and sodium sulfite. In addition there is sodium in water and in some medicines.

2000 to 3000 mg sodium d (87 to 130 mEq sodium) Mild sodium restriction. It is essentially a normal diet with moderate use of salt during cooking. No further addition of salt or other salty condiments is allowed at the table. Foods extremely high in sodium such as bacon, ham, salted crackers, and olives are not allowed.

1000 to 1500 mg sodium d (43 to 65 mEq sodium) Moderate sodium restriction often used as a maintenance diet for nephritis, toxemias of pregnancy, hypertension, and heart disease. Foods are prepared without added salt or sodium compound, and all processed foods high in sodium are not allowed.

500 mg sodium d (22 mEq sodium) Strict sodium restriction used in congestive heart failure with edema, hypertension, and ascites. It restricts the intake of foods naturally high in sodium content, such as meat, fish, eggs, milk, and vegetables high in sodium, i.e., beets, carrots, celery, and spinach. Prepared foods with added salt are not allowed. The diet thus requires the use of unsalted bread, unsalted butter, and other low sodium dietetic foods.

250 mg sodium d (11 mEq sodium) Lowest level of the sodium restriction prescribed for the acutely ill patient. It is used only for hospital patients with congestive heart failure, ascites, and severe hypertension. At this strict level of sodium restriction the intake of meats is limited to 5 ounces/day and dialyzed or low sodium milk is substituted for regular milk. Only those foods low in natural sodium content are allowed. The diet is therefore unpalatable and monotonous.

Diet, soft Diet consisting of foods that are soft in texture and easily digested without any harsh fibers and connective tissues; foods are prepared simply and not highly seasoned. It is an intermediate diet between the *regular* and the *full liquid* diet and bridges the gap between acute illness and convalescence stage. Many patients on admission are placed on this diet until diagnosis is made. Foods included are tender cooked or ground meat, fish and poultry, well-cooked vegetables, low fiber fruits eaten without skins and seeds, fine-grained breads and cereals, plain desserts, crisp, tender lettuce, and salad tomatoes.

Diet, space Bulk-free diet designed for use of astronauts in space travels. It requires little or no digestion and supplies calorie and other nutritional requirements. Foods developed for space travel must conform to weight and volume restrictions and be protected against chemical and biologic deterioration. Freeze-dried finger foods and beverage powders that easily rehydrate have been developed.

Diet, starch-restricted Diet limiting the intake of starch from bread, cereals, cereal products, and root crops. It is prescribed in cases of starch intolerance due to lack of pancreatic amylase. Foods allowed are milk, eggs, meats, fruits, and vegetables low in starch content. Carbohydrate in the diet is obtained from sugar, syrups, sweets, and fruits.

Diet, starvation Calorie-free diet designed to effect rapid weight reduction in a short period of time. Vitamin supplements are given to meet specific nutrient requirements and water intake is liberal to prevent dehydration. Loss in weight of 4 to 8 pounds/day in the early days of starvation is not rare. How long one should stay on this diet depends on several factors. Since severe complications may develop, starvation or fasting as a treatment for extreme obesity should be done in a hospital under strict medical supervision. With fat loss, the individual also loses nitrogen and goes into negative nitrogen balance. No method has been successful in losing fat without losing nitrogen.

Diet, sucrose-restricted Diet that limits the intake of sucrose because of intolerance to this disaccharide. All forms of sucrose are excluded from the diet, i.e., table sugar, jellies, jams, marmalades, preserves, corn syrup, maple syrup, other syrups, sweetened condensed milk, and other foods with added sugar. Most fruits, except for berries, lemons, and grapes, are given in limited amounts because they also contain sucrose. Vegetables high in sucrose content such as beets, green peas, sweet potatoes, navy beans, and soybeans are also restricted. Cereals, milk, egg, meat, fish, poultry, and vegetables low in sucrose are allowed in normal amounts. Sugar substitutes such as Sucaryl and saccharin may be used to sweeten foods.

Diet, synthetic Diet used for the diagnosis of food allergy. It contains amino acids, sugar, water, vitamin concentrates, salt mixtures, and, sometimes, emulsified fats. The mixture is given orally or by tube feeding. Persons who are allergic to food should show marked improvement with the synthetic diet; those who are allergic to substances other than food do not show any relief of symptoms. If allergy to food is ascertained, other foods may be added to the synthetic diet to determine which ones are allergenic.

Diet, taurine-restricted Protein modified diet prescribed for the treatment of psoriasis. Certain high protein foods are entirely eliminated; others are restricted as to amounts allowed per day. The daily food intake should not exceed ½ to 1 can evaporated milk diluted with an equal amount of water, 3 ounces chicken, turkey, beef, or veal, and ½ cup cottage cheese or 1 slice American or Swiss cheese. Fruits, vegetables, fats, sugars, and breads may be taken as desired. Foods that are to be avoided are eggs and dishes containing eggs, pasteurized and homogenized milk, ice cream, fish, cold cuts, organ meats, meat extractives, meat gravies, soups, and broths.

Diet, Taylor test Test diet consisting of egg whites, olive oil, and sugar given prior to urine analysis for chlorides.

Diet, therapeutic A normal diet adapted or modified to suit specific disease conditions; one designed to treat or cure diseases. See *Diet, modified.*

Diet, tube feeding Liquefied diet introduced into the stomach by means of a polyvinyl tube inserted through the mouth or nose. It is indicated in cases of inability or refusal to take food, as in obstruction of the esophagus, anorexia nervosa, severe burns, terminal malignancy, comatose condition, and following surgery of the mouth. It consists of liquid foods and/or selected nonfibrous solid cooked foods that may be liquefied in a blender. A satisfactory tube feeding formula must be nutritionally adequate, well tolerated by the patient, easily digested with no unfavorable reactions, and easily prepared. Some commercially prepared ready-to-use liquid formulas are now available. See Proprietary foods: composition, features, and uses, Appendix P-1.

Diet, tyramine-restricted Diet eliminating the intake of foods containing considerable amounts of tyramine. It is prescribed for patients receiving monoamine oxidase

(MAO) inhibitory drugs to prevent sudden hypertensive reaction to the amine. Foods with high tyramine content are alcoholic beverages such as ale, beer, and wine (particularly Chianti, sherry, sauterne, and Reisling); aged cheeses such as Camembert, Gouda, Parmesan, and Romano; liver; yogurt; herring; vanilla; and chocolate.

Diet, VMA test Diet given before and during the urinary collections for VMA (vanillylmandelic acid) in screening hypertensive patients with *pheochromocytoma*. Foods that give rise to phenoxy acids in the urine and give false positive results are limited, although they do not necessarily need to be omitted from the diet. These include bananas, chocolate, nuts, raisins, coffee, tea, and foods containing vanilla extract.

Diet, wheat-oat-rye-barley–free See *Diet, gliadin-free.*

Diet, Zen macrobiotic Diet promoted as a medical philosophy capable of curing or preventing any condition by diet alone without the use of medicine or surgery. The diet comprises 10 ways of eating, ranging from the lowest level, which includes cereals, vegetables, soup, animal products, salads, and fruits in certain definitive proportions, to the highest level, which is 100% cereals. The diet requires the use of natural foods and special cooking methods and does not allow industrialized and processed foods or plant foods produced with fertilizers or with added chemicals such as pesticides and insecticides.

Dietary allowances See *Recommended dietary allowances.*

Dietary counseling Process of providing individualized professional guidance to assist a person in adjusting his daily food consumption to meet his health needs. Success in dietary counseling depends on the dietitian's ability to explain scientific details in the simplest language considering the patient's background, socioeconomic needs, and personal preferences.

Dietary history Dietary study method used in evaluating or assessing dietary intakes of individuals. It is taken by 24-hour recall or repeated food records to lend information on the subject's past and present dietary habits, food likes and dislikes, usual food pattern, and type of meals normally eaten over a relatively long period of time. The dietary history is useful in food habit studies and furnishes data for classifying individuals into certain broad groups. See also *Dietary study.*

Dietary requirement *Minimum* amount of a specific nutrient that is needed by the body to attain a specified state of health. Unlike the *recommended dietary allowance,* it has no added margin of safety and is stated for *definite* (not average) conditions of age, weight, activity, and food intakes as well as physiologic status and pathologic state. There is variability and lack of precision in the assessment of nutritional requirement for the different nutrients. For this reason, the *minimum daily requirements* for certain nutrients are often stated as ranges, and average minimum dietary requirements should be considered only as close "approximates" and should not be interpreted as accurate and final.

Dietary standard Quantitative summary or compilation of nutrient allowances or requirements for various groups of people. It is used to formulate and evaluate food intakes of large population groups; it also serves as a rationale or yardstick for planning adequate nutrition and scheduling agricultural production. The establishment of a dietary standard is not easy because of the lack of available information about certain nutrients, the wide range of individual variation in nutrient requirement, and the lack of agreement among authorities setting the standard. The nutrients included in the standard are those that are apt to be absent or inadequate in the usual diet. Other nutrients, although required by the body, are not included in the tabulation. Either they are present in adequate amounts in the usual diet, or they are trace elements or vitamins for which there are insufficient data to serve as a basis for recommendation. Several countries have established dietary standards for their populations. One must recognize the philosophy behind the standard set in each country, and care must be taken to distinguish the use of such terms as *"standard," "requirement,"* and *"allowance"* in the interpretation for purposes of comparison or evaluation. See Comparative dietary standards for adults in selected countries and the FAO, Appendix A-2.

Dietary status Bodily condition resulting from the utilization of the essential nutrients available to the body. It depends not only on the dietary intake of these nutrients but also on the relative need of the body and the ability to utilize them.

Dietary study (survey) Method of determining or evaluating the dietary intake of an individual, group, or population at large. The adequacy of a given diet is determined by *qualitative* comparison with the basic food groups or by *quantitative* comparison with the recommended dietary standard of a particular country. A dietary study is used to detect adequacy or inadequacy of diets to give valuable information concerning food habits, menu preparation, and food procurement, availability, and distribution.

Dietary study methodology There are several methods of obtaining dietary information. These are generally classified into those applicable to individuals and those applicable to groups. Methods applicable to individuals include *estimation by recall,* with subject or parent of subject recalling food intake of previous 24 hours or longer; *food intake record,* which is a listing of all foods eaten (including between-meal intakes) for varying lengths of time, usually 3 to 7 days; *dietary history* taken by recall or repeated food records or both to discover the usual food pattern over relatively long periods of time; and *weighed food intake* of subject taken by a trained

person, parent of the subject, or the subject himself. Methods applicable to groups include *food account* or running reports of food purchased or produced for household use; *food list* or recall of estimated amounts of various foods consumed during the previous days, usually the past 7 days; *food record* or weighed inventory of foods at the beginning and end of the study, with or without records of kitchen and plate wastes. See Methods of research in nutrition: dietary survey, Appendix M-2.

Dietetic foods Processed foods for therapeutic purposes. In the United States, a wide array of different dietetic foods are commercially available. The most common are products containing nonnutritive (artificial) sweeteners such as low calorie soft drinks, canned fruits and juices, puddings and gelatin desserts, confectionery, and baked goods. Other dietetic foods are labeled, e.g., "diabetic" foods; low sodium products marked with the phrase "no salt added"; and products with "no fat or oil added."

Dietetic integrated program A new program that combines college course work and the practical training of an internship. On completion of this 4-year baccalaureate program the graduates are accepted as members of the American Dietetic Association. The first program of this type was established in medical dietetics at Ohio State University.

Dietetic intern One who is a recipient of a bachelor's degree with a program in dietetics from an accredited school, college, or university and is undergoing a dietetic internship in an accredited institution.

Dietetic internship A period of practical training in any accredited hospital, college, business or industrial organization which provides opportunities to acquire knowledge and skills in dietetics.

Dietetics Combined science and art of regulating the planning, preparing, and serving of meals to individuals or groups under *various conditions of health and disease* according to the principles of nutrition and management with due consideration for economic, social, cultural, and psychologic factors. The science consists of knowledge of nutrition, food, and the dietary constituents needed in different states of health and disease. The art consists of knowledge of the practical planning and preparation of meals at various economic levels as well as attractive and pleasing service of food so that an individual, well or ill, will be encouraged to eat the food and adhere to the diet.

Dietitian (dietician) 1. As defined in the *Dictionary of Occupational Titles,* a dietitian is a professional person who "plans and directs food service programs in hospitals, schools, restaurants, and other public or private institutions; plans menus and diets providing required food and nutrients to feed individuals and groups; directs workers engaged in preparation and service of meals; purchases or requisitions food, equipment, and supplies; maintains and analyzes food cost control records to determine improved methods for purchasing and utilization of food, equipment, and supplies; inspects work areas and storage facilities to insure observance of sanitary standards; instructs individuals and groups in application of principles of nutrition to selection of food; and prepares educational materials on nutritional value of foods and methods of preparation." 2. A person who has followed a prescribed academic program resulting in a baccalaureate degree from an accredited school, college, or university with a program in dietetics and who has satisfactorily completed a dietetic internship in an accredited institution.

Administrative d One who plans, organizes, develops, and directs food service programs within budgetary limitations and according to principles of nutrition and management; who develops standards of food procurement, production, and service; who maintains sanitary standards and safety methods in the department; who analyzes and keeps up-to-date job descriptions and specifications for all positions; who standardizes recipes and supervises their use; who supervises selection and training of nonprofessional food service personnel; who assists in the maintenance of records for department planning and financial management; and who evaluates work procedures, employee utilization, and physical layout and equipment.

Chief d Also called dietary director; one who plans, organizes, and directs all activities of the department, including educational and research programs. These activities include establishment of short- and long-range programs of the department in accordance with the goals of the institution; formulation of department policies and standards; planning for effective personnel utilization and budget management; organization, direction, and evaluation of the whole food service department; participation in conferences and general staff meetings in the hospital as well as in professional and community activities; delegation of responsibilities to all concerned in the service of food; formulation and execution of educational programs for dietetic interns, and medical, nursing, and dental students, interns, or residents; development and implementation of research programs in administration, food production, normal and therapeutic nutrition, and education; and lastly, coordination of dietary services with those of other departments. Although the word "chief" or "director" implies a department that employs a staff of dietitians, the activities mentioned above also apply to an "only dietitian" who is, at the same time, also designated head or chief dietitian.

Consultant d Also called a dietary consultant or nutrition consultant; one who advises and assists public and private establishments (such as child care centers, hospitals, nursing homes, and schools) on food service management and nutritional problems in group feeding; who plans, organizes, and conducts such activities as in-service training courses, conferences, and institutes for food service managers, food handlers, and other workers; who develops and evaluates informational materials; who studies food service practices and facilities and makes recommendations for improvement; and who confers with architects and equipment personnel in planning for building or remodeling food service units.

Dial-a-Dietitian "Dietitian" who communicates nutrition facts in response to a client's telephoned questions pertaining to normal nutrition and dietary modifications. The Dial-a-Dietitian program originated in Detroit in 1958. By means of public service time on radio and television and space in newspapers, a telephone number is published in order that people in the community may call for information on normal nutrition. A telephone-answering service records the question with the caller's name, address, and telephone number. The questions are then referred to members of the regional dietetic association for answering, usually within 24 to 48 hours, and the telephone-answering service answers in the name of the dietetic association. Specific questions relating to clarification of a therapeutic diet, such as preparation, purchasing, selection, or substitution of specific foods, are answered. However, requests for therapeutic diet prescriptions are first referred to a physician and then a hospital dietitian; the detailed dietary instructions are not given by telephone.

Registered d Member of the American Dietetic Association who has passed an examination and paid a registration fee. A registered dietitian (R.D.) must participate in 75 clock hours of professional education every 5 years to maintain his registration.

Teaching d One who plans, organizes, and teaches courses or conducts educational programs related to normal and therapeutic nutrition; who coordinates and integrates current principles of normal and therapeutic nutrition into teaching programs for patients and educational curricula of dietetic interns and medical, nursing, and other professional students; who directs and participates in staff development and in-service education and training of dietary personnel; and who prepares manuals, brochures, visual aids, and other materials used in teaching. Occasionally a teaching dietitian also engages in research and gives dietary counseling to patients in hospital or public health centers.

Therapeutic d One who plans and directs preparation and service of modified diets prescribed by the physician; who consults with physicians concerning dietary prescriptions and implements these through meals adapted to the needs of individual patients; who consults with nursing and social service staffs concerning problems affecting patients' food habits and needs; who formulates menus for therapeutic diets and maintains standards of palatability and appearance of patient meals; who prepares and reviews materials on modified diets for use by the department and other educational programs for professional students; who interviews and teaches patients about ways to meet their nutritional needs, assisting them to meet these needs by careful planning of prescribed diets for home use; and who may engage in research and teaching of nutrition and diet therapy to dietetic, medical, and nursing students.

Dietogenetics Term suggested for the interrelationship between genetics and dietary response.

Diet therapy Also called dietotherapy; the branch of dietetics that is concerned with the use of food for therapeutic purposes. Its goals are to maintain good nutritional status, correct deficiencies that may have occurred, afford rest to the whole body or to certain organs that may be affected by disease, adjust the food intake to the body's ability to metabolize the nutrients, and bring about changes in body weight whenever necessary. A therapeutic diet is planned on the basis of a normal diet; essential nutrients should be provided as generously as the limitation of the diet allows. The diet must be flexible and adapted to the patient's food preferences, eating habits, economic status, religious beliefs, and social customs. Foods included should be acceptable to the patient and should emphasize natural and commonly used items that are available and easily prepared at home. A correctly planned diet is successful only if the food is eaten.

Diffusion Redistribution of material by random movement; spreading out. *Simple diffusion* is movement of solutes from higher to lower electrochemical potential. *Facilitated diffusion* is carrier-mediated movement of solutes also down their electrochemical potential, but the rate of movement is faster than could be accounted for by simple diffusion.

Digestibility Extent to which a foodstuff is digested and absorbed from the digestive tract and not excreted in the feces. The fecal residue excreted is primarily indigestible materials, secretions, linings shed from the digestive tract, and microorganisms with their end products.

Apparent d Measure of the difference between food intake and output in the feces without consideration of fecal excretion not due to food eaten.

True d Measure of the difference between food intake and fecal output, with allowances for linings shed from the intestinal tract, bacteria, and residues of digestive juices that are not part of indigestible food fecal output.

Digestion The mechanical and chemical breakdown of complex substances into their constituent parts; the conversion of food into smaller and simpler units that can be absorbed by the body. See Summary of digestive enzymes, Appendix J-1.

Digitalis A powerful heart stimulant from the dried leaves of the common foxglove.

Digitonin A plant glycoside of the steroid digitogenin, in which the sugar residues are attached to the —OH group at the third carbon atom. It forms insoluble compounds with cholesterol and other sterols.

Diglyceride Glyceride containing two molecules of fatty acid.

Diguanide Compound capable of reducing blood sugar levels. Commercial preparations are metformin and phenformin. See *Oral hypoglycemic agents.*

Dihydrocoenzyme I DPNH or NADH, the reduced form of *coenzyme I.*

Dihydrocoenzyme II TPNH or NADPH, the reduced form of *coenzyme II.*

Dihydroxyacetone A ketotriose derivable from glycerol or glucose. As dihydroxyacetone phosphate, it is produced in the splitting of fructose-1,6-diphosphate by the enzyme aldolase during the anaerobic metabolism of glycogen.

Diiodothyronine Intermediate product in the synthesis of the thyroid hormone triiodothyronine. See *Thyroid gland.*

Diiodotyrosine Iodinated tyrosine, a precursor of *thyroxine,* a thyroid hormone. See *Thyroid gland.*

Diketogulonic acid Product resulting from the oxidation of *dehydroascorbic acid.* It has no vitamin C activity.

Dinitrophenol Potent but toxic metabolic stimulant; has been suggested in the treatment of myxedema and obesity but is toxic in large amounts and causes acute hepatitis, skin eruptions, agranulocytosis, and profuse sweating.

Diodrast Complex organic iodine compound that is opaque to roentgen rays; used in roentgenologic examination of the urinary tract. It is also useful in kidney function tests. By determining the amount of Diodrast excreted and the plasma content after a standard dose, the functional activity of the glomeruli or kidney tubules may be estimated. This is known as the *Diodrast clearance test.* See also *Clearance test.*

Diose Glycolic aldehyde; the simplest monosaccharide containing only two carbon atoms.

Dipeptidase An exopeptidase that hydrolyzes peptide linkages containing free amino and carboxyl groups.

Dipeptide Product formed by the combination of two amino acids or by hydrolysis of proteins.

Diphosphoglyceric acid Glyceric acid ester with two molecules of phosphoric acid; an important intermediate in carbohydrate metabolism.

Diphosphopyridine nucleotide (DPN) See *Coenzymes I and II*.

Diphosphothiamin (DPT) See *Cocarboxylase*.

Dipsesis (dipsosis) Extreme thirst.

Dipsomania Uncontrollable craving for alcoholic drinks.

Disaccharidase Enzyme that hydrolyzes disaccharides. Examples are *lactase, maltase,* and *sucrase*.

Disaccharide Sugar containing two monosaccharides joined in glycosidic linkage with the elimination of a molecule of water. The most common are *lactose, maltose,* and *sucrose*.

Disaccharide intolerance Inability to absorb certain disaccharides because of lack in certain specific disaccharidases such as maltase, lactase, sucrase, and isomaltase. The condition may also be acquired from secondary surgical operations, infectious enteropathies, celiac disease, and other malabsorption states. Diarrhea is the principal symptom. Other clinical features include flatulence, abdominal pain, vomiting, and excretion of large amounts of volatile fatty acids. Exclusion of the poorly tolerated disaccharide from the diet results in disappearance of symptoms. See *Diet, lactose-free; Diet, maltose-free;* and *Diet, sucrose-restricted*.

Disaster feeding See *Emergency feeding*.

Disease 1. A sickness, malady, or ailment. 2. A disturbance in the performance or structure of a part or organ of the body. 3. A specific entity that is the result of one or several pathologic processes going on in the body. 4. Any disorder or unhealthy condition of the mind or body.

Dismutation Reaction resulting in simultaneous oxidation and reduction of the same compound, yielding two products, one oxidized and the other reduced.

Dispersion 1. Act of scattering or separating. 2. Incorporation of the particles of a substance into another, whether in true solution, suspension, or colloidal solution. Particles or materials that are subdivided into very small units and scattered through another substance are called dispersed materials; the substance through which the dispersed materials are scattered is called dispersion medium or continuous phase; and the particles in dispersion are referred to as dispersed phase or discontinuous phase.

Dissolution 1. Liquefaction. 2. Death or decomposition. 3. Loosening or separation of a compound or body into its parts by chemical action.

Distillation Process of vaporization and subsequent condensation; used principally to separate liquids from nonvolatile substances.

Diuresis Increased excretion of urine. Any agent that causes diuresis is called a *diuretic*.

Diverticula Herniations or outpouchings of the mucous membrane through gaps or weak spots in the circular muscle of the colon. Diverticula may be single or multiple and occur most frequently in the distal descending portion of the colon. They are formed because of unusually high intraluminal colonic pressures.

Diverticulitis Inflammatory condition of a diverticulum (or diverticula) characterized by nausea, vomiting, fever, abdominal tenderness, distention, pain, and intestinal spasm. The inflammatory process may eventually lead to intestinal obstruction or perforation, necessitating surgery. See Dietary management of selected disorders, Appendix O.

DMF Refers to the total number of decayed, missing, and filled teeth. It is often used in surveys to determine the amount of *caries* present in a community or given population. Teeth, however, may be missing for other reasons, including removal because of local custom.

DNA Abbreviation for *deoxyribonucleic acid*.

D/N ratio Abbreviation for dextrose/nitrogen ratio. See *Glucose/nitrogen ratio*.

DOCA Abbreviation for *deoxycorticosterone acetate*.

Dopa 3,4-Dihydroxyphenylalanine, an intermediate product in the formation of *melanin* from tyrosine.

Dopamine 3,4-Dihydroxyphenylethylamine, an intermediate product in tyrosine metabolism and the precursor of norepinephrine and epinephrine. It is present in the central nervous system and is localized in the basal ganglia.

Douglas bag Portable rubber bag for measuring respiratory exchanges; often used in energy determination involving exercise or activity. It has a capacity of 60 to 100 L. Expired air is collected for a period of 3 to 10 minutes. The air in the bag is then measured in a gas meter and analyzed for carbon dioxide content.

DPN Abbreviation for *diphosphopyridine nucleotide*. See *Coenzyme I* under *Coenzymes I and II*.

DPPD Chemical antioxidant that has been found to be effective in preventing fetal resorption in animals; it can replace some functions of *vitamin E*.

DPT Abbreviation for *diphosphothiamin*. See *Cocarboxylase*.

Dropsy Abnormal accumulation of fluid in a body cavity or cellular tissue.

Dryco Half skim milk formula with added vitamins; it is high in protein and low in fat. (Borden.) See Proprietary foods: composition, features, and uses, Appendix P-1.

Duct An enclosed channel or tube for passage of secretory or excretory products.

Ductless gland See *Endocrine*.

Dulcin Synthetic sweetening agent 250 times as sweet as sugar; has toxic effects and is not allowed as a food additive.

Dulcitol Six-carbon sugar alcohol formed by the reduction of galactose. It accumulates in the lens of experimentally induced cataracts in rats fed a high galactose diet.

Dumping syndrome Postgastrectomy syndrome that develops during or shortly after a meal; characterized by epigastric discomfort, sweating, weakness, pallor, nausea, and rapid pulse. It is due to the sudden reduction in blood plasma volume in the peripheral circulation secondary to the drawing of large quantities of fluid from the bloodstream into the intestine following the rapid introduction of large quantities of hypertonic food in the jejunum. Dietary treatment consists of small frequent feedings and the avoidance of liquids during meals and of substances with high osmotic effect such as sugars. See *High protein, low carbohydrate diet* under *Diet, protein modified*. See also Dietary management of selected disorders, Appendix O.

Duodenum The first portion of the small intestine, extending from the pylorus to the jejunum. It is about 8 to 10 inches long. It is in the duodenum that pancreatic juice and bile are secreted.

Dwarfism Abnormal stunted growth or development of the body; a state of being smaller than the average for the species. It is primarily due to hypofunction of the pituitary gland. Dwarfism is sometimes associated with malformation or disproportion of parts.

Dymelor Trade name for acetohexamide, an *oral hypoglycemic agent*.

Dynamic state Continuous metabolism or turnover (i.e., synthesis, degradation, and replacement) of body constituents even at constant composition; a state of flux. Bodily constituents are constantly and simultaneously being broken down and rebuilt, and the apparent stability of the organism is the result of a balance between the rates of synthesis and degradation of its constituents.

Dynamometer Apparatus for measuring and recording maximum grip strength and grip strength endurance. *Maximum grip strength* is the value obtained when a person applies the strongest hand pressure.

Grip strength endurance is the average strength exhibited in 1 minute.

Dysentery Inflammation of the intestines, primarily the colon, characterized by abdominal pain, tenesmus, and severe diarrhea containing blood and mucus. It is caused by various agents. Two types of dysentery having public health significance are transmitted by insect vectors, contaminated food and drink, or by hand-to-mouth transfer of contaminated materials; these are amebic dysentery, caused by *Entamoeba histolytica,* and bacillary dysentery, caused by *Shigella* genus.

Dysgeusia Taste perversion associated with a generalized decrease in taste acuity.

Dyspepsia Gastric indigestion; a wide variety of complaints referable to the upper gastrointestinal tract following the ingestion of food. Typical symptoms are heartburn, nausea, epigastric pain, abdominal discomfort, belching, distention, and flatulence. It may be the result of an organic disease of the gastrointestinal tract, such as esophagitis, gastritis, or peptic ulcer, or may be functional in nature and occur in the absence of any demonstrable organic lesion. Dyspepsia is also due to rapid eating, inadequate chewing, swallowing of air, or emotional stress.

Dysphagia Difficulty in swallowing.

Dysplasia Abnormal development or growth.

Dyspnea Difficult or labored breathing; a common symptom in cardiac disease.

Dyssebacia Disorder of the sebaceous follicles; plugging of sebaceous glands. Nasolabial dyssebacia is often seen in *riboflavin* deficiency.

Dystonia Lack of tonicity of muscles brought about by lesions of the lenticular nuclei of muscles or by certain diseases.

Dystrophy Abnormal development; degeneration; defective or faulty nutrition.

Dysuria Painful or difficult urination; often associated with certain diseases of the kidney.

E

EAA Abbreviation for *essential amino acid*.

ECG Abbreviation for *electrocardiogram*.

Eclampsia Condition usually occurring during the latter half of pregnancy characterized by edema, high blood pressure, albuminuria, and convulsions, usually ending in coma. The condition is referred to as preeclampsia in the absence of convulsions and/or coma. Both terms, eclampsia and preeclampsia, are collectively called *toxemia of pregnancy*.

Ectomorph Description given to a tall, thin individual with underdeveloped muscles and large subcutaneous tissue and surface areas with respect to body mass.

Ectopic Out of the normal place, as ectopic pregnancy, in which the ovum lodges outside the uterus, usually in the fallopian tube.

Eczema Inflammatory skin disease usually accompanied by itching, watery discharge, exudative lesions, and development of scales and crusts; of varying types and causes.

Edema Presence of an abnormally large amount of fluid in the tissue spaces of the body due to a disturbance in the mechanisms involved in fluid exchange. Factors that tend to increase the volume of interstitial fluid include reduction in plasma osmotic pressure, rise in capillary blood pressure, increase in permeability of the capillary membrane, and obstruction of the lymph channels. Edema is seen in association with malnutrition (such as in beriberi and protein deficiency), cardiac failure, renal disease, liver disease, or simple allergy.

Edestin Simple protein of the globulin type found in beans, peas, and seeds of hemp.

Edible portion (EP) Part or portion of the food that is fit to eat and customarily eaten.

EDTA Abbreviation for *ethylenediaminetetraacetic acid*. A powerful chelating and sequestering agent that forms water-soluble complexes with many different cations in solutions. Salts of the acid are used for their solubilizing and stabilizing actions.

EEG Abbreviation for *electroencephalogram*.

EFA Abbreviation for *essential fatty acid*.

Effector Nerve end organ that serves to distribute impulses that activate gland secretion and muscle contraction; opposite of *receptor*.

Efferent Sending or conveying impulses away from a center, as efferent nerves.

Effervescent Giving off gas bubbles; bubbling.

Egg white injury Condition characterized by exfoliative dermatitis, muscle pains, anorexia, and emaciation as a result of prolonged and excessive intake of raw egg white. This is actually a biotin deficiency as caused by the presence of *avidin* in raw egg white which combines with biotin, rendering it unavailable for use. Cooking the egg destroys avidin.

EKG Abbreviation for *electrocardiogram;* from the German word *elektrokardiogram*.

Elaidic acid Monounsaturated fatty acid with 18 carbon atoms; the double bond is in the *trans* configuration. The *cis* isomer is called oleic acid.

Elastase Proteolytic enzyme present in the pancreatic juice that is capable of dissolving elastin.

Elastin An albuminoid, the characteristic protein of yellow elastic fibers abundant in ligaments, lung matrix, and blood vessel walls. It is insoluble in water and digestible by the enzyme *elastase,* but it is not hydrolyzed to gelatin by boiling.

Electrocardiogram (**ECG**) Graphic tracing by a machine called an *electrocardiograph* that measures and records the electric current produced in various parts of the heart muscle during its cardiac cycle. The electrocardiogram provides important information in the diagnosis of heart disorders.

Electroencephalogram (**EEG**) Graphic record of the changes in electrical potential in the brain by means of pad electrodes applied to the scalp or needle electrodes placed in contact with the membrane covering the skull in the various regions of the brain. The electroencephalogram is useful in the diagnosis of various conditions of the brain such as trauma, tumors, epilepsy, etc.

Electrolysis Decomposition of a chemical compound by direct use of electric current; passage of electricity through an electrolyte.

Electrolyte A substance that, in solution, conducts an electric current and ionizes into an electrically charged particle.

Electron Negatively charged particle.

Electron transport chain Process that occurs in the mitochondria of the cell where hydrogen and then electrons from a substrate are passed from nicotinamide adenine dinucleotide (NAD) to flavin adenine dinucleotide (FAD) to coenzyme Q_{10} to cytochromes and then to oxygen to form water. The series of electron carriers are reduced and oxidized and thus provide for the regeneration of NAD and FAD. As this occurs, the energy released is trapped

by adenosine diphosphate (ADP) to form adenosine triphosphate (ATP). This is called oxidative phosphorylation. See *Phosphorylation* and the Electron transport system and coupled oxidative phosphorylation, Appendix F-4.

Electrophoresis Migration of charged colloidal particles in an electric field at a definite pH toward the oppositely charged electrode. It is a useful method in the determination of molecular weights of protein and separation of the various protein components of a mixture as well as in defining the homogeneity or heterogeneity of a given protein. It is also a valuable tool in the examination of blood proteins for diagnostic purposes, and *paper electrophoresis* is widely used in the study of minute amounts of biologic mixtures.

Elution 1. Separation and removal of impurities by washing. 2. Process of extracting an adsorbed substance from the solid adsorbent medium, as in chromatography. The solvent used in elution is called *eluant,* and the extract obtained is called *eluate.*

Emaciation Extreme leanness; wasting away of body flesh.

Embden-Meyerhof pathway Anaerobic phase of glycogen (or glucose) metabolism. See *Glycolysis.*

Embolus Any bit of matter foreign to the blood as air, blood clot, tissue cells, fat, and clumps of bacteria, or any foreign body that gains entrance into the bloodstream until it lodges in a blood vessel. The obstruction of a blood vessel by an embolus is called *embolism.*

Embryo Early stage of a developing organism. In the human the embryo is the developing individual from the time of conception up to the end of the second month. *Embryology* is the science dealing with the embryo and its development; a specialist in this field is an *embryologist.*

Emergency feeding Consideration of feeding in times of disaster, either natural or man-made, e.g., flood, fire, volcanic eruption, or war. First concern is to allay hunger and maintain morale. Problems such as lack of water and of cooking and refrigeration facilities must be considered. Canned and ready-to-eat packaged food must be provided. This is especially so after a nuclear attack to avoid the hazards of radioactive contamination of food and drink. When an emergency is of more than a few days' duration, meeting nutritional needs must be considered.

Emetic Any agent or drug that causes vomiting (emesis).

Emigration Escape or outward passage of leukocytes through the walls of small blood vessels.

Emphysema Abnormal presence of air or gas in the body tissues or overdistention of the air spaces in the lungs due to rupture of the pulmonary alveoli.

"Empty" calories Refers to carbohydrate-rich foods such as sugars, syrups, jellies, and other sweets that contribute mainly calories with either no or insignificant amounts of the other nutrients.

Empyema Accumulation of pus in a cavity or body space such as the gallbladder, heart sac, and chest wall.

Emulsification Process of lowering surface tension or breaking up large particles of an immiscible liquid into smaller ones that remain suspended in another liquid. An agent that has this ability is called an emulsifier, e.g., bile salts and lecithin. Emulsification of fat by the action of bile salts facilitates its digestion.

Emulsoid Lyophilic *colloid* in which the dispersed phase has an affinity for the dispersion medium.

Enamel The hard, compact, and calcified substance that covers and protects the crown of the tooth. See *Tooth.*

Enantiomorphs Isomers whose molecules are mirror images of each other and that rotate around the plane of polarized light to the same degree.

Encephalitis Inflammation of the brain; may be due to viral infection, poison, or other diseases and injury involving the brain.

Encephalomalacia Softening of the brain because of a deficient blood supply; characterized by uncoordinated muscle movement, tremors, and retraction of the head; seen in vitamin E–deficient chickens.

Encephalon The brain. Any degenerative disease of the brain is called *encephalopathy.*

Endemic Prevalent in a particular region or locality. An endemic disease is one that has a low incidence but is more or less constantly present in a given population.

Endergonic reaction Reaction requiring an input or supply of energy to push the reaction; usually associated with anabolism.

Endocarditis Acute or chronic inflammation of the inner lining of the heart and its valves; generally associated with rheumatism and other acute febrile diseases.

Endocardium Endothelial membrane lining the heart chambers.

Endocrine Secreting internally or into the bloodstream. The *endocrine glands* are ductless glands producing internal secretions called hormones that are discharged directly into the bloodstream. See Summary of endocrine glands, Appendix K.

Endocrinology Study of the structure and function of the endocrine glands and their internal secretions.

Endogastritis Inflammation of the mucous membrane of the stomach.

Endogenous Originating or coming from within or inside the cell or tissue.

Endometrium Mucous membrane that lines the interior wall of the uterus.

Endomorph Description given to a stocky, fat individual with round body features, prominent abdominal viscera, large trunk and thighs, and tapering extremities.

Endopeptidase Proteolytic enzyme that splits centrally located peptide bonds of protein. Examples are pepsin, trypsin, and chymotrypsin.

Endoplasmic reticulum *Organelle* of the cell,

which consists of a series of canals in the cytoplasm connecting the nucleus with the membrane. The rough endoplasmic reticulum contains *ribosomes*. The smooth endoplasmic reticulum is thought to be the site of hormone synthesis.

Endosperm Portion of the seed that surrounds the embryo. It contains mainly starch, a reserve food supply.

Endothelium Membrane that lines the closed cavities of the body such as the heart, blood vessels, and lymph vessels.

Endothermic Chemical reaction requiring the uptake or absorption of heat.

End point Point at which a sudden change in some property of a solution takes place. For example, in titration the indicator will change color at the end point.

Energy Capacity to do work. It exists in five forms: kinetic, potential, thermal, nuclear, and radiant or solar. Energy is needed by the body for muscular activity, to maintain body temperature, and to carry out metabolic processes. Energy comes from the oxidation of foods and is measured in terms of *calories*. See *Food, energy value; Basal metabolism;* and *Metabolizable energy.* See also Utilization of food energy, Appendix D-4.

Energy balance Also called caloric balance; the equilibrium between energy intake and energy output. When energy intake exceeds energy needs, the extra energy is stored, leading to an increase in body weight (positive balance). When energy intake is less than energy needs, the body utilizes its own reserves, resulting in loss of weight (negative energy balance).

Enfamil Commercial milk preparation for routine infant feeding; made of nonfat milk with added corn and coconut oils, lactose, and vitamins. Also available with iron. (Mead Johnson.) See Proprietary foods: composition, features, and uses, Appendix P-1.

English disease See *Rickets.*

Enolase Enzyme that catalyzes the conversion of 2-phosphoglyceric acid to phosphoenol-

pyruvic acid, with the formation of an energy-rich phosphate bond.

Enrichment 1. Addition of vitamins and minerals (thiamin, niacin, riboflavin, and iron) to cereal products such as flour, bread, rice, crackers, macaroni, and spaghetti to restore those lost in milling and processing. Minimum and maximum levels for addition have been set. 2. In countries other than the United States this refers to the addition of vitamins, minerals, amino acids, or protein concentrates to foods to improve their nutrient content. See *Fortification.*

Ensure Lactose-free liquid nutritional product for tube or supplemental feeding; contains caseinate and soy protein isolates, corn syrup, sucrose, corn oil, vitamins, and minerals. (Ross.) See Proprietary foods: composition, features, and uses, Appendix P-1.

Enteric Pertaining to the intestines.

Enteritis Acute or chronic inflammation or irritation of the intestinal mucosa, chiefly the small intestines. It may result from overeating, food or chemical poisoning, ingestion of irritants, or bacterial or protozoan invasion. Often accompanied by diarrhea and abdominal pain.

Enteroclysis Injection of a liquid preparation of a nutrient or medicine into the rectum.

Enterocolitis Inflammation of the small intestine and colon.

Enterocrinin Hormone produced by the intestinal mucosa that stimulates the glands of the small intestine to secrete digestive fluid.

Enterogastrone Hormone produced by the duodenum that inhibits gastric secretion and motility on ingestion of fat.

Enterokinase Enzyme of the intestinal juice that converts inactive trypsinogen to active trypsin.

Enzyme Organic catalyst produced by living cells that is responsible for most of the chemical reactions and energy transformation in both plants and animals. Many enzymes are simple proteins, often existing as inactive *proenzymes* or *zymogens;* other enzymes require, in addition to the protein molecule, another factor in order to exhibit full activity. This *cofactor* may be an inorganic element such as zinc, or it may be an organic molecule such as a vitamin or its derivative. Some enzymes are thus described in terms of their protein portion or *apoenzyme* and their cofactor portion is designated as *coenzyme, prosthetic group,* or *activator.* See also Summary of enzymes, Appendix J-2.

Eosinophil Type of white blood cell that has an affinity for a red-staining dye known as *eosin.* Under the microscope such white cells show many red grains within them.

Eosinophil count Normal eosinophil count ranges from 0.5% to 4% of the total number of leukocytes in 1 mm³ of blood. Eosinophil count is now employed as a rapid and simple method for the study of adrenocortical function. Administration of cortisone or corticotropin (ACTH) results in a decline in circulating eosinophils. Failure to produce a fall of more than 50% is an indication of adrenal insufficiency.

EP Abbreviation for *edible portion.*

Epidemic Occurrence in a community or region of a disease or illness that is spreading rapidly or in excess of normal expectancy.

Epidemiology Study of the occurrence, frequency, and distribution of a disease. A specialist in this field is an *epidemiologist.*

Epidermis Outermost layer of the skin; the cuticle. It is composed of several layers of cells: horny, nucleated, granular, pigmented, and columnar cells.

Epigastric Pertaining to the epigastric region or *epigastrium,* the upper and middle portion of the abdomen in front of the stomach.

Epiglottis Lidlike elastic cartilage that covers the larynx or voice box and closes on swallowing to prevent food from going into the voice box.

Epilepsy Nervous disorder characterized by episodes of motor, sensory, or psychic dysfunction with or without unconsciousness and/or convulsions. The most common are grand mal, Jacksonian, petit mal, and psychic or psychomotor epilepsies.

Grand mal e Characterized by sudden loss of consciousness, stiffening of the body, bluing of the skin, muscle spasm with the eyes turned up, frothing at the mouth, and often accompanied by passage of urine, confusion, and deep sleep. The person awakens with no memory of the episode.

Jacksonian e Attacks of muscular spasm localized to one area or side of the body often without loss of consciousness in the beginning, but as the disease progresses the spasms may become general, ending in unconsciousness.

Petit mal e Characterized by very short lapses into unconsciousness that may appear as a sudden momentary pause in movement or conversation, rarely lasting 30 seconds; the person rarely falls or has muscular spasm. Frequent in children and may occur as often as 200 times a day.

Psychic or psychomotor e Characterized by automatic movements such as chewing, smacking the lips, "dreamy" feeling of unreality, confused mental state, and other automatic acts of which the patient is quite unaware and does not remember after the attack.

Epileptiform seizures Fits or seizures similar to attacks of epilepsy.

Epimer Either of a pair of isomeric aldoses that differ only in the configuration of a single carbon atom, as glucose and mannose are epimers with respect to carbon atom 2, and glucose and galactose are epimers with respect to carbon atom 4.

Epinephrine Adrenaline, the major hormone of the adrenal medulla. It is secreted in response to stimulation of nerve fibers by a variety of factors, including fear, anger, pain, hypoglycemia, hemorrhage, muscular activity, and anesthetic drugs. Its action is varied, causing dilatation of the skeletal muscles as well as coronary and visceral vessels and resulting in *increased* blood flow in these regions, *constriction* of the capillaries of the skin and arterioles of the kidney, *elevation* of respiratory quotient with increase in oxygen consumption and carbon dioxide production, and *acceleration* of glycogenolysis with formation of glucose in the liver and lactic acid in the muscles. See also *Norepinephrine.*

Epiphysis Bone at the end of the shaft. It is initially separated from the bone by cartilage but when growth is complete it becomes part of the bone.

Epithelium Covering of the skin and internal mucous membrane lining the body cavities, including vessels and passages. It consists of cells joined by small amounts of cementing substances. Vitamin A is believed to maintain the health of these cells.

Epsom salt Magnesium sulfate, substance used as a purgative. It increases the bulk of the feces because its osmotic pressure causes retention of water in the intestine.

Equivalent weight Relative weight of a substance that will react with one gram atomic weight of hydrogen or is chemically equal to 8 parts by weight of oxygen. Also defined as the weight of a molecule or of an atom or radical divided by its valence.

Erepsin Former term given to the various peptidases of the intestinal juice that act on peptide bonds adjacent to a free amino or carboxyl group.

Ergastoplasm Rough endoplasmic reticulum that contains the ribosomes.

Ergin Former term for vitamin. See *Vitamin.*

Ergocalciferol Name for vitamin D_2 or irradiated ergosterol; formerly called *calciferol* or *viosterol.* See also *Vitamin D.*

Ergon One of the early names given to vitamins.

Ergosterol Provitamin D_2, a sterol found chiefly in yeasts and widely distributed in plants and certain animal tissues. It is converted to *ergocalciferol* or vitamin D_2 on irradiation or exposure to ultraviolet light.

Ergot Fungus that grows on grasses and cereal grains, especially rye. It can contract arterioles and smooth muscles and is used in medicine to hasten labor, arrest internal hemorrhage, or check bladder paralysis and spinal congestion. Excessive intake of ergot, either as a medicine or by eating ergot-infected rye flour, causes poisoning called *ergotism.* The condition is characterized by muscular spasm and cramps or by a kind of dry gangrene.

Ergothioneine One of the three histidine compounds found in the body. It occurs principally in red blood cells and liver. The other two compounds, *carnosine* and *anserine,* occur in muscles.

Erucic acid Monounsaturated fatty acid containing 22 carbon atoms; found in rape seed, mustard seed, and other vegetable seed oils. When given to rats, it increases the cholesterol content of the adrenal gland.

Eructation Belching or casting up gas or acid from the stomach.

Erythema Redness of the skin due to congestion of the capillaries.

Erythrobic acid D-Ascorbic acid, a form not utilized by humans to any appreciable extent. It is used as a preservative in the meat industry.

Erythroblast Nucleated cell occurring normally in the bone marrow from which the red blood cell develops.

Erythroblastosis fetalis Hemolytic disease of the newborn due to isoimmunization of an Rh-negative mother against an Rh-positive fetus, the fetal blood characteristic having been inherited from the father. It is characterized by jaundice, progressive hemolytic anemia, enlargement of the liver, massive edema, and kernicterus. Death of the fetus may occur even in the uterus. See *Rh factor.*

Erythrocruorin An iron porphyrin conjugated to protein; occurs in the blood and tissue fluids of some invertebrates and is similar in function to hemoglobin.

Erythrocuprein A copper-containing protein found in the red blood cells. It contains two atoms of copper per mole and accounts for most, if not all, of the copper in the red cell.

Erythrocytes Also called red blood cells; the pigmented biconcave and nonnucleated disks that transport oxygen to the tissues in combination with hemoglobin, the blood pigment responsible for the red color of fresh blood. Normal RBC count is 4 to 6 million/mm^3.

Erythrocyte maturation factor See *Vitamin B$_{12}$*.

Erythrocytosis Increase in the number of red blood cells.

Erythrodextrin Dextrin formed by the partial hydrolysis of starch; gives a red color with iodine.

Erythropoiesis Formation or development of erythrocytes from the primitive cells to the mature erythrocytes. See *Hemopoiesis*.

Erythropoietin Hormone produced by the kidney that stimulates the production of red blood cells. See *Hemopoiesis*.

Erythrose A tetrose, a 4-carbon aldose sugar occurring in the body as an intermediate product of metabolism.

Erythrulose A 4-carbon ketose.

Esophagus A hollow muscular tube measuring about 2 cm in diameter and 25 to 30 cm in length, extending from the pharynx to the stomach. *Esophagitis* is the inflammation of the esophagus.

ESR Abbreviation for *erythrocyte sedimentation rate*. See *Sedimentation rate*.

Essential amino acid (**EAA**) See under *Amino acid*.

Essential fatty acid (**EFA**) See under *Fatty acid*.

Ester Compound formed from an alcohol and an acid by elimination of water; the process is called *esterification*.

Esterase Enzyme that catalyzes the hydrolysis of an ester into an alcohol and an acid. See Summary of enzymes, Appendix J-2.

Estradiol The primary estrogenic hormone; regarded as the follicular hormone; occurs in the placenta and urine during pregnancy. It exists in the isomeric forms—alpha and beta. See also *Estrogen*.

Estrin Former term for *estrogen*.

Estriol The second estrogenic hormone iso-lated from the urine of pregnant women. See *Estrogen*.

Estrogen Collective term for the natural or synthetic female sex hormones. The three naturally occurring estrogens—*estradiol, estrone,* and *estriol*—are produced principally by the maturing follicles in the ovary, although they are also formed in the placenta and adrenal cortex. Two synthetic estrogenic compounds of therapeutic importance are *ethynylestradiol* and *stilbestrol*. The estrogens are responsible for the development of the female sex organs, growth of the genitalia and mammary glands, and development of secondary sex characteristics such as alteration in body contour and growth of axillary and pubic hair. In addition, estrogenic hormones also have profound effects on calcium and phosphorus metabolism and probably are related to bone metabolism, lipid metabolism, and skin or related structures. See Summary of endocrine glands, Appendix K.

Estrone The first estrogenic hormone isolated in a chemically pure state from the urine of pregnant women. See *Estrogen*.

Estrus (oestrus) 1. Mating period of animals, especially the female, marked by intense sexual urge. 2. Menstrual cycle occurring during reproductive life.

Ethanol Ethyl alcohol, the form of alcohol that is ingested in alcoholic drinks. See *Alcohol* and *Fermentation*.

Ethanolamine Beta-aminoethyl alcohol, a basic component of certain cephalins. It may be formed by reduction of glycine or decarboxylation of serine and forms choline when methylated by methionine. A lipotropic agent, it can prevent the formation of fatty livers.

Ethnic Pertaining to people and races, their traits, and their customs.

Ethylation Introduction of an ethyl group (C_2H_5) into a compound.

Ethylene A colorless gas with a sweetish taste and odor; used as an inhalation anesthetic and to facilitate ripening of fruits.

Etiology Study and theory of the causes of disease.

Eugenics Science concerned with the improvement of the human race.

Eupepsia Normal digestion; presence of a normal amount of pepsin in the gastric juice.

Euphoria Bodily comfort; absence of pain or distress. In psychology, the exaggerated sense of well-being.

Eupnea State of ordinary, quiet breathing as seen in a normal person at rest.

Euthanasia Painless killing of people suffering from a painful, incurable disease; an easy or merciful death.

Eutrophia Healthy state of nutrition; normal nutrition.

Ewald test diet See *Diet, Ewald test.*

Exacerbation Increase in severity of any symptom or disease.

Excelsin Simple protein of the globulin type found in Brazil nuts.

Exchange list Classification or grouping of common foods on the basis of similarity of nutrient composition. Each food within the list has approximately the same food value and may be used interchangeably.

Excision Cutting out or removing a part or foreign body from an organ or tissue.

Excrement The feces; fecal matter.

Excreta Waste materials discharged from the body.

Exergonic reaction Reaction accompanied by a release of energy; usually associated with catabolism.

Exhalation Expiration; to breathe out. The giving off in the form of vapor.

Exocardia Congenital displacement of the heart.

Exogenous Coming from or originating from the outside; not from within; due to an external cause.

Exopeptidase Proteolytic enzyme that acts on peptide bonds adjacent to a free amino or carboxyl group. Among the principal exopeptidases are aminopeptidase and carboxypeptidase.

Exophthalmic goiter Goiter characterized by protruding eyeballs. See *Goiter.*

Exophthalmos Abnormal protrusion of the eye.

Exosmosis Diffusion or passage of a liquid from within outward.

Exothermic reaction Reaction associated with liberation of heat or energy.

Expanded Nutrition Program Funds were provided by the Department of Agriculture in 1969 for the Extension Service to train nutrition aides. The aides work with low-income families and help them with home-making skills and provide nutrition information.

Expectorate To spit or expel by coughing materials from the lungs and trachea.

Expiration To breathe out or expel air from the lungs.

Expire To breathe out; to die; to end.

Extensor Muscle that enables extension, stretching, or straightening out of a limb or part, as opposed to flexor.

Exteroceptor Receptor or end organ in or near the skin and mucous membrane receiving stimuli from the external environment.

Extravasation Escape or discharge of fluid out of its proper place, as of blood from a ruptured vessel into the surrounding tissues.

Extrinsic factor Literally, a substance originating from the outside. In nutrition, this refers to the extrinsic factor of Castle or vitamin B_{12} obtained from food. See *Vitamin B_{12}.*

Exudative diathesis Condition seen in vitamin E–deficient chickens that is characterized by generalized edema with collection of fluids in the subcutaneous tissues, particularly the breast and abdomen.

F

Fabricated foods New foods or imitations of natural foods synthesized from agricultural products in order to obtain certain nutritional and organoleptic properties. Soy proteins have been made to look like a conventional food. See *Textured protein*.

Factor Any constituent that tends to produce a result. In nutrition, it refers to an essential or desirable element in the diet that has some effect on growth, reproduction, or health of organisms. It may be a vitamin, a mineral, or any other nutrient. The structure of the factor may be identified or it may remain unidentified.

FAD Abbreviation for *flavin adenine dinucleotide*. See *Flavin nucleotide*.

Failure to thrive Also called failure to grow; infants fail to thrive because of inadequate intake of food, unusually high energy requirements, excessive losses as in diarrhea and excessive vomiting, or a combination of two or more of these factors. Failure to thrive frequently affects the child who has been deprived of adequate maternal love and attention.

Fair Packaging and Labeling Act This act, passed in 1966, set regulations for labeling and packaging consumer commodities such as food, drugs, devices, and cosmetics as defined in the Food, Drug, and Cosmetic Act. Meat, meat products, poultry, poultry products that are not canned, and prescription drugs do not come under this law. See *Nutrition, labeling*.

Falling disease Condition seen in grazing cattle characterized by staggering, falling, and sudden death. It is caused by a chronic copper deficiency resulting from a low content of the mineral in the herbage.

Fallopian tube Tube that serves to transport the ovum from the ovary to the uterus.

Fanconi's syndrome Condition characterized by a low renal threshold for amino acids. A generalized aminoaciduria occurs even with normal levels of amino acids in the blood. This leads to withdrawal of calcium from the bones to neutralize the acids. As a result, conditioned rickets or osteomalacia may occur.

FAO Abbreviation for *Food and Agriculture Organization*.

Farnoquinone Vitamin K_2, a naphthoquinone derivative. Originally isolated from putrid fish meal; it is synthesized by a large number of intestinal bacteria. See *Vitamin K*.

Fastidium cibi Aversion to food or to eating.

Fat In the strictest sense the term means *neutral* or *true fat*, which is a mixture of glyceryl esters of fatty acids. Dietary fat is an example of a *lipid*.

Fat, body There are two types of body fat: element constant and element variable. Element constant is protoplasmic fat, which is part of the essential structure of cells. In addition to neutral fat, it contains other lipids such as phospholipid, cholesterol, and cerebroside. Protoplasmic fat is of constant composition and is not altered by variations in food intake, hence it is not reduced during starvation. Element variable is depot fat or *adipose tissue*, which is the fuel store of the body and found mainly in the subcutaneous tissue and around visceral organs. This fat store is filled up or depleted, depending on the balance between the energy value of food eaten and expended.

Fat functions Fat is a concentrated source of energy, yielding about 9 calories/gm. It is a carrier of fat-soluble vitamins, adds palatability and satiety value to the diet, and has protein-sparing action. In addition, fat also acts as a shock absorber, serves as a padding around vital organs, and insulates the body against the loss of heat.

Fat, neutral Triglyceride or true fat; an organic ester of three molecules of fatty acid combined with one molecule of glycerol. This is the form in which fats occur chiefly in foodstuffs and in fat depots of most animals. Neutral fat may be *soft* or *hard,* depending on the length of the fatty acid chain; or it may be *liquid* or *solid,* depending on the degree of saturation or unsaturation of the fatty acids. See *Fatty acid.*

Fat soluble Generally refers to substances that cannot be dissolved in water but can be dissolved in fats and oils or in fat solvents such as ether and chloroform. The fat-soluble vitamins are vitamins A, D, E, and K.

Fatty acid (FA) An organic acid containing carbon, hydrogen, and oxygen; generally consists of a carbon chain that terminates in a —COOH group. It is found in abundance in ester linkage in several lipid compounds, or it may exist as a free or nonesterified fatty acid. With a few exceptions, those occurring in natural fats contain an even number of carbon atoms (4 to 24 carbon atoms). Fatty acids are generally classified according to the number of carbon atoms or degree of saturation between the carbon atoms.

Essential FA Polyunsaturated fatty acids that are necessary for growth, reproduction, health of the skin, and proper utilization of fats. According to this definition, three fatty acids may be considered *physiologically essential:* linoleic, linolenic, and arachidonic acid. An essential dietary fatty acid is one that cannot be synthesized in the body or cannot be synthesized in sufficient amounts and must exist preformed in the diet. According to this definition, only *linoleic acid* may be considered a dietary essential because it serves as a precursor for the other two physiologic essential fatty acids.

Free FA Also called nonesterified fatty acid; plasma free fatty acids (FFA) such as oleic, palmitic, stearic, and linoleic acids are bound to serum albumin as part of the lipoproteins. They are believed to aid in the transport of fat, both from alimentary sources and from fat depots, for oxidation in various tissues. During fasting, FFA from depot fat increases, whereas glucose and insulin administration decrease the movement of depot fatty acids to plasma FFA. In fats and oils the amount of free fatty acids is a measure of the degree of hydrolytic rancidity.

Long-chain FA Those containing 12 or more carbon atoms. The most prevalent in foods are stearic acid (18 carbon atoms) and palmitic acid (16 carbon atoms).

Medium-chain FA Those containing 8 to 10 carbon atoms. Although not prevalent in foods, medium-chain fatty acids are more readily absorbed than the long-chain fatty acids. Examples are caprylic acid (8 carbon atoms) and capric acid (10 carbon atoms).

Monounsaturated FA Also called monoenoic fatty acids; those with only one unsaturated linkage or double bond, having two hydrogen atoms less than the saturated form. The most abundant monounsaturated fatty acids in animal fats are oleic and palmitoleic acids.

Nonesterified FA See *Free fatty acid* under *Fatty acid.*

Polyunsaturated FA Those having two or more unsaturated linkages or double bonds and classed as dienoic, trienoic, and tetraenoic. Of greatest interest are linoleic acid (two double bonds), linolenic acid (three double bonds), and arachidonic acid (four double bonds). See *Essential fatty acid* under *Fatty acid*.

Saturated FA Those having all the carbon atoms of the molecule linked to hydrogen so that only single bonds exist. Saturation of fatty acids accounts for the firmness of fats at room temperature. The most common in animal fats are palmitic and stearic acids.

Short-chain FA Those containing four to six carbon atoms. These are not abundant in food fats and yield only about 5 calories/gm compared to 9 calories/gm of the longer chain fatty acids. Examples are caproic acid (six carbon atoms) and butyric acid (four carbon atoms).

Unsaturated FA Those containing one or more double bonds between one or more of the carbons in the chain. Unsaturation alters certain properties of fatty acids. In general the melting point is greatly lowered and the solubility in nonpolar solvents is enhanced. All the common unsaturated fatty acids in nature are liquid at room temperature. They are abundant in vegetable oils such as olive oil, corn oil, cottonseed oil, and soybean oil. See also *Monounsaturated fatty acid* and *Polyunsaturated fatty acid* under *Fatty acid*.

Fatty liver Accumulation of fatty deposits rich in cholesterol esters in the liver. This may be the result of a number of causes, including lack of *lipotropic factors;* liver poisoning by phosphorus, chloroform, and other chlorinated compounds; and following chronic infectious diseases such as tuberculosis, metabolic disorders such as diabetes, or various nutritional disorders such as kwashiorkor, chronic alcoholism, and vitamin E deficiency.

Favism Fava bean poisoning caused by the ingestion of fava beans or even the inhalation of its pollens by susceptible individuals. Symptoms include vomiting, dizziness, prostration, acute hemolytic anemia, and jaundice. It is due to a deficiency of the enzyme glucose-6-phosphate dehydrogenase.

FCT Abbreviation for *Food Composition Table*.

FDA Abbreviation for *Food and Drug Administration*.

Febrile Having fever.

Fecal marker A substance that is used in metabolic studies to indicate the start and end of the collection of feces.

Feces Excrement from the intestines; composed of undigested food residues, intestinal secretions and shed linings, casts and dead cells, and bacteria or their products.

Federal Trade Commission (FTC) Federal agency of the United States government that protects the consumer from false advertising.

Feed Generally refers to food given to animals.

Feeding, artificial Manner of introducing food, nutriment, or medicine other than by the natural way of eating or oral administration. The most common method is the use of a polyvinyl tube, which is passed through the mouth or nose until it reaches the stomach or the duodenum. The tube is sometimes introduced through the rectum when it is unwise or impractical for patients to have the tube pass through the esophagus, as in cancer or obstruction in the esophagus. *Parenteral* administration of nutrient or medicine is via the subcutaneous, intramuscular, intravenous, or intraperitoneal route. Nutriments generally introduced this way include dextrose solution, amino acid solution, vitamin preparations, physiologic saline solution, blood serum or plasma, and plasma expanders such as dextran. Artificial feeding is indicated when the patient is unable or refuses to take food following operations, accidents, or unconsciousness. It is also indicated when part of the body has to be resected as in carcinoma of the esophagus, and parenteral feeding is often used as a supplement to oral or tube feeding. See also *Diet, tube feeding*.

Fehling's test Test for reducing sugars. Fehling's solution (an alkaline copper sulfate solution with potassium sodium tartrate) gives a red precipitate of cuprous oxide in the presence of a reducing sugar.

Fels Parent Specific Standards Set of height standards for boys and girls that takes into account the height of the parents.

Fermentation Also called glycolysis; the enzymatic oxidation of carbohydrate under anaerobic or partially anaerobic conditions.

Acetic f Formation of acetic acid from the oxidation of alcohol by the vinegar bacterium *Acetobacter aceti* in the presence of oxygen.

Alcoholic f Anaerobic formation of alcohol by the action of yeast on sugar.

Lactic f Formation of lactic acid by lactic acid bacteria.

Fermented foods Foods prepared by the fermentation action of bacteria, yeast, or molds. Examples are cheese, yogurt, wine, and beer.

Ferriprotoporphyrin Also called *hemin;* a complex of ferric iron and protoporphyrin with a net positive charge.

Ferritin An iron-protein complex found chiefly in the liver, spleen, bone marrow, and reticuloendothelial cells. It contains 23% iron and is believed to be the chief storage form of iron in the body. When ferritin storage capacity is exceeded, iron accumulates in the liver as *hemosiderin.*

Ferroprotoporphyrin Also called *heme;* a complex of ferrous iron and protoporphyrin.

Fetor hepaticus Foul breath resembling the odor of rotten liver and characteristic of liver insufficiency, as in hepatic coma.

Fetus Unborn offspring from the end of the third month until birth. Before this period (i.e., conception to the third month) the proper term is *embryo.*

Fever 1. Elevation in body temperature above normal (98.6° F or 37° C); pyrexia. 2. Any disease characterized by a marked increase of temperature, acceleration of basal metabolism, and increase in tissue destruction. It may be *acute* such as in

influenza, chickenpox, and pneumonia or *chronic* as in tuberculosis.

FFA Abbreviation for *free fatty acid.*

FFHC Abbreviation for *Freedom from Hunger Campaign.*

FH$_2$ Abbreviation for *dihydrofolic acid.*

FH$_4$ Abbreviation for *tetrahydrofolic acid.*

Fiber Threadlike, elongated structure of organic tissue such as muscle fiber and nerve fiber. In diet therapy, the term *fiber* includes indigestible organic tissues such as ligaments and gristle in meats and indigestible carbohydrates such as cellulose, hemicellulose, and lignin found in fruits, vegetables, and cereals.

Fibrillation Spontaneous contraction of individual muscle fibers that are no longer under control of the motor nerve, such as cardiac (auricular or ventricular) fibrillation.

Fibrin The colorless insoluble protein mainly responsible for the blood clot. It is formed from the interaction between a soluble precursor, *fibrinogen,* and an enzyme, *thrombin.* Fibrin serves as the essential network in which blood cells are enmeshed to form the clot. Dissolution of fibrin by enzyme action is called *fibrinolysis.*

Fibrinogen The soluble protein precursor of fibrin present in blood plasma which, by the action of *thrombin,* is converted into *fibrin,* thus forming the blood coagulum.

Fibrinolysin Also called *plasmin;* a proteolytic enzyme that dissolves fibrin and inactivates fibrinogen. Present in the plasma as the inactive precursor *profibrinolysin,* it is converted under certain circumstances to its active form by a second substance, *fibrinokinase,* present in the tissue. Activation can also be brought about by chloroform and by streptokinase.

Fibroblast Connective tissue cell; a spindle-shaped cell with a thin layer of cytoplasm and a large, oval, flattened nucleus. It forms the fibrous tissues in the body.

Fibrosis Formation of tough fibrous connective tissue in an organ beyond the amount normally present.

Fibrositis Also called muscular rheumatism; a condition characterized by pain and stiffness of the muscles, particularly of the neck, shoulders, back, and buttocks. Results from a number of causes such as exposure to cold and damp atmosphere, poor posture, excessive or unaccustomed muscular activity, infections, injury to muscles and tendons, and metabolic or endocrine disorders.

Ficin Proteolytic enzyme found in the milky sap of the fig tree; used in the clotting of milk and as an active anthelmintic against *Ascaris* and *Trichuris*.

FIGLU Abbreviation for *formiminoglutamic acid*.

Filter Apparatus that separates one or more components of a mixture from the others. The liquid that has passed through a filter is called a *filtrate*, and the process is known as *filtration*. Sometimes filtration is accomplished by a difference in pressure on either side of the membrane, either by producing a positive pressure on the liquid to be filtered or a negative pressure on the filtrate.

Filtrate factor See *Pantothenic acid*.

Fish protein concentrate (FPC) A tasteless, odorless powder prepared from whole fish that contains approximately 80% protein of high biologic value. FPC is used as a supplement in various foods to increase the protein quality.

Fish skin Dry skin that comes off in fine or rough scales. See *Xeroderma*.

Fission 1. Sexual reproduction in which the cell simply divides into two or more parts. 2. Splitting of the nucleus of an atom with the release of a tremendous amount of kinetic energy.

Fissure 1. Crack in the skin or ulcers in the mucous membrane. 2. Groove or deep fold in various organs, as in the skull or brain.

Fistula 1. Artificial opening or tubelike passage in the body. 2. Deep ulcer, often leading to an internal hollow organ, as a result of incomplete healing of a wound, an abscess, or other disease conditions.

Flaky-paint dermatosis Also called *crazy-pavement dermatosis;* extensive, often bilateral hyperpigmentation of the skin that peels off, leaving a hypopigmented skin with superficial ulceration. Occurs as patches, usually on the buttocks and back of the thighs.

Flatulence Distention of the stomach or the intestines with air or gases.

Flatus 1. Gas in the digestive tract. 2. Air expired in breathing; act of expelling air from the lungs.

Flavin Any one of a group of yellow pigments widely distributed in plants and animals, including *riboflavin* and Warburg's *yellow enzymes*. It is derived from *isoalloxazine* and has an intense green fluorescence.

Flavin nucleotide Derivative of the vitamin *riboflavin* that participates as a coenzyme in many oxidation-reduction reactions.

Flavin adenine dinucleotide (FAD) Riboflavin-5-phosphate attached by a pyrophosphate linkage to adenosine monophosphate. FAD arises from flavin mononucleotide by reaction with adenosine triphosphate and an enzyme found in yeast and animal tissues.

Flavin mononucleotide (FMN) Riboflavin-5-phosphate; consists of a three-ring system, *isoalloxazine,* attached to the corresponding alcohol of ribose, *ribitol,* which in turn is phosphorylated. FMN arises from riboflavin by reaction with ATP and the enzyme *flavokinase.*

Flavokinase Enzyme that catalyzes the phosphorylation of riboflavin to riboflavin-5-phosphate by adenosine triphosphate.

Flavonoid Flavone derivative, including *citrin, hesperidin,* and *rutin,* that reduces capillary fragility not corrected by administration of ascorbic acid. It has been called vitamin P. See also *Bioflavonoid*.

Flavoprotein Flavin-containing protein that constitutes the yellow enzyme; has as a prosthetic group either a phosphoric acid ester of riboflavin (flavin mononucleotide) or the latter combined with adenylic acid (flavin adenine dinucleotide).

Fletcherism System advocating thorough chewing of food (for as much as 30 times) to obtain greater satisfaction from food flavors, to induce more effective secretion of digestive juices, and hence to enhance digestion and utilization of food. It is also claimed that chewing for a long time satisfies the appetite with much less food, thus reducing the total amount of food ingested.

Flexical A low residue elemental diet preparation made from casein hydrolysates, sucrose and corn syrup, and soy and MCT oil, with added vitamins and minerals. (Mead Johnson.) See Proprietary foods: composition, features, and uses, Appendix P-1.

Fluorapatite Crystals in which the hydroxy group of hydroxyapatite has been replaced by fluorine. This may occur during tooth formation if fluorine is available.

Fluorescence Property certain substances have, after exposure to light, of emitting light of longer wavelength than the light that is absorbed.

Fluoridation Addition of small amounts of fluorine (about 1 to 2 ppm) in drinking water to reduce the incidence of dental caries in young children. Fuoridation of water is now adopted as routine procedure in many countries. A substitute method for the prevention of dental caries is the direct topical application of stannous fluoride on the teeth or the rinsing of the child's mouth twice a week with a solution containing 0.2% sodium fluoride. Studies have shown that the mouth-rinse method can reduce tooth decay by 50% during the first year and 80% in the second year. The addition of stannous fluoride in toothpaste is also an added step in the prevention of tooth decay. See also *Dental caries*.

Fluorine A trace mineral regularly present in human tissues, particularly in the teeth, bones, thyroid gland, and skin. Current interest in this trace mineral is centered on its role in the prevention of *dental caries*

and *osteoporosis*. At present there is no evidence that fluorine is indispensable in other tissues, although its role has not been established. Fluorine is present as a normal constituent in all diets, being widely but unevenly distributed among foods. For further details, see Summary of minerals, Appendix H.

Fluoroscopy X-ray examination of deep tissues in the body. The form and motion of internal structures can be seen.

Fluorosis Condition arising from excessive intake of fluorine, particularly excessive fluoridation of water (over 2.5 ppm). The incidence and severity of the condition increases as the levels approach 10 to 20 ppm. See also *Mottled enamel*.

FMN Abbreviation for *flavin mononucleotide*. See under *Flavin nucleotide*.

Folacin Generic name for folic acid and related compounds exhibiting qualitatively the biologic activity of folic acid.

Folic acid Pteroylglutamic acid (PGA), a water-soluble vitamin. The generic name "folic acid" was originally applied to a number of compounds having the same biologic property as PGA. This vitamin was first recognized as a factor necessary for normal growth and hemopoiesis of certain microorganisms and animals and has been given various names such as vitamin M, vitamin B_c, vitamin B_{10} and B_{11}, rhizopterin, citrovorum factor, *Lactobacillus casei* factor, norite eluate factor, and factors R, S, U, and SLR. When the substance was finally isolated from spinach, it was called folic acid because of its great abundance in dark green leaves (foliage). As a coenzyme, folic acid plays an important role in single-carbon metabolism. Deficiency occurs only in man, chickens, and monkeys, since most animals are able to synthesize the vitamin. However, induced folic acid deficiency in animals is possible by incorporation of sulfonamides in the diet or by administration of a folic acid antagonist. Folic acid is widely distributed in plant and animal tissues. For further details, see

Summary of vitamins, Appendix I-1. See also *Pteroylglutamic acid*.

Folinic acid N^5-formyltetrahydrofolic acid, a reduced form of folic acid with a formyl group on carbon 5 and regarded as the biologically active form of the vitamin. This is the name given to citrovorum factor, a substance in the liver required for the growth of *Leuconostoc citrovorum*.

Folinic acid-S.F. Also called leucovorin; a crystalline synthetic material resembling citrovorum factor or folinic acid in biologic action. It is prepared by reducing and formylating folic acid.

Follicle Excretory or secretory sac or gland such as the *graafian follicles* and hair follicles.

Follicle-stimulating hormone (FSH) Anterior pituitary hormone that stimulates the growth of the graafian follicles of the ovary in the female and of the sperm-forming tissue of the testes in the male.

Folliculosis Condition characterized by dry and rough skin, especially in the area of the shoulder and back of the arm. The follicles are raised above the surface, giving the superficial appearance of chronic gooseflesh. It is seen in vitamin A deficiency but should not be confused with follicular keratosis as no horny plugs project from the follicular orifices. See *Keratosis.*

Food Anything that, when taken into the body, serves to nourish, build and repair tissues, supply energy, or regulate body processes. Aside from its nutritional function, food is valued for its palatability and satiety effect as well as the varied meanings attached to it (emotional, social, religious, etc.) by different individuals, groups, or races.

Food account Method used in dietary studies and surveys involving groups or population at large. It consists of running reports of food purchased (or produced) for household use. It is useful in checking trends in purchasing certain foods or food groups. See also *Dietary study methodology* and Methods of research in nutrition: dietary survey, Appendix M-2.

Food additive Any substance, other than the basic foodstuff but not including chance contaminants, present in food as a result of any aspect of food production, processing, storage, or packaging. Generally classified as *intentional additives* (or those added to perform a specific function such as improvement in nutrient value, flavor, color, etc.) and *accidental additives* (or those which unavoidably become part of the product through some phase of production, processing, or packaging).

Food adulterant Any substance such as a toxic organism, filth, pesticide residue, or poisonous substance found in foods that is harmful to health or any substance added to increase the bulk or weight of a product.

Food allergen Food that produces allergic manifestations. The most common food allergens are wheat, milk, egg, shellfish, chocolate, nuts, and onion. Food allergy, however, may develop with any kind of food. Allergic symptoms may appear within a few minutes, a few hours, or 1 to 3 days after ingestion of the food allergen. Symptoms are varied, generally affecting the nasobronchial, ocular, nervous, vascular, gastrointestinal, and cutaneous tissues. See also *Allergen.*

Food analog Fabricated food that is made to look like a traditional food such as bacon or meat.

Food analysis Quantitative or qualitative determination of food components using different techniques. The general method of food analysis is by proximate determination of water, nitrogen (protein), ether extract (fat), ash, and carbohydrate (by difference). Specific mineral and vitamin components are determined by different methods. The *Official Methods of Analysis* published by the *Association of Official Agricultural Chemists* (AOAC) is a good reference for accepted methods. See also *Proximate analysis.*

Food and Agriculture Organization (FAO) International organization of the United Nations directly concerned with the production, distribution, and consumption of foods to improve nutrition and raise standards of living of the people of all countries. It provides technical assistance through five divisions: agriculture, economics, fisheries, forestry, and nutrition.

Food and Drug Administration (FDA) Agency of the Department of Health, Education, and Welfare that enforces legislation concerning food, drugs, and cosmetics.

Food and Nutrition Board Board of the National Academy of Sciences/National Research Council that was established in 1940 to serve as an advisory body. It publishes the recommended dietary allowances (RDA), which are revised approximately every 5 years.

Food balance sheet Measure of the food available per person. It is calculated by dividing the total food for the year by the number of people in the country.

Food-borne disease Disease caused by the ingestion of food that contains bacteria, parasites, naturally occurring toxicants, chemical poisons, or radioactive fallout.

Food Composition Table (FCT) Handbook Number 8, *Composition of foods—raw, processed and prepared,* published by the U. S. Department of Agriculture. It was originally issued in 1950 and revised in 1963. Food values are given in this table in terms of 100 gm edible portion (EP) and 1 pound as purchased (AP) of the foods. There are 2483 food items included. Information is given about the energy value and content of water, protein, fat, saturated fatty acids, unsaturated fatty acids (oleic acid and linoleic acid), carbohydrate, calcium, iron, vitamin A, thiamin, riboflavin, niacin, and ascorbic acid.

Food, Drug, and Cosmetic Act Law passed in 1938 to provide for safe, effective drugs and cosmetics, pure wholesome foods, and honest labeling and packaging. Recent amendments are concerned with pesticides, food additives, and color additives. The Food and Drug Administration enforces this act and its amendments.

Food, energy value Also called fuel value of food; oxidation of foodstuffs in the *bomb calorimeter* yields on the average 4.15, 9.40, and 5.65 calories/gm of pure carbohydrate, fat, and protein, respectively. However, the *physiologic fuel* values of foods when burned inside the body are somewhat lower because of incomplete digestion of the three nutrients and incomplete oxidation of protein. Experiments conducted by Atwater on the typical American mixed diets showed that the digestibility of carbohydrate was 98%; protein, 92%; and fat, 95% and that the urinary energy loss for incomplete oxidation of protein was 1.25 calories/gm protein. On the basis of these observations, the *Atwater values* for the available energy of the three foodstuffs were derived. Later experiments showed that each food has a specific coefficient of digestibility, making the fuel value specific for each type of food. The Nutrition Division of FAO therefore proposed the use of *specific fuel factors* for estimating the caloric value of foods. See *Atwater values* and *Specific fuel factor.*

Food exchange list See *Exchange list.*

Food extender A substance or diluent added to stretch or make food go farther as well as to reduce costs. It is important that extenders also contribute valuable nutrients and do not contain offending materials. Examples of meat extenders are legumes, nuts, and soybean cakes.

Food fad Idea associated with food that has become fashionable for a time to meet the needs of a current trend, usually at the sacrifice of important nutrients. According to Fleck (1971), a food fad may be identified as a "food or combination of foods that are declared to be beneficial or to serve as a cure-all." It may also be an exaggerated truth about a food. Food fads are usually short-lived and remain popular only until they are replaced by another fad. Diets for weight reduction are probably the most common fad.

Food fallacy False belief about food; misrepresentation, misinterpretation, or misinformation about a food fact. A *fact* implies a scientific basis, and facts about food are the result of research.

Food for Freedom Program Program administered by the Agency for International Development that uses agricultural surpluses to feed the world's hungry people.

Food group Classification of various foods into groups on the basis of similarity in nutrient content of the members of each group. It is a practical guide in planning diets that will satisfy nutrient allowances by merely defining the number of servings to eat from each of the groups. See the Four basic food groups and Food grouping systems in different countries, Appendices B-1 and B-2.

Food habit Manner or pattern by which an individual or group selects, prepares, and consumes food as a result of cultural, social, and religious influences.

Food infection Result of the ingestion of food that has been contaminated with bacteria such as *Salmonella, Shigella,* and *Clostridium perfringens.*

Food intoxication Poisoning due to the ingestion of toxins in food, such as those produced by the botulinus and staphylococcus organisms. Usually results from improper refrigeration or inadequate processing. Symptoms include vomiting, abdominal cramps, diarrhea, and weakness.

Food inventory Method of recording food intake of a group or family. It consists of a weighed inventory of foods at the beginning and close of the study together with day-to-day records, with or without records of kitchen and plate wastes. Nutrients are calculated from food tables or by laboratory analysis of the foods. See also *Dietary study methodology.*

Food list Method used in dietary studies applicable to groups. The subject reports an estimated quantity (by weight, retail unit, or household measure) of various foods consumed in previous days, usually the past 7 days. A list of foods may be used to aid in the recall. See also *Dietary study methodology* and Methods of research in nutrition: dietary survey, Appendix M-2.

Food patterns Types of foods consumed by people in a country, culture, or locale.

Food poisoning See *Food infection* and *Food intoxication.*

Food record Method used in dietary studies. It consists of taking records of food (including in-between meals) for varying lengths of time, usually 3 to 7 days. Accuracy of the method depends on the ability of the subjects to estimate quantities of foods and the correct application of food tables. See also *Dietary study methodology* and Methods of research in nutrition: dietary survey, Appendix M-2.

Food Stamp Program Means of providing additional food for persons on a limited income. Eligible individuals or families whose income is below a certain level may purchase food stamps at a discount price. The eligibility of persons for the program is determined according to state and local welfare standards.

Foodstuff Any material made into or used as *food.*

Foot drop Condition in which the foot hangs or falls down due to paralysis of the lower limbs, as seen in polyneuropathy of beriberi.

Force-feeding Food that is brought to the stomach by other than normal means, e.g., by a nasogastric tube.

Formaldehyde (HCHO) Methanal; substance used as a disinfectant.

Formil Commercial milk product for routine infant feeding; made of cow's milk with partial butterfat replacement (corn and coconut oil), lactose, and vitamin supplements. Also available with added iron. (Pet.) See Proprietary foods: composition, features, and uses, Appendix P-1.

Formiminoglutamic acid (FIGLU) A metabolite of histidine seen in the urine of folic acid–deficient individuals. It is also seen in children with acute leukemia receiving folic acid antagonist therapy, e.g., *aminopterin.*

Formula 2 Ready-to-use blended food product for tube feeding; contains nonfat milk, beef, egg yolk, corn oil, and strained vegetables, fruit, and cereal with added vitamins and minerals. (Cutter Laboratories.) See Proprietary foods: composition, features, and uses, Appendix P-1.

Formulated foods Imitation foods such as imitation dairy products, fruit juices, and meats or new types of food.

Fortifex Protein food mixture developed in Brazil; contains maize, defatted soybean flour, DL-methionine, calcium carbonate, vitamin A, thiamin, and riboflavin.

Fortification Addition of one or more nutrients such as vitamins, minerals, amino acids, or protein concentrates to food so that it contains more of the nutrients than were originally present. For example, the addition of vitamin A to margarine, vitamin D to milk, lysine to bread, and iodine to salt.

FPC Abbreviation for *fish protein concentrate.*

Freedom From Hunger Campaign (FFHC) Program of the FAO to bring to the attention of the world the problems of world hunger and the means of alleviating them. The aim is to assist hungry people in helping themselves. This involves training programs to promote increased food production and better use of food.

Free fatty acid (FFA) Unesterified fatty acid. See under *Fatty acid.*

Friedman test *Pregnancy* test using the rabbit as a test animal. The test urine is injected into an ear vein, and the ovaries are examined 24 hours later for ruptured or hemorrhagic follicles.

Fröhlich's syndrome Disturbance in fat deposition usually occurring in children before puberty; characterized by the presence of superficial fat in the body and the external genitalia. It may be the result of an inherent defect in the pituitary gland or atrophy of the secretory cells by tumor injury or some infectious disease.

Fructofuranose The furanose form of fructose. In sucrose, fructose is found in the furanose form.

Fructokinase Enzyme that catalyzes the phosphorylation of fructose to fructose-1-phosphate.

Fructopyranose *Fructose.* See *Pyran.*

Fructosan Also called *levan;* a polysaccharide yielding fructose on hydrolysis. Inulin is a fructosan.

Fructose Levulose or fruit sugar. A 6-carbon monosaccharide found in fruits and honey and obtained from hydrolysis of sucrose to glucose and fructose. It is an essential intermediate in carbohydrate metabolism.

Fructose intolerance Inborn error of metabolism characterized by the inability to utilize fructose because of a lack of the specific enzyme fructose-1-phosphoaldolase. Clinical symptoms include fructosuria, nausea and vomiting, hypoglycemia, and convulsions and coma, leading to death. Strict avoidance of foods containing fructose or sucrose is necessary.

Fructosuria Presence of fructose in the urine.

Fruitarian Person whose diet consists chiefly of fruits. See also *Vegan.*

FSH Abbreviation for *follicle-stimulating hormone.*

Fuel factors Energy values per gram of carbohydrate, protein, and fat. See *Food, energy value; Atwater values;* and *Specific fuel factor.*

Fumarase Enzyme that catalyzes the conversion of fumaric acid to malic acid.

Fumaric acid Transethylene dicarboxylic acid, an intermediate product in carbohydrate metabolism.

Fundus Base or part of an organ farthest from the mouth or opening, as the fundus of the stomach.

Furan Organic cyclic compound with one oxygen and four carbon atoms.

Furanose Cyclic structural formula of a sugar in which the oxygen ring bridges carbon atoms 1 and 4 in aldoses or carbon atoms 2 and 4 in ketoses.

Furuncle Nodule or boil due to an infection of a hair follicle.

G

Galactan Also called galactosan; a polysaccharide that yields galactose on hydrolysis.

Galactoflavin An analog of riboflavin that is a potent inhibitor; D-galactose replaces D-ribose in the molecule.

Galactogogue A substance that promotes the flow of milk. Foods such as candy, beer, and garlic have been said to stimulate lactation.

Galactokinase Specific enzyme that catalyzes the phosphorylation of galactose to galactose-1-phosphate.

Galactolipid Compound lipid that yields D-galactose, 4-sphingenine, and a fatty acid on hydrolysis. It is found in large amounts in the myelin sheaths of nerves.

Galactosamine An amino sugar; galactose containing an amino group in carbon atom 2. It is found in the polysaccharide of cartilage, chondroitin (as chondrosamine), and in the structural material of the skeletons of arthropods.

Galactosan *Galactan.*

Galactose A 6-carbon sugar differing from glucose only in the position of the hydroxyl group on carbon atom 4. It is seldom found free in nature; occurs mainly linked with glucose to form lactose (milk sugar) ; also a constituent of cerebrosides and certain polysaccharides such as agar and flaxseed.

Galactosemia Presence of galactose in the blood. It is an inborn error of metabolism characterized by the inability to convert galactose to glucose because of the absence of the enzyme *galactose-1-phosphate uridyl transferase*. Symptoms are varied and include jaundice, enlarged liver and spleen, anorexia, loss of weight, vomiting, diarrhea, cataract formation, and mental retardation. Treatment is dietary in nature and consists of the elimination of galactose-containing foods from the diet. See Dietary management of selected disorders, Appendix O.

Galactoside A glycoside containing galactose.

Galactosuria Presence of galactose in the urine.

Galactowaldenase Enzyme that catalyzes the interconversion of galactose and glucose.

Galacturonic acid A sugar acid resulting from the oxidation of the primary alcohol group of galactose to a carboxyl (—COOH) group. It occurs in various vegetable sources such as pectins and certain plant gums.

Gallbladder Pear-shaped organ with a thin, flaccid wall and a capacity of 30 to 50 ml. It is attached to the right lobe of the liver for the storage and concentration of bile. See *Bile.*

Gallstones Stones in the gallbladder or biliary ducts. See *Cholelithiasis.*

Gamma ray Electromagnetic radiation similar to an x-ray but more energetic and penetrating. It has no electric charge and no detectable mass. May be produced in atomic reactors from heavy atoms such as uranium.

Ganglion Pl. ganglia. Collection of nerve cells usually located outside the brain and spinal cord; serves as a relay station for impulses transmitted to or from the nerves.

Ganglioside Glycolipid occurring in the nervous tissue that contains a substance called neuraminic acid in addition to fatty acids, 4-sphingenine, and hexoses (glucose or galactose).

Gangrene Decay or death of a part of the body due to failure of the blood supply as a result of disease or injury. Causes other than injury include diabetes, hardening of the arteries, blood clots, and other similar conditions.

Gargoylism Also called Hurler's syndrome; an inborn error of metabolism characterized by excessive excretion of chondroitin sulfate B, dwarfism, stiff joints, cloudy cornea, enlarged liver and spleen, and mental deficiency.

Gastralgia Paroxysmal epigastric pain in the absence of gastric lesions; probably caused by incorrect eating habits and anemia.

Gastrectasis Dilatation of the stomach.

Gastrectomy Surgical removal of all or part of the stomach.

Gastric Pertaining to the stomach or gastric glands.

G acidity Amount of hydrochloric acid in the stomach, which may be present in two forms—as *free acid* or as *combined acid* (in combination with protein of the food, regurgitated duodenal secretion, saliva, and mucus). The sum of the free and combined acid is termed *total acidity.*

G analysis Measurement of the amount of acid produced in the gastric secretion either as free acid or total acidity. It consists of withdrawing a sample of the gastric contents followed by ingestion of a simple test meal (e.g., Ewald or Boas test meal), dilute alcohol, meat extractives, or subcutaneous injection of histamine to stimulate gastric secretion. The specimens are titrated as to the content of free and total acid.

G enzymes Pepsin, rennin, and gastric lipase. See Summary of digestive enzymes, Appendix J-1.

G gavage Introduction of food in a liquid form directly into the stomach through a tube by way of the mouth, nose, or an artificial opening in the gastrointestinal tract.

G glands Collection of cells (*parietal, chief, argentaffin,* and *mucous*) arranged around a central canal in the stomach wall.

G juice Thin colorless secretion of the gastric gland containing mucus, hydrochloric acid, enzymes, and an intrinsic factor.

G lavage Washing out the stomach.

G resection Surgical removal of a segment or part of the stomach.

Gastrin Hormone elaborated by the pyloric mucosa that stimulates hydrochloric acid secretion by the parietal cells.

Gastritis Acute or chronic inflammation of the mucous lining of the stomach. Due to a variety of causes, including allergy, ingestion of poison or irritants, and dietary indiscretion, i.e., rapid eating, overeating, or large intakes of fibrous or highly seasoned foods. Gastritis may also accompany cancer.

Gastroenteritis Inflammation of the stomach and intestine, usually due to viral infection; characterized by diarrhea, vomiting, and abdominal pain with or without fever.

Gastroenterology Study of the stomach and the intestines and their diseases. A specialist in this field is called a *gastroenterologist.*

Gastroenterostomy Surgical formation of a communication between the stomach and the small intestine, usually performed to short-circuit the food around a stomach ulcer.

Gastrointestinal tract (GIT) Refers to the whole of the digestive tract from the mouth through the stomach, intestines, and anus.

Gastrostomy Establishment of an opening in the stomach from the outside, usually for artificial feeding.

Gaucher's disease Disturbance in lipid metabolism characterized by the accumulation of *kerasin* in the liver, spleen, bone marrow, and lymph nodes.

Gavage Feeding by insertion of a stomach tube through the mouth into the stomach.

Geiger-Müller counter Instrument used in

the detection and counting of ionizing radiations.

Gel A colloidal system that does not pour but is like a solid. *Gelation* is the formation of a gel or the solidification of a sol.

Gelatin Product obtained from the partial hydrolysis of collagen derived from cartilage, bones, tendons, and skin. Although a protein of animal origin, it is of poor biologic value and considered an *incomplete protein*. It lacks tryptophan and is low in cystine and tyrosine. See also *Protein quality*.

Gelatinase Enzyme found in various molds, yeasts, and bacteria that is capable of liquefying gelatin.

Gene Unit in the *chromosome* that carries the hereditary characteristics. Its function involves a transfer of DNA "template" or specificity to RNA, which in turn is responsible for protein synthesis characteristic of the species.

Genetics Study of heredity.

Genital Pertaining or relating to the genitalia or organs of reproduction. The male has two testes with their ducts, the prostate gland, the penis, and the urethra. The female has the vaginal lips and canal, the ovaries, the fallopian tubes, and the uterus.

Genitourinary Relating to the genitalia and the organs of urine formation and excretion (kidneys, ureters, bladder, and urethra).

Gentiobiose A glucosyl-glucose disaccharide with a 1,6-beta-glucosidic bond.

Geophagia The practice of eating earth. It usually occurs in poverty-stricken populations, although the habit is not limited to the poor. The cause is unknown.

Gerhardt's test Test that detects the presence of diacetic acid in urine as a result of incomplete utilization of fat. In the presence of diacetic acid, urine forms a wine red color with ferric chloride that fades on heating.

Geriatrics Field of medicine devoted to the treatment of the problems and diseases of old age. See *Nutrition, geriatrics*.

Germfree animals Also called gnotobiotes; animals born and raised under sterile environmental conditions. Nutrient requirements are different due to the lack of microorganisms in the intestinal tract that normally provide some nutrients for the host.

Gerontology Study of the aging process.

Gestation Pregnancy; period of fetal development.

Gevral High protein, low fat nutritional supplement with added vitamins and minerals. It is relatively low in sodium and is useful in high protein, sodium restricted diets. (Lederle.) See Proprietary foods: composition, features, and uses, Appendix P-1.

GFR Abbreviation for *glomerular filtration rate*.

Giantism (gigantism) Unusual height and size due to oversecretion of the growth hormone as a result of a pituitary disorder before or during puberty, prior to the closure of the epiphysis.

Gibberellin Plant growth hormone isolated from certain species of fungi; stimulates rapid growth and elongation of rice seedlings and other plant stems.

Gibbs-Donnan equilibrium Solute concentrations of two solutions separated by a membrane, which is freely permeable to both solvent and solute, will be the same when equilibrium is established. Thus both the osmotic pressure and chemical composition of the two solutions will be equal.

Gilbert's disease Rare congenital abnormality of the liver resulting in intense jaundice because of a lack of the enzyme *uridine diphosphate glucuronate transferase*.

Gingivitis Inflammation of the gums (gingiva). Gingivitis seen in association with vitamin C deficiency is characterized by spongy, swollen gums that bleed readily. This may result in a high susceptibility to infection; teeth may even become loose if the condition is not corrected.

GIT Abbreviation for *gastrointestinal tract*.

Gland Cell, tissue, or organ that produces a product used by the body (secretion) or eliminated from the body (excretion). Examples of glands that *secrete* are adrenal and thyroid glands; glands that *excrete* are sweat and oil glands.

Glare blindness See *Hemeralopia.*

Glaucoma Eye disease characterized by increased intraocular pressure resulting in unusual hardness of the eyeball, restricted field of vision, depression of the optic disk, colored halo around artificial lights, and decrease in sight that may eventually lead to blindness. The condition is primarily due to lack of drainage of the fluid from within the eyeball.

Gliadin Glutamine-bound fraction of protein in wheat, oat, rye, and barley; a simple protein of the prolamine type. It lacks lysine and is classified as a partially incomplete protein. See also *Gluten.*

Globin A colorless basic protein often found in combination with other proteins; soluble in water, acid, or alkali and coagulable by heat. See Classification of proteins, Appendix C-2.

Globulins Group of plant and animal proteins sparingly soluble in water but soluble in salt solution; an important component of human blood. Fractionation of plasma globulins by electrophoresis gives alpha, beta, and gamma globulins. See Classification of proteins, Appendix C-2.

Glomerular filtration rate (GFR) Number of milliliters of blood that is passed through the glomerulus in 1 minute. The normal GFR is approximately 130 ml/minute. A polysaccharide such as *inulin* can be used to measure the GFR since it is filtered but not reabsorbed by the kidney tubules. The amount of inulin in the urine corresponds to the amount that has been filtered from the plasma. This test can be used to estimate the degree of function of the kidney.

Glomerulonephritis Inflammatory disease of the kidneys affecting chiefly the glomeruli. It may be acute or chronic and generally follows streptococcal infection of the respiratory tract such as tonsillitis, sinusitis, pneumonia, and influenza. Symptoms include nitrogen retention, presence of albumin and blood in the urine, and varying degrees of hypertension, edema, and uremia preceding convulsions and death. See also *Nephritis* and Dietary management of selected disorders, Appendix O.

Glomerulus Pl. glomeruli. A coil or cluster of blood vessels projecting into the expanded end of each secreting tubule of the kidney.

Glossitis Inflammation of the tongue (glossa); usually due to biting, burning, or injuring the tongue. It may also be a symptom of a gastrointestinal disorder or deficiency in one or more of the B complex vitamins. See also *Tongue.*

Glucagon A hyperglycemic-glycogenolytic factor of the pancreas; protein in nature and regarded by some as a hormone; also found in gastric and duodenal mucosa as well as in some commercial insulin preparations. It increases the blood sugar level by stimulating the breakdown of glycogen in the liver.

Glucoascorbic acid An analog of ascorbic acid containing an extra CHOH group. It acts as an antivitamin C and can cause scurvy even in animals that do not normally require the vitamin in their diet.

Glucocorticoids Steroid hormones of the adrenal cortex that affect carbohydrate metabolism. Examples are *cortisone* and *corticosterone.*

Glucofuranose Cyclic form of glucose in which carbon atoms 1 and 4 are bridged by an oxygen atom, forming a furanose structure.

Glucogenesis Formation of glucose; may arise from any of the intermediates in glycolysis or from glucogenic substances such as glycerol and some of the amino acids that can be converted into one of the intermediates in carbohydrate metabolism.

Glucokinase Specific enzyme that catalyzes the phosphorylation of glucose to glucose-1-phosphate.

Glucola Trade name of a drink that may be used in place of a 100 gm carbohydrate meal for a glucose tolerance test. A 7-ounce bottle contains the equivalent of 75 gm of glucose. It consists of a partial hydrolysate of cornstarch dissolved in a cola-flavored solution that is also carbonated.

Glucolysis Metabolic breakdown of glucose. See *Glycolysis*.

Gluconeogenesis Formation of glucose or glycogen from noncarbohydrate sources such as glycerol and glucogenic amino acids.

Gluconic acid Acid derived from glucose by oxidizing the aldehyde group on carbon atom 1 to the carboxyl level.

Glucopyranose Cyclic form of glucose in which carbon atoms 1 and 5 are bridged by an oxygen atom, forming a pyranose structure.

Glucosamine Amino sugar in which carbon atom 2 of glucose contains an amino group. Results from the hydrolysis of chitin and occurs in various mammalian polysaccharides, including heparin, hyaluronic acid, and several bacterial polysaccharides.

Glucose Also called dextrose, grape sugar, or blood sugar; a 6-carbon monosaccharide occurring naturally in plant tissues and obtained from the complete hydrolysis of starch. It is the chief form in which carbohydrate is absorbed into the bloodstream. Physiologically glucose is considered the most important sugar. It is the major source of energy for the brain and nervous tissues and the form in which carbohydrate is circulated in the blood. See also *Blood sugar level*.

Glucose/nitrogen ratio (G/N ratio) Formerly called D/N ratio. The ratio between the amount of glucose and the amount of nitrogen excreted in the urine of an animal rendered diabetic by phlorizin. It is an indication of the proportion of sugar that can be derived from protein. The ratio varies with the severity of the diabetes, reaching a maximum value of about 3.65.

Glucose tolerance factor (GTF) The biologically active form of chromium, which is bound to an organic compound that has

not yet been identified. It is believed that this factor binds insulin and thus increases the uptake of glucose by the cell.

Glucose tolerance test (GTT) Test that measures the ability of the body to utilize a known amount of glucose. It is performed after a 12-hour fast. The subject is given orally from 50 to 100 gm of glucose or an allowance of 1.75 gm/kg body weight. Blood samples for glucose analysis are obtained before the glucose is taken and then $\frac{1}{2}$, 1, 2, 3, and 4 hours after ingestion. A normal individual shows a rise in blood sugar about $\frac{1}{2}$ hour after ingestion of glucose, but the blood sugar level returns to normal after 2 hours. A diabetic person shows a much higher rise in blood sugar after $\frac{1}{2}$ hour that continues to rise even higher after 2 hours and remains higher than normal after 4 hours. The plotted results of blood sugar values form the *glucose tolerance curve*.

Glucoside A glycoside of glucose. An enzyme that splits a glucoside is called a *glucosidase*.

Glucostatic mechanism Theory that serves to explain the mechanism of hunger. According to this theory, the "feeding" and "satiety" centers in the *hypothalamus* are influenced by the difference between the level of glucose in the arterial and venous blood (called Δ-glucose). Following a meal, the Δ-glucose reaching the brain is high, causing inhibition of hunger. When the difference between arterial and venous glucose is small, the feeding center is stimulated, causing hunger sensations.

Glucosuria Former term for *glycosuria;* the presence of glucose in the urine.

Glucuronic acid A sugar acid resulting from the oxidation of the primary hydroxyl group of glucose to COOH. It is present in various complex polysaccharides, and many toxic substances in the body are excreted in combination with glucuronic acid as *glucuronides*.

Glutamic acid Alpha-aminoglutaric acid, a nonessential amino acid that is a constituent of *folic acid*. It is involved in transamination and deamination reactions and in the synthesis of glutathione and glutamine. The monosodium salt of glutamic acid (MSG) is widely used as a flavoring agent.

Glutamine Compound formed from glutamic acid and ammonia in the liver, brain, and kidneys. It plays an important role in transamination reactions and serves as source of ammonia in the kidneys for base conservation. Glutamine can cross the blood-brain barrier, thus providing a source of glutamic acid for brain oxidation. The splitting of glutamine to glutamic acid and ammonia is catalyzed by the enzyme *glutaminase*.

Glutathione A tripeptide composed of glutamic acid, cysteine, and glycine; widely distributed in nature and isolated from yeast, muscle, and liver. It is the prosthetic group of glyceraldehyde phosphate dehydrogenase and is believed to help maintain the sulfhydryl-containing enzymes in the reduced state that is essential for their activity.

Glutelin A simple protein found in cereals; insoluble in water and neutral solutions but soluble in dilute acids and alkalies. Examples are *glutenin* in wheat, *oryzenin* in rice, and *hordein* in barley. See Classification of proteins, Appendix C-2.

Gluten Protein fraction of wheat and other cereals that gives flour the elastic property that is essential for breadmaking. It is composed of two fractions: *glutenin* and *gliadin*. It is believed that the gliadin portion is responsible for the malabsorption syndrome in susceptible individuals with gluten-induced enteropathy. The condition is corrected by eliminating wheat, oats, rye, and barley from the diet.

Glutenin The *glutelin* of wheat. See also *Gluten*.

Glyceraldehyde Glyceric aldehyde, the simplest form of carbohydrate—containing only three carbon atoms. In the form of phosphate ester it acts as an intermediate product in the anaerobic breakdown of carbohydrate; also serves as precursor of glycerol.

Glycerol Also called glycerin; trihydroxypropane, a trihydroxy alcohol. It is a clear, colorless, sweetish, and viscous liquid obtained from the hydrolysis of fats and oils. Esters of glycerol with fatty acids are called *glycerides*. Glycerol possesses three hydroxy groups; it can combine with three molecules of fatty acid to form a *triglyceride* or simple fat.

Glycerose A triose; a 3-carbon sugar derived from the corresponding alcohol, glycerol.

Glycine Also called glycocoll; aminoacetic acid, the simplest amino acid. It is an essential constituent of body tissues, a precursor of bile acid, and a participant in the detoxication mechanism and synthesis of purine, creatine, glutathione, and porphyrins. Not considered a dietary essential except for growing chickens.

Glycinin The chief protein of soybeans.

Glycinuria Condition characterized by excessive excretion of glycine in the urine and elevated blood levels accompanied by metabolic acidosis, respiratory distress, seizures, hematologic abnormalities, and mental retardation, leading to death. It is considered an inborn error of metabolism, although the specific enzyme defect has not been identified; probably due to failure of conversion of glycine to glyoxalate. Symptoms have been controlled by a low protein diet with arginine and pyridoxine supplementation.

Glycocholic acid One of the *bile acids* yielding glycine and cholic acid on hydrolysis.

Glycocoll Obsolete name for *glycine*.

Glycogen Animal starch; a branched-chain polysaccharide composed of glucose units. It is the chief carbohydrate storage material in animals, especially in the liver and muscles. In a well-nourished adult, glycogen is about 2% to 8% of the weight of the liver. Although muscle contains less glycogen (approximately 1%) than the liver, the greater mass of the muscle accounts for a considerable quantity of this storage form of carbohydrate. The amount of reserve glycogen stored in the liver and muscle depends largely on the nature of the diet and the amount of exercise. Fasting results in a rapid depletion of liver glycogen, and muscle glycogen is depleted during continuous or violent exercise.

Glycogenesis Formation or synthesis of glycogen. Glycogenic substances are hexoses as well as a wide variety of other compounds, e.g., glycogenic amino acids, glycerol derived from lipids, intermediates in glycolysis such as lactic acid and pyruvic acid, and products structurally related to hexoses.

Glycogenolysis Breakdown or splitting up of glycogen as opposed to glycogenesis. The interconversion of glycogen to glucose occurs in several steps involving phosphorylation, rearrangement, dephosphorylation, and condensation or hydrolysis, with each step requiring a specific enzyme.

Glycogenosis Type II glycogen storage disease characterized by extreme deposition of glycogen in the heart. The heart enlarges to as much as five times its normal weight. Infants affected by this condition usually die of heart failure before the age of 2 years. They resemble cretins or mongoloids, have poor appetites, and fail to grow. The specific enzyme deficiency has not been clearly identified.

Glycogen storage disease Group term used to describe a number of hereditary abnormalities in metabolism that result in the deposition of either too much or too little glycogen in the tissues. The condition is due to a deficiency in one or more of the following enzymes involved in the interconversion of glycogen and glucose: *glycogen synthetase, glucose-6-phosphatase, branching enzyme, debranching enzyme, myophosphorylase,* and *hepatophosphorylase.* See Inborn errors of metabolism, Appendix G.

Glycolipid Lipid that yields a carbohydrate, a fatty acid, and an alcohol on hydrolysis.

Glycolysis Also called Embden-Meyerhof pathway; a series of reactions involving the anaerobic breakdown of glycogen (or glucose) in the tissues, with lactic or pyruvic acid as the end product. The net result is the synthesis of two molecules of adenosine triphosphate (ATP) per mole of glucose catabolized; oxygen is not consumed in the overall process. In the presence of oxygen, pyruvic acid is completely oxidized to carbon dioxide and water in the mitochondria by way of the Krebs tricarboxylic acid cycle and its associated oxidative phosphorylation. Although the yield of ATP from glycolysis is small compared to the net yield of 38 moles of ATP/mole of glucose by complete oxidation, glycolysis provides a means of rapidly obtaining ATP (hence energy) in a relatively anaerobic organ such as muscle. See also Embden-Meyerhof pathway, Appendix F-1.

Glyconeogenesis Former term for *gluconeogenesis.*

Glycoprotein Conjugated product composed of a polysaccharide bound to protein such as ovomucin in egg white.

Glycosidase Group name for hydrolytic enzymes that attack glycosidic linkages of carbohydrates. The enzymes are specific for their particular substances.

Glycoside Carbohydrate or sugar molecule joined in acetal linkage to a nonsugar moiety known as the *aglycon.* The glycoside is named after the parent sugar, as glucoside, galactoside, etc.

Glycosuria Presence of sugar in the urine. It may be due to *diabetes mellitus,* lowered renal threshold for glucose without any accompanying blood glucose elevation, brain tumor or injury, or temporarily due to emotional tension or worry.

Glymidine Sulfonylpyrimidine derivative that has a hypoglycemic action; used for the oral treatment of diabetes mellitus.

Gnotobiotes See *Germfree animals.*

G/N ratio Abbreviation for *glucose/nitrogen ratio.*

Goiter Enlargement of the thyroid gland

due to lack of iodine (simple goiter), over-production of the thyroid hormone in hyperthyroid states (exophthalmic goiter or thyrotoxicosis), or decreased production of the thyroid hormone in hypothyroid states (cretinism and myxedema).

Exophthalmic g Also called thyrotoxicosis, Grave's disease, or Basedow's disease; results from hyperthyroidism and is characterized by a high basal metabolic rate leading to loss of weight, excessive nervousness, protruding eyeballs (exophthalmos), and enlarged thyroid gland. See also *Hyperthyroidism*.

Simple g Enlargement of the thyroid gland producing no symptoms either of hypothyroidism or hyperthyroidism. It may be due to a deficiency in iodine, a constituent of the thyroid hormone *thyroxine*, or to antithyroid agents such as *goitrogens* in food, thiourea, thiouracil, or some of the sulfonamides that interfere with the synthesis of thyroxine by the thyroid gland.

Goitrogens Substances present in some foods that are capable of producing goiter by interfering with the production of the thyroid hormone. These have been identified as *arachidoside,* present in the red skin of peanuts, and *thiooxazolidone,* present in plants of the *Brassica* genus, e.g., cabbage, cauliflower, and turnip. Goitrogens are destroyed by heat.

Golgi apparatus An organelle of the cell consisting of a complex tubular system that seems to connect directly to the endoplasmic reticulum. The functions of these organelles are not completely understood. The Golgi bodies may function as storage vesicles for compounds synthesized in the cell.

Gonadotropic hormones Also called gonadotropins; hormones secreted by the anterior pituitary that influence the gonads. These are follicle-stimulating hormone (FSH), luteinizing hormone (LH), and lactogenic hormone (prolactin). In the female they are responsible for the growth, maturation, and expulsion of the ova. In the male they stimulate spermatogenesis and production of androgen.

Gonads Ovary in the female and testes in the male.

Gooseflesh Also called goose pimples; term given to rough skin characterized by erection of the hair follicles, as from cold or shock. Also seen in vitamin A deficiency. See *Keratosis*.

Gossypol Bright yellow pigment of undetermined composition found in cottonseed oil; must be removed before the seedcake can be used as foodstuff; has produced toxic symptoms in cattle fed the oil cake.

Gout Hereditary disease occurring mostly in males characterized by a disturbance in purine metabolism and a high uric acid level in the blood. In its acute form there are sudden attacks of severe pain in a joint, generally of the big toe, frequently following an exceptionally large meal or some other stress. The joints affected swell and become red and tender. In its chronic form the condition is characterized by deposition of sodium urate in the joints, cartilages, and soft tissues with visible deposits (tophi) on the helix of the ears and joints of the fingers and toes. Repeated gouty attacks may result in deformity. See *Diet, purine-restricted*.

Graafian follicles Follicles in the ovary.

Granulocyte Leukocyte or white blood cell with irregular nuclei and granules either as eosinophil, basophil, or neutrophil.

Granum Pl. grana. A *chloroplast* that contains hundreds of molecules of mixed phosphatide per molecule of chlorophyll.

Grape sugar Glucose or dextrose. See *Glucose*.

GRAS list Food additives classified by the FDA as *g*enerally *r*ecognized *a*s *s*afe. Included in the list are additives considered harmless as commonly used in foods such as salt, spices, flavorings, and emulsifiers.

Grave's disease Another name for exophthalmic goiter. See *Exophthalmic goiter* under *Goiter*.

Gross energy value See *Heat of combustion*.

Ground substance A gelatinous substance composed of mucopolysaccharides that provides the framework for collagen. This makes up the matrix of the bone. See *Bone.*

Growth hormone See *Somatotropin.*

GTF Abbreviation for *glucose tolerance factor.*

GTT Abbreviation for *glucose tolerance test.*

Guanine One of the major purines of nucleic acids. It is hydrolyzed to xanthine and ammonia by *guanase,* a highly specific deaminase found in animal tissues such as liver, spleen, and kidneys.

Guanosine The guanine nucleoside; guanine linked to ribose.

Gulonic acid A sugar acid resulting from the reduction of glucuronic acid or oxidation of the primary hydroxyl group of gulose to COOH.

Gulose An aldohexose; an isomer of glucose.

Gynolactose One of the sugars found in milk. It contains nitrogen and may very well be one of the components of the *bifidus factor.*

H

Haldane apparatus Open-circuit type of respiration apparatus that applies the principle of *indirect calorimetry*. A small animal placed in the chamber is weighed before and after the experiment. The difference in weight represents carbon dioxide and water eliminated and oxygen consumed. The first two are directly measured by weighing the flasks containing soda lime and sulfuric acid that absorbed them. Oxygen consumed is indirectly determined by subtracting the sum of carbon dioxide and water losses from the total weight loss of the animal.

Half and half Mixture of equal volumes of table cream and whole milk; has 12% butterfat.

Half-life Time during which the radioactivity originally associated with an isotope will be reduced by one half through radioactive decay. This period is a constant for a given radioactive isotope. Some examples are carbon 14, 5700 years; tritium, 12.26 years; strontium 90, 28 years; phosphorus 32, 14.3 days; potassium 42, 12.5 hours; and iodine 125, 60 days.

Halibut liver oil Expressed oil from fresh halibut liver standardized to contain approximately 100 times the amount of vitamin A and 10 to 30 times the amount of vitamin D.

Hallucinations Sensory perceptions that are not realistic, such as seeing objects that are not actually present, hearing unreal sounds, or sensing a certain taste, smell, or touch that is nonexistent. Hallucinations may occur in extreme hunger, hysteria, and a variety of neurotic disorders.

Hand-Schüller-Christian disease Form of *xanthoma*. Yellow nodules are formed in the cranium and other bones. They contain large amounts of cholesterol and cholesterol esters.

HANES Abbreviation for *Health and Nutrition Examination Survey*.

Haptoglobin (Hp) Serum mucoprotein that binds hemoglobin. The major role appears to be the conservation of body iron by binding hemoglobin and preventing its loss from the body. Increased levels of Hp are found in individuals with inflammatory or neoplastic disease. Plasma levels are decreased in acute hepatitis and hemolytic conditions.

Harelip Congenital cleft or defect in the upper lip, usually due to failure of the median nasal and maxillary processes to unite.

Harris-Benedict formula Formula for predicting basal metabolism based on body weight and standing height. It is written as follows:

BMR (men) =
$$66.473 + 13.752\ W + 5.003\ H - 6.755\ A$$

BMR (women) =
$$66.096 + 9.563\ W + 4.676\ H - 4.676\ A$$

where W is weight in kilograms, H is standing height in centimeters, and A is age in years.

Hartnup disease Also called H disease; a hereditary abnormality in the metabolism

110

of tryptophan characterized by gross aminoaciduria, pellagra-like skin rash, intermittent cerebellar ataxia, and mental deterioration. It is ascribed mainly to niacin deficiency, either because of the malabsorption of tryptophan in the intestines or due to a metabolic defect in the transformation of tryptophan to niacin.

Hay fever Acute conjunctivitis with nasal catarrh due to sensitivity to pollens and other allergens.

Hb Abbreviation for *hemoglobin.*

Head Start See *Project Head Start.*

Health State of physical, mental, and emotional well-being and not merely the freedom from disease or the absence of any ailment.

Health and Nutrition Examination Survey (HANES) The National Center for Health Statistics is conducting nutritional status surveys of the United States' population on a 2-year cycle. The sample consists of persons from age 1 through 74 years who are not institutionalized. There is an oversampling of groups that are prone to nutritional difficulties such as poor children of preschool age, women of child-bearing age, and the aged. The survey includes household interviews, questionnaires, physical measurements, physical examinations, tests and procedures, and biochemical determinations on blood and urine samples. These examinations are being done in mobile examination centers.

Health Maintenance Organization (HMO) In the publication *Health maintenance organizations. The concept and structure* (1971), the U. S. Department of Health, Education, and Welfare describes the basic structure of HMO as "an organized system of health care which accepts the responsibility to provide or otherwise assure the delivery of an agreed upon set of comprehensive health maintenance and treatment services for a voluntarily enrolled group of persons in a geographic area and is reimbursed through a pre-negotiated and fixed periodic payment made by or on behalf of each person or family unit enrolled in the plan." The HMO provides comprehensive care with major emphasis on prevention, care continuity, and maximum health service at a reasonable cost. The American Dietetic Association has proposed that nutritional care be a basic service of HMO.

Heart A hollow muscular contractile organ; the center of the circulatory system. It is divided into four cavities: a left and a right atrium (or auricle) and a left and a right ventricle. The heart lies in a loose-fitting sac called the *pericardium* and is covered by a serous membrane called the *epicardium.* The muscular walls of the heart are known as the *myocardium,* and the layer of squamous epithelium lining the chambers of the heart is called the *endocardium.* The main function of the heart is to pump blood throughout the body. If this stops for even a short time, irreversible changes occur and death quickly ensues.

Heartburn Epigastric pain just below the sternum often accompanied by regurgitation of acid and presence of gas in the stomach. It may occur 10 to 15 minutes after eating a heavy meal, especially when the person is in a recumbent position. It is a common symptom of many disorders such as hiatal hernia and esophageal dysfunction. During pregnancy, heartburn results from upward displacement of the esophageal sphincter because of increased intra-abdominal pressure.

Heart failure See *Cardiac.*

Heat Sensation of an increase in temperature; measured as a quantity of energy. See *Calorie.*

Heat of combustion Amount of heat produced (usually expressed in calories) when a unit weight of a substance is oxidized.

Heat of solidification or crystallization Amount of heat released when 1 gm of liquid changes to its solid or crystalline state at constant temperature. At 0° C, 1 gm of water releases 80 calories when it changes to ice; this is the heat of crystallization.

Heat of vaporization Amount of heat needed to evaporate 1 gm of liquid at constant temperature. To change 1 gm of water at 100° C to vapor at the same temperature, 540 calories is required; this is the heat of vaporization.

Hebetude Mental dullness with impairment of the special senses, such as seen in asthenic fevers and chronic constipation.

Helium dilution The most common gasometric procedure for determining body density. The animal or man is enclosed in a chamber of known volume and a measured volume of helium gas is injected into the chamber. After a period of time long enough to allow for mixing of the helium and air in the chamber, a sample is removed and analyzed. The degree to which helium gas is diluted is inversely proportional to the volume or space occupied by the animal or man. The smaller the subject, the more diluted the helium gas will be.

Helminth Any parasitic worm or wormlike animal. *Helminthology* is the scientific study of worms.

Hemagglutination Clumping of the red blood cells. *Hemagglutinin* is an antibody that induces clumping of the red blood cells.

Hematin Ferriprotoporphyrin hydroxide, a neutral compound where iron is in the ferric state. It results from the precipitation of dissolved *hemin* in excess alkali followed by titration with excess acid.

Hematocrit The volume percentage of erythrocytes in blood. Originally the term meant a flat-bottomed centrifuge tube used to separate red blood cells. When normal blood is centrifuged in this tube, approximately 45% of the volume is separated as cells and the remaining 55% as plasma. It is useful in clinical analysis of blood and can detect decreases (hemoconcentration) or increases (hemodilution) in plasma volume.

Hematopoiesis See *Hemopoiesis*.

Heme Ferroprotoporphyrin or ferroheme, a nonprotein, iron-containing portion of hemoglobin with no net charge. Contains divalent iron and combines with various nitrogenous bases, forming hemochromogens.

Hemeralopia Glare blindness or day blindness; defective vision in bright light. Used to describe the condition of reduced *dark adaptation* resulting from vitamin A deficiency, although there may be other causes such as diseases of the retina.

Hemicellulose Indigestible polysaccharide found in plant cell walls, particularly in woody fibers and leaves. Hydrolysis by alkalies and acids yields xylose, a pentose sugar, other monosaccharides, and uronic acid. It may be digested to some extent by microbial enzymes. See also *Crude fiber*.

Hemin Ferriprotoporphyrin or ferriheme, a nonprotein, iron-containing portion of hemoglobin with a net positive charge. Contains trivalent iron and forms reddish brown crystals with chloride in glacial acetic acid.

Hemochromatosis Disorder of iron metabolism characterized by abnormal deposits of *hemosiderin* in the liver, spleen, and other tissues. The etiology is not clear; some believe that the primary cause is a faulty storage mechanism of iron due to an inborn error of metabolism, whereas others suggest dietary imbalances. Features of the disorder include bronzing of the skin, cirrhosis of the liver, and sclerosis of the pancreas.

Hemocuprein A bluish copper-protein compound found in the red blood cells of most mammals. It has a molecular weight of about 35,000 and contains two atoms of copper per molecule.

Hemocyanin A respiratory blue pigment; a copper-containing protein with a molecular weight of about 2,800,000. It is found in the blood of most mollusks and crustaceans.

Hemodialysis Blood is passed through a semipermeable membrane that is continually bathed in a hypotonic dialyzing fluid. In this way nitrogenous wastes can be removed from the blood. This method is used in acute and chronic kidney failure and in cases of poisoning where an overdose of a substance, usually removed by the kidneys, has been taken.

Hemodilution Increase in fluid content of the blood with a resulting decrease in the concentration of its solutes.

Hemoglobin (Hb) The oxygen-carrying pigment of red blood cells; a conjugated protein with the prosthetic group, *heme,* attached to the protein moiety, *globin.* A single red blood cell has about 280 million moles of Hb, each of which has a molecular weight of about 64,500. Of the 10,000 atoms of Hb, only four are iron atoms. The globin molecule accounts for "species specificity" of hemoglobin among animals. Types of human Hb have the same molecular weight and physical properties, but they differ in the globin portion because of a change in amino acid sequence. Hb A is the adult type; Hb F is for prenatal blood; Hb C, Hb G, Hb K, and Hb S refer to types of hemoglobin in certain blood disorders (e.g., Hb S is the type seen in sickle cell anemia). Normal Hb values for adults are about 14 to 16 gm/100 ml blood. The main function of hemoglobin is to carry oxygen from the lungs to the tissues and transport carbon dioxide back to the lungs. See also *Hemopoiesis* and *Blood.*

Carbamate h Also called carbaminohemoglobin; a compound of hemoglobin and carbon dioxide; the principal form in which carbon dioxide is transported from the tissues to the lungs.

Carboxyhemoglobin Carbon monoxide combined with the heme portion of hemoglobin. A cherry red compound more stable than oxyhemoglobin; it forms a complex several times stronger than that formed with oxygen. Thus, in carbon monoxide poisoning, carbon monoxide displaces oxygen, causing asphyxia.

Ferrihemoglobin Also called *methemoglobin;* iron is in the form of ferric ion.

Ferrohemoglobin Also called *reduced hemoglobin;* iron is in the form of ferrous ion.

Methemoglobin Also called ferrihemoglobin; produced by the oxidation of hemoglobin as when potassium ferricyanide is added. With the change in valence from the ferrous to the ferric state, *oxidized hemoglobin* loses its ability to combine with molecular oxygen and transport carbon dioxide.

Oxyhemoglobin Oxygenated hemoglobin. Oxygen is united loosely with ferrous iron in the lungs and is transported to the tissues.

Reduced h Also called ferrohemoglobin; can combine loosely with oxygen as *oxyhemoglobin* or transport carbon dioxide as *carbaminohemoglobin.*

Hemolysis Laking of the blood; destruction of red blood cells (RBCs) with the liberation of hemoglobin. May be brought about by various hemolytic agents such as bacterial toxins, bile salts, and the venoms of certain poisonous snakes or by the production in the body of specific *hemolysins,* a class of immune substances or antibodies elicited as a result of injection of incompatible blood. Placing the RBCs in a *hypotonic solution,* adding fat solvents such as ether and chloroform, irradiation, and alternate thawing and freezing are other hemolytic factors.

Hemophilia Hereditary hypoprothrombinemia characterized by delayed blood clotting; caused by a lack of factors VIII and IX required in thromboplastin regeneration. See *Blood clotting.*

Hemopoiesis (hematopoiesis) More appropriately termed erythropoiesis or the formation of red blood cells (RBCs). The average life-span of RBCs is 4 months or about 127 days. RBCs are continually destroyed or replaced. The process takes place mainly in the bone marrow and to some extent in the liver and spleen. The

113

primitive RBC matures by passing through several stages in the following order: *proerythroblast* (large cell with granular nucleus); *basophilic normoblast* (nucleus is more compact and less granular); *eosinophilic normoblast* (the cell acquires more hemoglobin and becomes acidophilic); *reticulocyte* (immature or young RBC devoid of nucleus but rich in ribosomes and nucleic acids); and finally, the mature RBC or erythrocyte. The hemoglobin (Hb) remains in the RBC through its life-span until the worn-out cell is removed from the circulation by cells of the *reticuloendothelial system* (bone marrow, liver, and spleen). On destruction, the heme portion of Hb is split into *bilirubin* and other pigments that are carried to the liver and secreted in the bile. The released iron can be reutilized to form Hb. Factors needed for normal hemopoiesis include a hormonal factor (erythropoietin, a hematopoietic hormone found in the plasma); a maturation factor (vitamin B_{12}); and other nutritional factors (good quality protein, folic acid, ascorbic acid, iron, copper, etc.). In general all nutrients plus sufficient calories are involved directly or indirectly.

Hemorrhage Bleeding; profuse escape of blood from the vessels, which may be due to various causes. There may be *pulmonary hemorrhage* (hemorrhage from the lungs); *primary hemorrhage* (bleeding as an immediate result of injury); *renal hemorrhage* (as in glomerulonephritis); or *spontaneous hemorrhage* (the bleeding of hemophilia), among others.

Hemorrhoid Pile or vascular tumor made up of enlarged and varicose veins in the lower portion of the rectum and the tissues around the anus.

Hemosiderin A dark yellow pigment of an iron-protein complex; a storage form of iron found mainly in the liver, spleen, and bone marrow. Unlike *ferritin*, which is a water-soluble complex of iron and protein, hemosiderin is insoluble and granular.

Hemosiderosis results when excess iron can no longer be stored as ferritin and hemosiderin storage has reached its normal limits.

Hemosiderosis Accumulation of hemosiderin in the liver and other tissues in quantities sufficient to destroy cells of the liver, other organs, and blood cells. It has been observed in patients with pernicious anemia or in hemolytic anemia after multiple transfusions. The latter is called transfusion siderosis.

Henry's law At constant temperature, the amount of gas dissolved in a liquid possessing no chemical affinity for the gas varies directly with the pressure of the gas in the surrounding medium.

HEP Abbreviation for *high-energy phosphate.*

Heparin A mucopolysaccharide with a molecular weight of about 18,000; it contains glucuronic acid, glucosamine, and sulfate ester groups. It acts as an anticoagulant by preventing the conversion of prothrombin to thrombin.

Hepatic Pertaining to the liver (hepatic gland).

Hepatic coma See under *Coma.*

Hepatic insufficiency Disorder that occurs in severe hepatic disease characterized by a tendency to hemorrhage. Prothrombin and fibrinogen levels are decreased, and blood clotting is delayed.

Hepatitis Inflammation of the liver. May be caused by infectious agents such as viruses and bacteria, toxic drugs such as arsenicals, or toxic solvents such as carbon tetrachloride. Main symptoms are marked anorexia, fever, headache, rapid and marked weight loss, jaundice, and abdominal discomfort. Chronic hepatitis may lead to *cirrhosis* of the liver. See Dietary management of selected disorders, Appendix O.

Hepatoflavin Name given to riboflavin isolated from the liver. See *Vitamin B_2.*

Hepatolithiasis Formation or presence of gallstones in the intrahepatic biliary duct.

Hepatomegaly Enlargement of the liver. It is seen in certain infections, in diseases of the liver, blood, and heart, and in some nutritional deficiency states such as kwashiorkor.

Herbivorous Subsisting on herbs and grasses. Ruminants are herbivorous animals.

Heredity Tendency of a living thing to reproduce the characteristics of its ancestors. The *genes* act as biologic units of heredity. See also *Deoxyribonucleic acid*.

Hernia Protrusion of a loop or part of an organ or tissue through an abnormal opening.

Herpes Inflammatory skin disease characterized by the formation of small vesicles or blisters on the skin or mucous membranes such as the cornea. There are many types, but the most common is an acute viral type called *herpes simplex*.

Hesperidin Flavone derivative found chiefly in pepper, lemon, and orange peels. One of the most active *bioflavonoids*.

Heteropolysaccharide Polysaccharide that yields mixtures of monosaccharides and derived products on hydrolysis. Examples are various vegetable gums and agar.

Hexokinase Enzyme that catalyzes the transfer of phosphate from adenosine triphosphate to hexoses, forming hexose-6-phosphates and adenosine diphosphate. Examples are *glucokinase* and *fructokinase*.

Hexosamine Nitrogenous sugar in which the amino group replaces a hydroxyl group. Examples are *glucosamine* and *galactosamine*. Found in certain glycoproteins, mucins, chitin, and heparin.

Hexosan Polysaccharide that yields hexose on complete hydrolysis. Cellulose, starch, and glycogen are important hexosans.

Hexose Class of monosaccharides of the general formula $C_6H_{12}O_6$. Contains six carbon atoms in the molecule. Examples are *fructose, galactose,* and *glucose.*

Hexose monophosphate shunt (HMS) Also called pentose phosphate pathway, Warburg-Dickens-Lipmann pathway, phosphogluconate shunt, or "oxidative" shunt; one of two major pathways of glucose metabolism; the other is anaerobic *glycolysis* or the Embden-Meyerhof (EM) pathway. HMS is an aerobic process whereas the EM pathway is anaerobic; the latter occurs almost exclusively in muscles whereas HMS is the major pathway in the mammary glands, testes, adipose tissues, leukocytes, and adrenal cortex. Both schemes occur in the liver simultaneously; about 50% of glucose is degraded by the EM pathway and the rest by the HMS. The HMS provides the pentoses, particularly ribose, needed for DNA and RNA synthesis. It yields NADPH (TPNH), which is needed for fat, steroid, and cholesterol synthesis and is important in photosynthesis. Many reactions and enzyme systems (e.g., transketolase, aldolase, dehydrogenase, and isomerase) involved in the HMS are identical with those observed in dark-reaction photosynthesis. See also *Photosynthesis.*

Hexose phosphate Mono- or diphosphoric acid ester of hexose formed during the breakdown of glucose and glycogen in mammalian tissues.

Hexuronic acid 1. Acid derived from a hexose sugar by the oxidation of the group on carbon atom number 6. The hexuronic acid derived from glucose is glucuronic acid. 2. Name originally given to a substance isolated from lemon juice, later identified as vitamin C.

HGF Abbreviation for *hyperglycemic-glycogenolytic factor.*

Hiccup (hiccough) Involuntary spasmodic contraction of the diaphragm in which a beginning inspiration is suddenly checked by closure of the glottis, thus causing a characteristic sound.

High blood pressure Abnormal pressure in the arteries at the height of the pulse wave. See *Hypertension.*

High-energy phosphate (HEP) Compound that contains a labile phosphate bond that yields free energy, varying from 5 to 12 kilocalories/mole, when the bond is dissociated. Examples are adenosine triphosphate, creatine phosphate, and acetyl phosphate. See also *Phosphate bond energy.*

Hill reaction Dissociation of free oxygen from water in the absence of sunlight and outside of intact green plants. Hill demonstrated that oxidation of water is not dependent on carbon dioxide fixation. Ferric oxalate (the "Hill reagent") can substitute for the carbon dioxide in ordinary photosynthesis. Later studies showed that other oxidizing agents (e.g., triphosphopyridine nucleotide, diphosphopyridine nucleotide, and benzoquinone) could oxidize water and release oxygen in the absence of carbon dioxide and sunlight. See also *Photosynthesis.*

Hippuric acid Conjugation product of benzoic acid and glycine; a normal constituent of the urine. Formed largely, if not solely, in the liver as a *detoxication* product of benzoic acid.

Hi-Pro Proprietary milk formula high in protein (38% dry weight).

Hirsutism Abnormal growth of hair in excessive amounts and unusual places, especially in women. Severe cases are suggestive of tumors of the adrenal cortex and ovaries; mild cases are seen during menopause.

Histaminase Enzyme capable of inactivating histamine. It has been used in the treatment of allergic dermatoses and intoxications. Widely distributed in tissues, especially kidney and intestinal mucosa.

Histamine Amine formed by the decarboxylation of histidine; occurs as a decomposition product of histidine and is prepared synthetically. It is a powerful vasodilator and can lower blood pressure. It can be useful in treating various allergies and as a stimulant for gastric and pancreatic secretion and visceral muscles. It is used as a diagnostic agent in testing gastric secretion (histamine test).

Histidase Enzyme of the liver that acts specifically on L-histidine, splitting it into ammonia, glutamic acid, and formic acid.

Histidine Beta-imidazole alanine, an *essential amino acid* for infants and children but not for adults. All animals need a dietary source of histidine. It was first isolated from sturgeon, and it may be obtained from any protein by sulfuric acid hydrolysis. It is a component of carnosine, anserine, and hemoglobin and a precursor of histamine.

Histidinemia Elevated blood level of histidine and its consequent excretion in the urine (histidinuria). The condition is associated with mental retardation and a defect in speech and hearing. It is believed to be an inborn error of metabolism, presumably due to lack of the enzyme *histidase.* See Inborn errors of metabolism, Appendix G.

Histidinuria Abnormal excretion of histidine in the urine. Attributed to restricted *histidase* activity in the liver.

Histology Branch of anatomy that deals with the minute structure, composition, and function of the tissues; microscopic anatomy.

Histone A simple, basic protein soluble in water and insoluble in dilute ammonia; found in cell nuclei in combination with nucleic acids. See Classification of proteins, Appendix C-2.

Hives Urticaria. Eruption of very itchy wheals with elevated centers; caused by contact with, inhalation of, or ingestion of an *allergen.*

HMO Abbreviation for *Health Maintenance Organization.*

HMS Abbreviation for *hexose monophosphate shunt.*

Holoenzyme The complete enzyme; composed of a nonprotein moiety or *cofactor* and a protein portion or *apoenzyme.*

Homeostasis "Constancy of the internal environment." The ability of the body to maintain balance of its physicochemical processes; these are dependent on *dynamic states* of metabolism. Homeostatic mechanisms in the body include fluid and pH balance, regulation of body temperature, blood sugar level, heart and pulse rates, and hormonal control.

Homocysteine A demethylated product of

methionine; a homolog of cysteine. Present in cells as an intermediate metabolite; capable of conversion to methionine by direct transfer of a methyl group from compounds such as choline and betaine.

Homocystinuria Inborn error of metabolism that is caused by a lack of the enzyme cystathionine synthetase in liver and brain. Plasma levels of methionine and homocystine are elevated, and homocystine is also excreted in the urine. The symptoms include mental retardation, a dislocated optic lens, glaucoma, cataracts, a shuffling gait, osteoporosis, and curvature of the spine. See Inborn errors of metabolism, Appendix G.

Homogenization 1. Process of rendering a substance uniform in structure, size, texture, and other quality factors. 2. In milk, homogenization is a mechanical process of forcing the liquid milk under high pressure through very small openings so that fat globules become emulsified (diameter of 1μ).

Homogentisic acid Intermediate product in the metabolism of phenylalanine and tyrosine. It is excreted in the urine in alkaptonuria and becomes oxidized to a blackish pigment on exposure of urine to air. See *Alkaptonuria.*

Homopolysaccharide Polysaccharide composed of only one kind of repeating unit which, on hydrolysis, yields only one type of carbohydrate. Examples are the *hexosans* (cellulose, starch, glycogen, and dextrans) composed wholly of glucose units and *levans* (or fructosans such as inulin) that yield only fructose units.

Homoserine Amino acid containing one more methylene group than serine.

HOP index Abbreviation for *hydroxyproline index.*

Hordein A simple protein of the prolamine type found in barley.

Hormone Organic substance produced by groups of cells or an organ and discharged directly into the bloodstream for specific regulatory action on other organs or tissues remote from its original source. With a few exceptions, hormones are generally manufactured by the endocrine glands. Certain hormones are protein in nature (e.g., parathormone and insulin); some are amino acid derivatives (e.g., thyroxine and epinephrine); and others are steroids (e.g., estrogens and androgens). For further details, see Summary of endocrine glands, Appendix K.

Hp Abbreviation for *haptoglobulin.*

Humectants Moistening agents; additives used to keep food from drying out.

Humerus Bone of the upper arm extending from the shoulder to the elbow.

Humidity Dampness; the degree of moisture, especially in the air.

Absolute h Percentage of water vapor in the air.

Relative h Actual amount of water vapor in the air as compared to the total amount the air would hold (i.e., at saturation) at the same temperature.

Humin A dark-colored substance formed during the acid hydrolysis of proteins; probably due to condensation of tryptophan with an aldehyde.

Hunger Craving for food more pronounced than appetite. A feeling of intermittent brief cramping sensations of pressure and tension in the epigastric region later accompanied by weakness and irritability.

Hyaluronic acid A viscous, high molecular weight mucopolysaccharide containing glucuronic acid and acetylglucosamine. It is found in connective tissue and acts as an intercellular cement that holds the cells together. It also binds water in the interstitial spaces and acts as a shock absorber in the joints.

Hyaluronidase Group of carbohydrases that hydrolyze *hyaluronic acid* polymers; found in bacteria, leeches, snake venoms, and testes. Called "spreading factor" because it promotes diffusion of injected medicine, since it can break down protective polysaccharide barriers.

Hycal A low protein, low electrolyte, high

carbohydrate liquid product made with demineralized glucose. It is ready to serve as a drink or as a dessert topping. (Beecham-Massengill.) See Proprietary foods: composition, features, and uses, Appendix P-1.

Hydrase Enzyme that catalyzes the removal or addition of water to a compound without hydrolyzing it.

Hydremia Excess water (fluid) in the blood in the absence of a proportionate increase in total amount of blood.

Hydrochloric acid HCl; muriatic acid. A compound composed of hydrogen and chlorine. It is a normal constituent of the gastric juice in man and other mammals. Its functions in digestion are to denature protein, activate pepsinogen to pepsin, provide an acid medium for absorption of iron, and stimulate the opening of the pylorus.

Hydrocortisone See *Cortisol*.

Hydrogen An inflammable, colorless, odorless, gaseous chemical element. It is the lightest of all known substances and has the smallest atomic weight. It is present in proteins, carbohydrates, fats, and water. It makes up approximately 10% of the body weight.

Hydrogenate To bring about a combination with hydrogen. Hydrogenation of oils is a process by which molecular hydrogen is added to double bonds in the unsaturated fatty acids of the glycerides. Thus oils are changed to solid fats, although the process reduces the biologic value of essential fatty acids when the polyunsaturated fatty acids become saturated.

Hydrogenolysis Cleavage of a molecule by adding hydrogen.

Hydrogen peroxide H_2O_2, a caustic liquid often used as a bleaching agent. Also used in medicine and surgery as an antiseptic agent and as a cleansing agent in mouthwashes, toothpastes, and toothpowders. Its antiseptic and cleansing action is due to the fact that it gives off sufficient oxygen to destroy bacteria; 1 volume can liberate approximately 10 volumes of oxygen.

Hydrolases New name given to a group of enzymes that hydrolyze a variety of compounds by the addition of water. Included in this group are lipase, peptidase, phosphatase, and amidase. To illustrate the new system of naming enzymes, "lipase" is now a trivial name; the systematic name is now "glycerol ester hydrolase."

Hydrolysis Splitting a substance into smaller units by reaction with water.

Hydrostatic pressure Pressure exerted by a liquid on the surfaces of the walls containing the liquid. In the body, it refers to the blood pressure, which maintains the fluid volume and circulation in the blood vessels.

Hydroxocobalamin Form of vitamin B_{12} in which the cyanide group is replaced by a hydroxyl group.

Hydroxyapatite A naturally occurring mineral crystal of the general formula $3Ca_3(PO_4)_2 \cdot Ca(OH)_2$. The minerals in *bone* are deposited in the organic matrix in crystal formation similar to that of hydroxyapatite except that the hydroxyl groups are partially substituted by other elements and radicals such as fluoride and carbonate.

25-Hydroxycholecalciferol (25-HCC) See *Vitamin D*.

Hydroxylysine Lysine to which a hydroxyl group has been added. It is found in the structural protein collagen.

Hydroxyproline Proline to which a hydroxyl group has been added. It is found in the structural protein collagen.

Hydroxyproline index (HOP index) Test that correlates the amount of urinary hydroxyproline and creatinine per kilogram of body weight. It can be used as a measure of malnutrition.

Hydroxyprolinemia Metabolic disorder due to lack of the enzyme hydroxyproline oxidase. Blood and urine accumulate large amounts of free hydroxyproline, and the condition may lead to mental retardation. At present no therapy is available. See Inborn errors of metabolism, Appendix G.

Hyper- Prefix meaning increased or greater

than normal. Examples are *hyperacidity* (increased acidity); *hypercholia* (excessive excretion of bile); *hypermotility* (increased motility); *hyperplasia* (abnormal multiplication of cells in a tissue); *hyperthermia* (fever or abnormally high body temperature); and *hypervolemia* (increased volume of circulating body fluids).

Hyperalimentation Administration, either orally or intravenously, of higher than normal amounts of nutrients. In parenteral hyperalimentation an indwelling catheter is passed into the superior vena cava. A hypertonic solution made up of glucose, protein hydrolysate, vitamins, and minerals can be administered continuously. Up to 4000 kilocalories can be given by this method. It is useful for patients who are unable to take food orally for a long period of time.

Hyperammonemia Metabolic disorder characterized by elevated blood ammonia levels. This is due to a deficiency of the enzyme ornithine transcarbamylase, which catalyzes the reaction between carbamyl phosphate and ornithine to form citrulline. The symptoms include ammonia intoxication and cerebral and cortical atrophy. A severe reduction of the protein intake results in a reduction of blood ammonia to near normal levels.

Hypercalcemia Excessive amounts of calcium in the blood; may occur in hyperparathyroidism and in patients with peptic ulcer under excessive alkali therapy and a milk diet over a period of years. Results in vomiting, anorexia, gastrointestinal bleeding, high blood pressure, and muscular weakness.

Hyperchlorhydria Excessive hydrochloric acid (HCl) in the stomach due primarily to increased secretion of the gastric juice.

Hypercholesterolemia Condition when blood cholesterol is above the normal limits (about 280 mg% or more). It is associated with atherosclerosis and other cardiovascular diseases, obstructive jaundice, lipoid nephrosis, excess ACTH, and hyperglycemia in diabetes mellitus. The etiologic factors for excess serum cholesterol are many and varied, but the exact mechanisms are not well understood. Hormonal, genetic, nutritional, and environmental factors have been implicated. See *Cholesterol* and *Sterols*.

Hyperglycemia Increased glucose concentration in the blood above normal limits. May occur in the following conditions: *diabetes mellitus* due to lack of insulin; increased *epinephrine* secretion; following ingestion of a very high carbohydrate intake (called "alimentary" hyperglycemia); *hyperthyroidism* due to increased hepatic glycogenolysis; increased intracranial pressure (as a result of skull fracture, cerebral hemorrhage, or brain tumor); administration of anesthetics such as ether, chloroform, and morphine; and *hyperpituitarism*. See also *Glucagon* and *Blood sugar level*.

Hyperglycemic-glycogenolytic factor (HGF) Also called simply *hyperglycemic factor;* another name for *glucagon*. A hormone secreted by the alpha cells of the islet of Langerhans of the pancreas and found in most insulin preparations. It accelerates glycogenolysis in the liver but has no effect on muscle glycogen. It is believed to increase the activity of the enzyme phosphorylase; hence it is similar to epinephrine in this respect.

Hyperinsulinism Condition of excessive insulin in the body. Caused either by an overdose of insulin (as in insulin shock) or overproduction of insulin by the pancreas. The latter is commonly known as *spontaneous hypoglycemia* or *functional hyperinsulinism*. See also *Hypoglycemia* and Dietary management of selected disorders, Appendix O.

Hyperkalemia Also called hyperpotassemia; increased potassium level in the blood. Toxic elevation of serum potassium is observed in cases of renal failure, advanced dehydration, shock, Addison's disease, and excessive intravenous administration of potassium. Symptoms, involving chiefly the cardiac and central nervous systems, include numbness, mental confusion, bradycardia, paralysis of the extremities, and ultimately cardiac arrest.

Hyperkeratosis 1. Hypertrophy of the horny layer of the skin, i.e., warts. 2. Hypertrophy of the cornea.

Hyperlipemia General term that refers to an excess of fat in the blood.

Hyperlipidemia Nonspecific term that refers to an elevation of one or more lipid constituents of the blood.

Hyperlipoproteinemia Elevation of blood lipoproteins, i.e., elevated plasma cholesterol and/or triglycerides. In 1967 Fredrickson, Levy, and Lees classified the disorder into five major types.

Type I Characterized by hyperchylomicronemia with normal or elevated cholesterol levels. It is extremely rare in occurrence.

Type II Consists of elevated beta-lipoproteins, elevated cholesterol, and normal triglyceride levels. It is one of the most common of the inherited forms and is also called familial hypercholesterolemia, familial xanthomatosis, familial hypercholesterolemic xanthomatosis, and xanthoma tuberosum multiplet.

Type III Identified by elevated prebetalipoproteins, elevated plasma cholesterol, and elevated triglycerides. It is relatively uncommon and is referred to as broad beta disease.

Type IV Characterized by elevated levels of prebeta-lipoproteins, elevated triglycerides, and normal or slightly elevated cholesterol levels. It is also called carbohydrate-induced or carbohydrate-accentuated hyperlipidemia or essential familial hyperlipemia. It is common in occurrence.

Type V Shows a plasma lipoprotein pattern of elevated hyperchylomicronemia and elevated prebeta-lipoproteinemia. Plasma cholesterol and triglycerides are also elevated. The disease is relatively rare and is also known as combined fat and carbohydrate–induced hyperlipemia.

Hypernatremia High levels of sodium in the blood.

Hyperoxaluria A rare metabolic disease characterized by an increased excretion of oxalate in the urine. The basic difficulty is the inability to metabolize glyoxylic acid. As a result, excess oxalic acid is produced and is precipitated as calcium oxalate in the kidney. The individual usually dies of renal failure in infancy. Calcium oxalate deposits may be found in other tissues.

Hyperparathyroidism Abnormally increased secretion of parathyroid hormone leading to withdrawal of calcium from the bones. Features of this endocrine disorder include tenderness of the bones, muscular weakness and pain, abdominal cramps, and spontaneous fractures.

Hyperpituitarism Pathologic condition due to increased activity of the *hypophysis* (pituitary gland). Symptoms vary, depending on the pituitary cells affected and the type of hormone secreted in excessive amounts. *True hyperpituitarism* is an overactivity of the eosinophilic cells (excess growth hormone) resulting in *gigantism* in children and *acromegaly* in adults.

Hyperpnea Condition in which the rate and depth of breathing are increased.

Hyperprolinemia Disorder in the metabolism of proline probably resulting from a lack of the enzyme proline dehydrogenase. Symptoms include fever, vomiting, diarrhea, drowsiness, frequent convulsions, and hearing loss. Fasting levels of blood plasma proline are three to five times normal; urinary levels of proline, hydroxyproline, and glycine are also elevated.

Hypertensinogen Former name for *angiotensinogen*. It is the protein substrate on which *renin* acts to produce angiotensin. See *Angiotensin*.

Hypertension Also called high blood pressure; elevation of *blood pressure* above normal. Blood pressure varies considerably among individuals, depending on many factors such as age, physical constitution, occupation, and health. For adults the average systolic/diastolic pressure is about 120/80 mm Hg. Hypertension may occur at any age, but more frequently in persons over

40 years old. About 85% to 90% of cases involve so-called *essential hypertension* (hypertension of unknown cause), which is an accompanying symptom of many renal and cardiovascular disorders, tumor of the adrenals, and emotional disturbances. Hypertensive persons usually suffer from dizziness, frequent headaches, impaired vision, shortness of breath, chest pain, failing memory, and sometimes gastrointestinal disturbance. A *sodium-restricted diet* is beneficial.

Hyperthyroidism Endocrine disorder caused by excessive secretion of the thyroid hormone as a result of overmedication with potent thyroid drugs, hyperactivity of the thyroid gland, or tumor (toxic adenoma of the thyroid). The clinical syndrome is generally called *exophthalmic goiter* because two thirds of the patients show exophthalmos, i.e., protruding eyes with widely open lids. Other symptoms include thyroid enlargement, increased BMR and pulse rate, nervousness and muscle tremors, and loss of weight.

Hypertrophy Morbid enlargement or overgrowth of an organ or part due to an increase in size of its constituent cells.

Hypervitaminosis Vitamin toxicity, a condition in which the level of a vitamin in the blood or tissues is high enough to cause undesirable symptoms. Hypervitaminosis has long been associated with excessive intake of the fat-soluble vitamins, especially A and D, which are not generally excreted from the body. Recently toxic effects have been observed for some of the water-soluble vitamins, especially niacinamide and folic acid, when these are taken in excessively high therapeutic doses. See Summary of vitamins, Appendix I-1.

Hypo- Prefix denoting below normal or reduced quantity. Examples are *hypoacidity* (lowered HCl secretion), *hypocupremia* (copper deficiency in the blood), and *hypoplasia* (defective development).

Hypogeusia (hypogeusesthesia) Diminution in the sense of taste.

Hypoglycemia Condition characterized by blood glucose levels below normal (about 50 mg%). *Spontaneous hypoglycemia,* which occurs without the administration of exogenous insulin, is brought about by any of the following etiologic factors: *hyperinsulinism* (as in tumor or hypertrophy of the pancreas), *hepatic disease* (toxic hepatitis and von Gierke's disease), *adrenal hypofunction* (as in Addison's disease), *pituitary hypofunction* (e.g., Simmond's disease), and certain *inborn errors of metabolism* (e.g., sugar malabsorption and leucine-induced hypoglycemia). Severe exercise, intense lactation, fasting, inanition, and cachexia also cause hypoglycemia. The symptoms are characteristic of those seen in *insulin shock* and include extreme hunger, nervousness, flushing of the skin with profuse sweating, dizziness, palpitation, and apathy. On the basis of dietary management, hypoglycemias are grouped into fasting and stimulative types.

Fasting h Blood sugar is below 60 mg% before breakfast or after a fasting condition. This may also occur in adrenal or pituitary hypofunctions, liver diseases, and other conditions. In contrast to the stimulative type, fasting hypoglycemia becomes more severe if carbohydrate is restricted. Thus the dietary treatment consists of readily available glucose (high carbohydrate, high protein diet), which should be constantly and regularly supplied (frequent meals with snacks).

Stimulative h Also called *functional hyperinsulinism;* hypoglycemia in the absence of an organic lesion. Carbohydrate stimulates the pancreas to secrete higher than normal levels of insulin. As a consequence, hypoglycemia occurs 2 to 4 hours after meals; there is no hypoglycemia following fasting and omission of meals. The condition is prevented by restricting the dietary intake of carbohydrate to levels below 100 gm; calories are supplied by protein and fat. In order that absorption from the intestines will be gradual, the daily food allowance is divided into six meals, using part of the regular meals for midmorning, midafternoon, and bedtime snacks.

Hypoglycemic agents Substances that lower blood glucose level such as *insulin* and *oral hypoglycemic agents*. See also *Blood sugar level*.

Hypokinesis "Deconditioning" of the body due to lack of exercise or physical activity. Prolonged physical inactivity results in stiffness, fatigue, weakness, sensitivity, incoordination, instability, muscular atrophy, asthenia, ataxia, myocardial ischemia, urolithiasis, and osteoporosis. See also *Nutrition, motor performance*.

Hypophysis Preferred name for *pituitary gland*. An endocrine gland about the size of a lima bean located beneath the brain and protected by a saddlelike depression called the *sella turcica*. It is composed of three portions: the anterior, intermediate *(pars intermedia)*, and posterior lobes. According to anatomic origin, the anterior and middle lobes make up the buccal component or the *adenohypophysis;* the posterior lobe and the neural stalk compose the *neurohypophysis*. Each lobe secretes important hormones that regulate vital processes in the body. The anterior lobe secretes *somatotropin, thyrotropin, gonadotropins (luteinizing hormone, FSH, luteotropic hormone),* and ACTH. The intermediate lobe elaborates the *melanocyte-stimulating hormone,* whereas the posterior lobe secretes *oxytocin* and *vasopressin*. The hypophysis is called the "master gland" or the "king of all glands" because it regulates the action of many of the other endocrine glands through the different hormones elaborated by its three lobes. See also Summary of endocrine glands, Appendix K.

Hypopituitarism Decreased activity of the *hypophysis* (pituitary gland) caused by a tumor, infarct, hemorrhage, or atrophy. Forms include *pituitary myxedema,* which is due to a lack of the thyroid-stimulating hormone (TSH) and is similar to myx-

edema of hypothyroidism; *panhypopituitarism,* which involves all the hormonal functions of the hypophysis (as in Simmond's disease); and *pituitary dwarfism,* which is characterized by cessation of growth and diminished metabolic activities.

Hypotension Reduced arterial systolic blood pressure below the normal. May result from injection of drugs that lower blood pressure, hemorrhage or shock, and suppression of renal blood flow. Primary hypotension is not a disease but is common among young asthenic women. Secondary hypotension is associated with diseases such as myocardial infarction, vascular accidents, cachexia, and fever. Postural hypotension may occur in some debilitated or elderly persons when they assume the upright position and there is exaggerated venous pooling.

Hypothalamus Area lying at the base of the brain just below the thalamus. It is responsible for the maintenance of body temperature, blood pressure, water regulation, control of satiety and appetite, and other basic functions necessary to life. Because of its close anatomic connection with the pituitary gland, it has been implicated in the control of endocrine gland function.

Hypothyroidism Endocrine disorder resulting from the decreased activity of the *thyroid gland*. The effects are *myxedema* in adults and *cretinism* in children.

Hypoxanthine A basic compound, 6-oxypurine, found in many plant and animal tissues; specifically associated with RNA. Hypoxanthine can be formed by the enzymatic conversion of *adenine* and is oxidized to *xanthine*.

Hysterectomy Partial or complete removal of the uterus performed either through the abdominal wall or through the vagina.

Hysteresis Phenomenon observed when a colloidal system is reproduced. A change in the properties of a colloid due to its history, e.g., previous handling, processing, aging, and heating. For example, a dried protein gel will not have the same rehydrating capacity as the original gel.

Hysteria Psychoneurotic condition in which the person lacks control over his actions and emotions. Characteristic symptoms include exaggerated response to sensory stimuli, choking sensation, anxiety, morbid self-consciousness, mild convulsions, hallucinations, and tonic spasms.

I

IAA Abbreviation for *indolacetic acid*.

IBC Abbreviation for *iron-binding capacity*.

IBW Abbreviation for *ideal body weight*. See *Weight*.

Ichthyosis Commonly called fish skin and alligator skin; a type of *dermatosis* characterized by dry, rough, and scaly skin, especially on the extremities, that becomes worse in cold weather.

ICNND Abbreviation for *Interdepartmental Committee on Nutrition for National Defense*.

ICSH Abbreviation for *interstitial cell–stimulating hormone*.

Icteric Pertaining to *icterus* or jaundice. See *Jaundice*.

Icteric index Measure of the yellow color in blood plasma; expressed by comparing the color of the serum with the color of a 1:10,000 potassium dichromate solution. The normal range is from 4 to 6. Values higher than 6 are indicative of *jaundice* or *icterus*.

Idiopathic 1. Without any known origin; self-originated. 2. Pertaining to disease of unknown cause, e.g., idiopathic celiac disease.

IEM Abbreviation for *inborn error of metabolism*.

IEP Abbreviation for *isoelectric point*.

Ileitis Acute or chronic inflammation of the lower ileum, although other parts of the intestine may also be affected by edema, fibrosis, and ulceration. Clinical symptoms include abdominal cramps, loss of weight, bloody diarrhea, and progressive anemia.

Ileum Third and last portion of the small intestine, extending from the jejunum to the large intestine.

IM Abbreviation for *intramuscular*.

Imbalance Pathologic condition brought about by a change in the proportion of the essential nutrients in the diet. See also *Amino acid balance-imbalance*.

Imbibition The taking up of fluid by a solid or a gel.

Immunity Security against any particular disease; power of an organism to resist or overcome infection. Immunity may be natural (inborn) or acquired by having the disease or by injection, inoculation, or vaccination with an *antigen*.

Impermeable Not permitting passage through; not capable of being penetrated. Commonly used in reference to a membrane or tissue.

Implantation Insertion of a tissue or part in another place of the body.

Inactivate To render inert or suspend biologic activity by the application of heat, irradiation, or other forms of energy.

Inanition Wasting of the body due to complete lack of food; a state of starvation.

Inborn error of metabolism (IEM) Metabolic defect due to missing genes that exists at birth and may persist throughout life. Examples are albinism, alkaptonuria, galactosemia, and phenylketonuria. See Inborn errors of metabolism, Appendix G.

Incaparina Protein-rich dietary supplement developed by the Institute of Nutrition in Central America and Panama (INCAP);

consists of cottonseed flour, ground corn, sorghum, *Torula* yeast, and added calcium and vitamin A.

Incidence Frequency of occurrence of a situation or a condition; the number of cases of a disease in relation to the unit population.

Incipient Beginning; commencing; about to appear.

Incomplete protein See *Protein classification* and *Protein quality.*

Incontinence Inability to restrain or control a natural discharge such as the urine or feces.

Incubation 1. Time between infection and the appearance of signs or symptoms of the disease. 2. Process of hatching eggs and culturing bacteria for growth studies.

Indican Potassium salt of indoxylsulfate, a derivative of *indole;* forms indigo blue when treated with ferricyanide. High urinary indican concentration is an indication of the extent of bacterial activity in the large intestines.

Indicator A substance or dye (such as litmus paper, methyl red, and phenolphthalein) used to determine the end point of a chemical reaction or the degree of acidity or alkalinity of materials by means of a change in color.

Indigestion Faulty or incomplete digestion of foods; often accompanied by heartburn, abdominal pain, and flatulence. May be due to nervous or emotional upsets, poor eating habits, or poor cooking methods.

Indolacetic acid (**IAA**) Product of decomposition of tryptophan by bacteria in the intestine; present in increased amounts in the urine of individuals with *phenylketonuria.* Considered the major phytohormone that occurs naturally in plant tissues and has been isolated or detected in bamboo shoots, coconut milk, oats, peas, and strawberries. See also *Indole plant hormones* and *Phytohormone.*

Indole A substance formed from the decomposition of tryptophan during intestinal putrefaction; partly responsible for the foul odor of feces. Eliminated as *indican* in the urine.

Indole plant hormones Group of naturally occurring plant hormones capable of inducing rooting, curvature of stems, production of hyperplasia and tumors, and suppression of flowering. Of the several indolic plant hormones identified, the most important are indolacetic acid, indolacetaldehyde, indolacetonitrile, and indole pyruvic acid.

Indoxyl Product formed from the oxidation of indole and skatole; excreted in the urine as indican.

Inedible Pertaining to that portion of food not fit for eating, such as tough skins and decayed or poisonous foods.

Infant feeding *Breast feeding* is generally accepted as the most desirable method of feeding an infant. Human milk is considered ideal. Except for iron and vitamin D, it contains adequate amounts of all nutritional factors needed by the newborn infant. It is also believed that human milk contains immune bodies that make the infant more resistant to infection. Although breast feeding is desirable, the following contraindications to maternal nursing should be considered: poor maternal health, past history of tuberculosis and severe chronic illness, mastitis and other acute infections, emotional and mental stress, another pregnancy, and insufficient milk production. *Artificial or bottle feeding* with cow's milk and other proprietary milk preparations is equally satisfactory for infants. Proper sterilization of the infant's formula makes artificial feeding safe, and various methods (such as heating, homogenization, and acidification) are employed in reducing the size of milk curds, making cow's milk more digestible. Artificial feeding is also indicated when the mother's milk does not agree with the infant or when the infant is unable to either digest or utilize milk because of a deficiency in certain enzymes in the body. *Mixed feeding* is a combination of breast and bottle feeding. It is generally carried out in either of two ways: as *complemental feeding* (the giving of a bottle to complete a single feeding at the breast) or as *supplemental feeding* (the substitution of the bottle for one or more of the breast feedings during the day). Complemental feeding is often used when the mother's milk is insufficient for the infant's needs. Supplemental feeding is used when the mother is away from home for periods longer than the feeding intervals; it is also advisable during the weaning stage when it is desired to allow the breast to dry up gradually. See Proprietary foods: composition, features, and uses, Appendix P-1.

Infantile paralysis See *Poliomyelitis*.

Infarction Necrosis or decay of tissues due to complete interference with the flow of blood.

Infection Transfer of disease; entrance and development of pathogenic microorganisms and parasites in the body. Any disease caused by growth of pathogenic microorganisms in the body is called an *infectious disease*. It may or may not be contagious.

Infestation Lodgment, development, and reproduction of arthropods such as insects, lice, mites, and ticks on the surface of the body.

Infiltration Diffusion of fluid or solid substances into a tissue, organ, or cell. These substances may be normal but present in an unusual amount, or they may be foreign.

Influenza An acute infectious viral disease characterized by fever, muscle pain, catarrhal inflammation of the nose, larynx, and bronchi, and prostration. Common complications are pneumonia and infection of the middle ear.

Infrared Long rays of radiant energy beyond the red end of the visible spectrum.

Ingestion 1. Eating; taking in of food or beverage. 2. Process by which a cell takes up foreign matter such as bacilli or smaller cells.

INH Abbreviation for *isonicotinyl hydrazide*. See *Isonicotinic acid hydrazide*.

Inhalation Breathing air or vapor into the lungs.

Inhibition Stopping or preventing the action of an organ, cell, or chemical by specific inhibitors such as a metal-complexing agent, substrate analog, and metabolic antagonist or antimetabolite.

Inhibition index Ratio of concentration of inhibitor to that of substrate required to produce a given degree of *inhibition*.

Innervation Amount of nerve stimulation to a part.

Inoculation Introduction of an organism or a substance into the body as a preventive measure against certain diseases.

Inorganic Denoting *mineral,* as distinct from animal and vegetable origins. Apart from carbonates and cyanides, inorganic chemicals are those that do not contain carbon and remain as *ash* when food is burned.

Inosine Decomposition product of *inosinic acid;* formed by the union of hypoxanthine and ribose.

Inosinic acid Nucleotide found in muscles but not in nucleic acids. Composed of hypoxanthine, ribose, and phosphoric acid and formed by the deamination of adenylic acid.

Inositol Water-soluble cyclic alcohol allied to the hexoses. It is found in muscles, liver, kidneys, brain, and other animal tissues and occurs in plants in combination with phosphoric acid as *phytic acid*. Its exact biologic significance is unknown; experimental deficiency in animals results in alopecia, retarded growth, fatty liver, and poor lactation. Although it enjoys vitamin status, inositol is not classified as a vitamin, since it is present in practically all plants and animal tissues in concentrations higher than those normally associated with vitamins. See also *Mesoinositol* and *Vitamin-like substances*.

Insensible perspiration Water lost through the skin that is not noticeable because evaporation takes place immediately. It is important for the maintenance of body temperature. This loss in body weight through vaporization of water can be measured within a short period of time using a sensitive balance. If taken under controlled conditions of temperature and humidity, the "insensible loss in body weight" may be used as an indirect method for ascertaining the basal heat production of an individual.

Insidious Coming on gradually, as the onset of a disease.

Inspiration Breathing air in; inhalation.

Inspiratory reserve volume See *Complemental air.*

Insulin Hormone secreted by the beta cells of the islets of Langerhans of the pancreas. It is a protein with a molecular weight of about 6000 and is composed of two polypeptide chains, A and B, containing 21 and 30 amino acid molecules, respectively, and joined at two points by disulfide bridges. The exact mechanism of insulin function is not yet established, although the following effects are noted after its administration: lowering of blood sugar levels, increase in liver and muscle glycogen formation, inhibition of gluconeogenesis in liver, and increase in the rate of glucose utilization by the tissues. Lack of insulin leads to *diabetes mellitus.*

Insulin preparations Insulin is commercially prepared in amorphous or crystalline form from beef, pork, and sheep pancreas. It is sold either unmodified as regular insulin or in combination with basic proteins (globin and protamine) or with crystalline zinc salts to make the compound less soluble and less absorbable, thus effecting a longer duration of action.

Globin i Insulin preparation modified by the addition of globin to make it more insoluble for prolonged action. This permits less frequent injections than when regular insulin is used. Duration of action is about 16 to 20 hours.

Isophane i Preparation of insulin combined with protamine in isophane ratio of approximately 0.5 mg protamine for each 100 units of insulin. NPH insulin is an isophane insulin.

Lente i Insulin preparation crystallized from an acetate buffer in the presence of zinc. By varying the conditions of preparation, it is possible to obtain insulin preparations of varying particle size and duration of action. *Semilente* is a suspension of amorphous insulin particles with a duration of action of 12 to 18 hours; *Lente* is a suspension of insulin crystals of small particle size, giving a duration of action of 24 hours; and *Ultralente* is a suspension of insulin crystals of large particle size, giving a duration of action of over 30 hours.

Neutral protamine Hagedorn (NPH) i An isophane insulin developed by Hagedorn; consists of crystals of insulin, protamine, and zinc suspended in a buffered medium. The duration of action is about 20 to 24 hours, which is longer than the duration of globin insulin and less than that of protamine zinc insulin (PZI).

Protamine zinc i (PZI) Preparation of insulin combined with zinc and protamine contained in the sperm of fish. This combination makes insulin more stable and produces a prolonged action (20 to 30 hours) because of its relative insolubility.

Regular i Also called amorphous, ordinary, or soluble insulin; it is an unmodified preparation now seldom used alone because of its very short duration of action (6 hours), requiring many injections each day. However, it becomes the insulin of choice in case of emergencies such as ketosis, infection, and surgery; also used in combination with the slow-acting insulins.

Insulin shock Also called insulin reaction; a reaction of the body due to a very low blood sugar level because of overdosage of insulin. It is characterized by a feeling of hunger, weakness, nervousness, double vision, shallow breathing, sweating, headache and dizziness leading to mental confusion, muscular twitching, convulsion, loss of consciousness, and eventually coma. Glucose or fruit juice must be given immediately. Death may occur if adequate treatment is not given.

Insulin unit The physiologic activity of insulin is expressed in international units (IU). One IU is equivalent to 0.125 mg of the international standard preparation or $\frac{1}{23}$ mg of a standard preparation of crystalline zinc insulin.

Integrating motor pneumotachograph (IMP) Electronic apparatus designed to measure very high rates of energy expenditure such as may occur during battle training or in athletic or sports activity.

Interdepartmental Committee on Nutrition for National Defense (ICNND) Organization formed by the ICA and the U. S. Departments of Defense, Health, Education, and Welfare, and Agriculture. Its purpose is "to assess, to assist, and to learn" about the food and nutrition situation in countries to which the United States is giving military support. Local specialists in each country assist personnel from the United States in defining the major nutritional problems.

Interfacial tension Tension existing where liquids come in contact or where a solid touches a liquid.

Interferon Protein formed in response to the entry of a virus into an animal cell. It can confer on similar animal cells resistance to infection.

Intermediary metabolism Synthesis (anabolism) and degradation (catabolism) of the cell constituents of living organisms. In the intact cell both processes go on simultaneously, and energy released from the degradation of some compounds may be utilized in the synthesis of other cellular components. In a broad sense, intermediary metabolism refers to the chemical reactions taking place inside the body, from the ingestion of foodstuffs to the discharge of ultimate chemical products and excretion of metabolic end products. See Utilization of carbohydrates, Utilization of proteins, and Utilization of fats, Appendices D-1, D-2, and D-3.

Intermittent Taking place at intervals, e.g., intermittent fever.

International Council of Scientific Unions Sponsors international congresses of nutrition every 3 years. It consists of sixteen unions, one of which is the International Union for Nutritional Sciences.

International Dietetic Association Organization whose aim is to raise the level of the dietetics profession in member countries.

International Union for Nutritional Sciences (IUNS) One of sixteen unions of the *International Council of Scientific Unions*. The aim of the union is to provide a means for international cooperation in the study of basic and applied nutrition. Information is exchanged at international congresses.

International unit (IU) Figure that represents the biologic activity of a nutrient or substance. It is a specific reference standard of known potency that produces in a laboratory animal specific effects over a specified period of time.

Interstitial Situated in the interspaces of tissue or between parts.

Interstitial cell–stimulating hormone (ICSH) Also called luteinizing hormone; a gonadotropic hormone secreted by the anterior pituitary gland. See *Luteinizing hormone*.

Intestinal juice Succus entericus. A straw-colored alkaline fluid secreted by the intestinal mucosa; contains enzymes that complete the hydrolysis of carbohydrate, protein, and fat. Mixed with it are the pancreatic secretions containing enzymes and the hormone enterokinase. See Summary of digestive enzymes, Appendix J-1.

Intestine Part of the digestive tract that extends from the stomach (pylorus) to the anus; divided into the small and large intestines.

Large i The last portion of the gastrointestinal tract, extending from the ileum to the anus. It is about 5 feet long and divided into three parts: *cecum, colon,* and *rectum.* Although no digestion takes place in the large intestine, it serves as the site for absorption of water and unabsorbed products of digestion and for temporary storage of feces until they are eliminated. The micro-flora inhabiting the large intestine can synthesize some vitamins (especially vitamin K) and can hydrolyze crude fiber to some extent. See also *Crude fiber*.

Small i That portion that extends from the pylorus to the large intestine at the cecum. It is about 20 feet long and divided into three parts: *duodenum, jejunum,* and *ileum.* The small intestine is the main site for the digestion and absorption of food.

Intima The innermost of the three coats of a blood vessel.

Intra- Prefix signifying within, e.g., *intracellular* (within the cell), *intramuscular* (within the muscle), *intravascular* (within the blood vessel), or *intravenous* (within the vein).

Intrinsic factor Chemical substance present in normal gastric juice that facilitates the absorption of the extrinsic factor (vitamin B_{12}) found in foods. A deficiency in this factor results in *pernicious anemia*.

Inulin Polysaccharide composed of *fructose* units; found in Jerusalem artichoke and dahlia tuber. It is used as a test for kidney function, since it is completely filtered by the glomerulus and not reabsorbed or excreted by the kidney tubules. See also *Kidney*.

Inversion Conversion of sucrose in solution into equal amounts of glucose and fructose by the action of acid or enzyme (invertase). The mixture is called *invert sugar*.

In vitro Observable in a test tube; refers to a process or reaction carried out in glass, culture dish, or test tube.

In vivo Within the living body; natural living conditions.

Iodinase Enzyme found in the cell-free extract of the thyroid tissue that catalyzes the incorporation of iodide into the organically bound form, monoiodotyrosine.

Iodine A trace mineral that is a dietary essential; an important constituent of the thyroid hormone thyroglobulin, which is necessary in the regulation of normal basal metabolic rate in the body. Found in seafoods and vegetables grown in soil con-

taining iodine. A deficiency in this mineral results in *simple goiter*. For further details, see Summary of minerals, Appendix H.

Iodine 131 Radioactive isotope of iodine. Useful in the diagnosis and treatment of thyroid gland disorders, determination of blood plasma volume and cardiac output, and as a diagnostic aid prior to surgery for the location of brain tumors.

Iodine number Also called iodine value; the number of grams of iodine taken up by 100 gm of fat. It is a quantitative value that reflects the amount of fatty acids and the degree of unsaturation of a fat or an oil. The value ranges from 10 for coconut oil to 200 for safflower oil.

Iodized salt Table salt that contains 1 part sodium or potassium iodide/5000 to 10,000 parts (or 0.01%) sodium chloride.

Iodopsin Visual violet; a light-sensitive violet pigment of the cones in the retina that is important for vision.

Iodothyroglobulin Globulin-iodine complex found in the thyroid gland; serves as the prosthetic group of *thyroxine*.

Ion Atom or chemical radical carrying an electric charge that is positive (cation) or negative (anion) or both (zwitterion).

Ion exchange Reversible exchange of ions in solution with ions present in a solid material. *Ion-exchange resins* such as Amberlite and Dowex can absorb ions under one set of conditions and release them under other conditions. These resins are used for purification of chemicals, recovery of metals, and analysis of compounds. An example of ion exchange is in softening water, where calcium ions are removed from the hard water by the resin and later liberated from the resin by the addition of salt.

Ionization Dissociation of a substance in solution into its constituent ions.

Iris The pigment diaphragm of the eye.

Irish moss See *Carrageenan*.

Iron A trace mineral essential to the body; occurs in hemoglobin of red blood cells of animals. In the body, iron is also present in muscle myoglobin, in various oxidative enzyme complexes such as cytochromes and oxidases, and stored in the tissues as *ferritin* and *hemosiderin*. Iron is necessary for the prevention of nutritional anemia and plays an important role in respiration and tissue oxidations. The hemoglobin of the red blood cells and the myoglobin of the tissue cells are vital for oxygen transport to the cells and storage within the cells, whereas the iron-containing enzymes within the cells are associated with metabolic enzymatic oxidations. Important dietary sources are liver, egg yolk, molasses, and dried fruits. For further details, see Summary of minerals, Appendix H.

Iron-binding capacity (**IBC**) Measure of the percent saturation of transferrin in the blood. Normal values for males, 150 to 285 μg/100 ml; for females, 144 to 322 μg/100 ml. In iron deficiency there is decreased saturation to less than 18%.

Irradiation Exposure to or treatment with ultraviolet rays from sunlight, roentgen rays, gamma rays, or radiation from radioactive materials such as cobalt 60. Has various uses, e.g., conversion of provitamin D to its active form, destruction of microorganisms in food, and therapeutic treatment of malignancies.

Irritability Property or ability to respond to a stimulus. The term usually applies to nerves.

Irritable colon Condition characterized by abnormal motor activity of the colon in the absence of organic lesions. The causes are varied, e.g., excessive use of laxatives and cathartics, dietary indiscretion, emotional upsets, and enteric infections. Symptoms include belching, abdominal distress and distention, flatulence, heartburn, and constipation or diarrhea.

Isanic acid A crystalline fatty acid containing 18 carbon atoms with one double bond and two triple bonds; found in *isano oil*. A strong purgative.

Ischemia Local and temporary anemia due to obstruction in the flow of blood.

Islets of Langerhans Cellular masses in the interstitial tissue of the pancreas from which *insulin* is secreted. Its impairment or destruction is associated with hyperglycemia and diabetes mellitus.

Isoagglutinin Also called *isohemagglutinin;* a substance normally present in most human serum or plasma that agglutinates or clumps corpuscles when mixed with incompatible blood.

Isoalloxazine A heterocyclic yellow flavin that is a constituent of *riboflavin* together with ribose.

Isoascorbic acid A geometric isomer of ascorbic acid with only slight vitamin C activity.

Isobar Any one of two or more atoms having the same atomic weight but different atomic numbers.

Isocaloric Of equal caloric or energy value.

Isocitric acid An intermediate compound in the *Krebs cycle* formed by the reversible interconversions of citric, *cis*-aconitic, and isocitric acids by the removal and addition of water.

Isoelectric Having the same electric charge.

Isoelectric point (**IEP**) The pH at which a dipolar ion such as an amino acid carries both negative and positive charges and bears a net charge of zero. At this pH, amino acids become electrically neutral, do not migrate in an electric field, and therefore precipitate from solution.

Isoenzyme Isozyme; multiple molecular form of an enzyme that catalyzes the same reaction. For example, lactic acid dehydrogenase occurs in five forms.

Isoionic point (**pI**) 1. The pH of a protein solution at which the ions are equally combined with or dissociated from the protein. 2. Point at which the number of protons dissociated from proton donors in a system equals the number of protons combined with proton acceptors.

Isoleucine Alpha-amino-beta-methylvaleric acid, an essential amino acid rarely limiting in foods.

Isomaltose An isomer of maltose obtained during the hydrolysis of certain polysaccharides with alpha-1,6 glucosidic linkage.

Isomer One of two or more compounds having the same kind and number of atoms but differing in the atomic arrangement in the molecule.

Isomerase 1. Enzyme that catalyzes the interconversion of aldose and ketose sugars. For example, *phosphohexose isomerase* catalyzes the interconversion of glucose-6-phosphate and fructose-6-phosphate. 2. Group term given to a large variety of enzymes that catalyze reactions involving isomerization. Examples are *epimerase, mutase, racemase,* and *transferase.*

Isomerization Process whereby an isomer, whether structural or spatial, is converted into another. Examples are the interconversion of glucose-6-phosphate and fructose-6-phosphate, UDP-glucose and UDP-galactose, and glucose-6-phosphate and glucose-1-phosphate.

Isomil A milk-free formula made with soy protein, soy and corn oils, corn sugar, sucrose, and added vitamins and minerals. (Ross.) See Proprietary foods: composition, features, and uses, Appendix P-1.

Isomorph One of two or more substances having the same crystalline form but of different composition.

Isoniazid Generic name for isonicotinic acid hydrazide.

Isonicotinic acid hydrazide (INH) Isonicotinyl hydrazide, an antituberculosis drug. Its prolonged administration induces pyridoxine deficiency by forming a hydrazone of pyridoxal and its phosphate, making the vitamin unavailable for enzyme reaction.

Isoriboflavin An isomer of riboflavin containing the two methyl groups in the 5,6 instead of the 6,7 positions. Acts as a metabolic antagonist and competes with the vitamin.

Isosmotic Having a uniform osmotic pressure.

An *isosmotic solution* contains the same number of particles per unit volume; hence it is capable of exerting the same osmotic pressure when separated from water by a membrane impermeable to the solute.

Isotonic Having a uniform tension; maintaining a normal state of tonus. In physiology, pertains to a solution in a tissue, especially red blood cells, that has the same osmotic pressure as the body fluids.

Isotopes Atoms or elements that have the same atomic number but different atomic weights. Of the element hydrogen, three isotopes are recognized: protium (^{1}H), deuterium (^{2}H), and tritium (^{3}H). Some isotopes occur in nature as minor constituents, whereas others are prepared in nuclear reactions as fission products of certain heavy elements or by bombardment of atoms by protons, neutrons, or alpha particles. See Applications of isotopes in biology and medicine, Appendix N.

Radioactive i Isotope with an unstable nucleus that undergoes spontaneous decomposition while emitting radiation. Radioactive isotopes occur in nature in trace amounts, but they are generally prepared by artificial means. Some radioactive isotopes of medical and biologic significance are iodine 131, phosphorus 32, gold 198, strontium 90, cobalt 60, and sodium 24. See also *Half-life.*

Stable i Isotope with a nucleus that does not undergo decay. These isotopes are used to prepare "tagged" or labeled compounds and are also helpful in studying biochemical reactions. Commonly used are deuterium, carbon 14, nitrogen 15, and oxygen 17.

Isozyme See *Isoenzyme.*

IU Abbreviation for *international unit.*

IV Abbreviation for *intravenous.*

❧ J ❧

Jaundice Icterus. The yellowish discoloration of the skin, mucous membranes, and certain body fluids due to the accumulation of bile pigments in the blood. It may be due to increased production of bile pigments from hemoglobin or may result from the failure of the liver to excrete bilirubin because of injury to the liver cells or obstruction to the flow of bile. Jaundice is generally classified into three types—hemolytic, obstructive, and toxic.

Hemolytic j Due to abnormally large destruction of red blood cells such as occurs in pernicious anemia, malaria, yellow fever, and other infections. There is increased production of bile pigments from hemoglobin in excess of the amount that can be excreted by the normal, healthy liver.

Obstructive j Due to complete or partial interference in the flow of bile anywhere along its course from the hepatic lobules to the duodenum. The obstruction may be due to the presence of gallstones, parasites, tumors, or inflammation or narrowing of the mucosa of the common bile duct.

Toxic j Due to damage or injury of the liver cells by toxic substances such as various poisons, drugs, and viral infections. The agent prevents the damaged liver from manufacturing bile and therefore causes a damming of the pigments into the bloodstream.

Jejunal A minimal residue *elemental diet* consisting of chemically pure amino acids, simple carbohydrates, trace of safflower oil, and added vitamins and minerals. (Johnson & Johnson.) See proprietary foods: composition, features, and uses, Appendix P-1.

Jejunostomy Creation of an artificial opening through the abdominal wall into the jejunum. *Jejunocecostomy* is the surgical formation of an anastomosis between the jejunum and the cecum. *Jejunocolostomy* is the surgical formation of an anastomosis between the jejunum and the colon. *Jejunojejunostomy* is the surgical formation of an anastomosis between two parts of the jejunum.

Jejunum The second portion of the small intestine between the duodenum and the ileum; it is about 8 feet long. *Jejunitis* is inflammation of the jejunum. *Jejunectomy* is the excision of all or part of the jejunum.

Joint *Junction* between two or more bones of the skeleton for articulation or movement. There are many types, depending on the kind of movement they permit, such as ball-and-socket joint (hip and shoulder), hinge joint (elbow, knee, and ankle), and pivot joint (head). The joints between the various bones in the skull are immovable.

Joule In the metric system, energy is measured in joules. One joule (J) equals 4.184 calories. The American Institute of Nutrition has proposed that the joule be used as the unit of energy in nutrition.

Junction Place of meeting or of coming together, as of two different organs or types of tissues.

Junket The precipitated protein of milk casein together with the fat but leaving behind the clear whey.

Juxtaposition Placing close together, side by side.

❦ K ❧

K 40 Potassium 40, a radioactive isotope naturally present in the body. Potassium 40 measurement is a new approach in the determination of body composition. It is based on the assumption that body potassium is found in constant concentration in the muscle and lean portions of the body but is not present in fat. Body potassium therefore becomes an index of lean body mass.

Kadji's test Test for *scurvy*. Blood is analyzed for ascorbic acid content before and after intramuscular injection of 200 mg ascorbic acid in saline solution. A rise in plasma concentration of less than 0.2 mg% 4 hours after administration of the vitamin is indicative of scurvy.

Kalemia Presence of potassium in the blood. See *Hyperkalemia*.

Kaolin A native hydrated aluminum silicate used externally as a dusting powder for skin diseases. Internally it is useful in various forms of enteritis because of its power to absorb moisture. *Kaopectate* is a proprietary adsorbent for intestinal disorders; it contains kaolin and pectin.

Karyotyping Mapping of the chromosomes of a cell.

Keloid Fibrous growth at the site of a scar that is sometimes tender and painful. It is usually elevated, firm, and whitish or pink with irregular borders; it tends to recur even after removal.

Kerasin A cerebroside occurring in the brain. On hydrolysis, it yields 4-sphingenine, galactose, and lignoceric acid (a fatty acid).

Keratin Insoluble protein of hair, hooves, nails, and feathers. Contains a large amount of sulfur and is a commercial source of the amino acid cystine. Not hydrolyzed by digestive enzymes of man.

Keratinization Process of becoming horny due to the development of *keratin*. In vitamin A deficiency, keratinization of epithelial tissue occurs throughout the body, first in the salivary glands and then in the respiratory tract, eyes, and skin. Secondary infections from keratinization of the respiratory tract lead to pneumonia; in the reproductive tract, keratinization leads to sterility in male rats and resorption gestation in female rats; in the eyes, it leads to *xerophthalmia*.

Keratitis Inflammation of the cornea. May be due to infection, vitamin A deficiency, allergy, or injury to the eye.

Keratoconus A cone-shaped deformity of the cornea. The etiology is not established, although it has been shown that lack of vitamin E in the diet of rats occasionally causes keratoconus as well as other ocular disturbances. Treatment with calcium and vitamins E and D has been reported to benefit some patients with progressive keratoconus; however, the results have not been confirmed.

Keratomalacia Softening and necrosis of the cornea of the eye. The earliest sign is dryness of the conjunctiva, which may lead to ulceration and blindness. This eye lesion is associated with vitamin A deficiency.

Keratosis Any skin disease characterized by

horny growth. *Follicular keratosis* is characterized by dry, rough, scaly skin with appearance of goose pimples or prominent projections about the hair follicles. The follicles are blocked with plugs of keratin derived from their epithelial lining, which has undergone squamous metaplasia. This is seen in vitamin A deficiency.

Keratosulfate A mucopolysaccharide found in nails.

Kernicterus Deposition of bile pigment in the basal nuclei of the brain accompanied by degeneration of the nerve cells. Often associated with *erythroblastosis fetalis.*

Keto- Prefix denoting the presence of the ketone or carbonyl group (C=O). A *keto acid* is a compound that contains both the carbonyl group (C=O) and the carboxyl group (—COOH).

Ketogenesis Formation of ketone bodies or acetone bodies in the liver. Ketone bodies formed in the liver are oxidized in other tissues, especially in the muscles. When ketogenesis exceeds ketolysis (i.e., oxidation), ketone bodies accumulate and cause *ketosis.*

Ketogenic Capable of being converted into ketone bodies. The ketogenic substances in metabolism are the fatty acids and certain amino acids. See also *Ketogenic amino acid* under *Amino acid;* and *Diet, ketogenic.*

Ketogenic-antiketogenic ratio Ratio between those substances in the diet that give rise to ketone bodies (ketogenic factors) and those substances that tend to prevent the accumulation of ketone bodies (antiketogenic factors). The *ketogenic factors* are precursors of ketone bodies such as fatty acids and the ketogenic amino acids. The *antiketogenic factors* are precursors of glucose; these include the carbohydrates, glucogenic amino acids, and the glycerol portion of fat. For clinical purposes, the following simplified ratio may be used:

$$\frac{\text{Ketogenic factors}}{\text{Antiketogenic factors}} = \frac{0.5\ P + 0.9\ F}{0.5\ P + 0.1\ F + 1.0\ C}$$

where P, F, and C represent, respectively, the grams of protein, fat, and carbohydrate metabolized. A ketogenic/antiketogenic ratio of 3:1 will produce a state of ketosis.

Ketogenic hormone Hormone that increases the production of acetone or ketone bodies. It is said to lower the level of blood lipids, depress the metabolic rate, and increase the specific dynamic effect of protein.

Ketohexose A monosaccharide consisting of a 6-carbon chain (hexose) and a ketone group. Examples are fructose and sorbose.

Ketolysis Oxidation of ketone bodies to completion, i.e., carbon dioxide and water.

Ketone Compound containing the carbonyl group (C=O); derived from the oxidation of a secondary alcohol.

Ketone bodies Also called acetone bodies; collective term given to the intermediate products of fatty acid degradation. These are *acetoacetic acid, beta-hydroxybutyric acid,* and *acetone,* which are believed to stem from acetoacetyl CoA. They are present in the blood in very small amounts under ordinary conditions. Ketone bodies formed in the liver are normally oxidized in other tissues. However, ketone bodies tend to accumulate when the rate of production becomes so excessive that the organism cannot burn them at a sufficiently rapid rate. See *Ketosis.*

Ketonemia Presence of ketone (acetone) bodies in the blood above normal levels.

Ketonil A commercially prepared product free of phenylalanine.

Ketonuria Presence of ketone (acetone) bodies in the urine.

Ketose Carbohydrate containing the ketone group. Fructose is a ketose.

Ketosis Clinical condition in which *ketone bodies* accumulate in the blood and appear in the urine; characterized by a sweetish acetone odor of the breath. Ketosis may be caused by a disturbance in carbohydrate metabolism (as in uncontrolled diabetes mellitus), by a dietary intake quite low in carbohydrate but very high in fat (as in ketogenic diet), or by a diminution in carbohydrate catabolism with consequent high mobilization of body fats (as in starvation). Uncontrolled ketosis leads to *acidosis*. It causes a decrease in the alkali reserve in plasma, hyperventilation and a low CO_2 tension in alveolar air, an increase in urinary ammonia, and in advanced states a low blood pH.

Ketoxylose Xylulose; one of the few L-sugars found in nature. It is excreted in the urine of humans with a hereditary abnormality in pentose metabolism.

Kidney One of a pair of bean-shaped organs located in the back of the abdominal cavity on either side of the spine just below the spleen on the left and the liver on the right. The functioning unit is the *nephron,* which consists of a *glomerulus,* or tuft of capillaries, that is surrounded by *Bowman's capsule.* This capsule is attached to a long winding *tubule* through which passes the fluid from the blood contained in the glomerulus. Urine is produced in the nephron and emptied into the *pelvis* of the kidney. From here, urine flows into the *ureter,* which is a muscular tube extending from the kidney to the *urinary bladder.* The chief functions of the kidney are to maintain a constant blood composition and volume by its unique filtering system; to maintain a normal pH of body fluids, which is accomplished by excreting an acid urine and by synthesizing ammonia whenever necessary; and to excrete body wastes or metabolic by-products. See also *Urine.*

Kidney clearance test Test of *kidney function* by measuring the ability to excrete waste products such as urea, inulin, or dye in the urine. The quantity excreted per minute divided by the amount present in 1 ml of plasma is the urinary clearance.

Kilocalorie See *Calorie.*

Kinase A substance that activates an enzyme. The term also refers to the enzyme that catalyzes the transfer of phosphate from adenosine triphosphate to an acceptor.

Kinematics Science of motion, including the movements of the body.

Kinetic Pertaining to motion; producing motion. *Kinetic energy* is the capacity to do work as a result of motion.

Kinin Type of naturally occurring plant growth factor, often classed as a *phytohormone.* Can stimulate cell division and has been isolated from tobacco and apple fruitlets.

Kjeldahl method Method of determining the amount of nitrogen in an organic compound by digestion with sulfuric acid and conversion to ammonia. Nitrogen is calculated by measuring the amount of ammonia formed. In foodstuffs, most of the nitrogen comes from protein (about 16% nitrogen). Thus the *crude protein* content in foods may be determined by multiplying the total "Kjeldahl nitrogen" by the factor 6.25.

Knoop theory Also called beta-oxidation theory; a theory of fatty acid oxidation as formulated by Knoop. It maintains that fatty acids are oxidized at the beta carbon. See *Beta oxidation.*

Koagulations vitamin See *Vitamin K.*

Kofranyi-Michaelis respirometer Lightweight portable *respirometer* that makes possible the systematic measurement of energy expenditure during work. The instrument weighs only about 5 pounds and can be worn on the back.

Koilonychia Spoon-shaped nails; a nail deformity in which the outer surface becomes concave.

Koladex Cola-flavored beverage containing 100 gm dextrose/10-ounce bottle. It is used for the standard glucose tolerance test.

Korsakoff's syndrome Set of symptoms characterized by confusion, loss of memory, and irresponsibility. Seen in chronic alcoholism; probably due to nutritive deficiency, particularly thiamin.

Kosher foods Foods used in accordance with the dietary laws of Orthodox Judaism. Milk and meat are not consumed at the same meal. Meat must be prepared by an ordained slaughterer (shochet) and cleaned (koshered) by soaking in water, salting, and washing. Meat from cloven-hooved animals that chew their cud such as cows, sheep, and goats may be eaten. Fish that have fins and scales may be consumed. Pork, shellfish, and fish without scales and fins cannot be eaten.

Krebs cycle Tricarboxylic acid cycle (TCA) or citric acid cycle. It is a cycle of reactions in which acetylcoenzyme A combines with oxalacetate, forming seven intermediary products—*citrate, cis-aconitate, isocitrate, alpha-ketoglutarate, succinate, fumarate,* and *malate*—and eventually reforming *oxalacetate,* which is set free to unite with another molecule of acetylcoenzyme A, thus repeating the cycle. The Krebs cycle is considered the final common pathway in the oxidation of carbohydrate, protein, and fat to carbon dioxide and water with the release of energy. The acetylcoenzyme A that unites with oxalacetate may come from the anaerobic phase of carbohydrate metabolism, from fatty acid breakdown, and indirectly from ketogenic amino acids. Some of the intermediate products in the cycle may also be formed from glucogenic amino acids and during fatty acid breakdown. For details, see Interrelationship of carbohydrate, protein, and fat, Appendix E.

Krebs-Henseleit cycle Also called ornithine cycle in urea formation. See *Ornithine* and *Urea.*

Kreis test Test for oxidative rancidity of fats. A fat sample is treated with a solution of phloroglucinol in ether and hydrochloric acid. Rancid fat develops a pink color due to the presence of epihydrin aldehyde or malonaldehyde.

Kwashiorkor Nutritional deficiency disease due to inadequate intake of protein; occurs principally in children shortly after weaning to a diet high in starch and low in protein. It is characterized by retarded growth, anemia, edema, fatty infiltration of the liver, pigmentary changes of the skin and hair, gastrointestinal disorders, muscle wasting, and psychomotor changes. Recent studies have shown that nutrients other than protein are involved. Magnesium and potassium depletion may be serious. Nonnutritional factors such as infections, parasites, and faulty food habits due to cultural reasons are other etiologic agents.

Kynureninase Enzyme present in mammalian liver that catalyzes the cleavage of kynurenine to yield *anthranilic acid* and *alanine.*

Kynurenine An intermediate product in tryptophan metabolism. Kynurenine in mammalian liver may be hydrolyzed to anthranilic acid and alanine, requiring pyridoxal phosphate as a cofactor. Large amounts of kynurenine are excreted in the urine in pyridoxine deficiency. It is found in normal urine in trace amounts but may be temporarily increased after tryptophan administration.

Kyphosis Also called *humpback.* Abnormal curvature of the spine. Often the result of bad posture, vitamin D deficiency, or certain types of arthritis.

L

Labeled substance A substance that is marked or tagged using the isotope tracer technique to permit the scientist to follow its fate in metabolic reactions. Isotopes of common elements such as carbon, nitrogen, oxygen, and hydrogen are usually employed. See also *Isotopes.*

Labile Unstable.

Lactalbumin One of the milk proteins; the others are casein and lactoglobulin. It is identical to serum albumin and is not easily precipitated by acids. The soft flocculent curds are easier to digest in contrast to the large hard curds of casein. Thus the higher ratio of lactalbumin to casein in human milk (one half of human milk protein is lactalbumin) is an advantage for infant feeding. Although the total amount of protein in cow's milk is about two times that of human milk protein, the ratio of lactalbumin to casein is only 1:5. Also the higher lactose/protein ratio in human milk is favorable. See *Lactose* and *Infant feeding.*

Lactase Enzyme that splits lactose to glucose and galactose. It is present in the intestines of all young mammals but may be lacking in mature mammals and in individuals with certain disorders such as tropical sprue and celiac disease. See also *Lactose intolerance.*

Lactation The period of milk secretion; the secretion of milk by the mammary gland. The amount of milk produced is affected by several factors, including nutritional status of the mother, frequency of sucking by the young, ingestion of medicinal or food *galactogogues,* and hormonal control. See *Estrogen, Oxytocin,* and *Luteotropic hormone.*

Lacteals Tiny vessels in the villi of the wall of the small intestine through which chylomicrons are absorbed. These ducts empty into the lymphatic system.

Lactic acid $CH_3CHOH \cdot COOH$; an acid produced by fermenting lactose (milk sugar); also formed from sucrose, glucose, or maltose by the action of lactic acid bacteria. In mammalian tissues, lactic acid is formed by the reduction of pyruvate when oxygen is lacking and pyruvate cannot be oxidized and channeled into the *Krebs cycle.* It is also produced in the tissues during muscle contraction when energy needs are met by the glycolysis of glycogen to lactic acid. See also *Cori cycle.*

Lactic dehydrogenase (LDH) Enzyme that reversibly catalyzes the reduction of pyruvic acid to lactic acid or the oxidation of lactic acid to pyruvic acid. It is present in the tissues and released into the blood when there is tissue necrosis, as in liver damage, myocardial infarction, and renal tubular necrosis.

***Lactobacillus bifidus* factor** See *Bifidus factor.*

***Lactobacillus bulgaricus* factor (LBF)** A growth factor for certain microorganisms identical to pantothenic acid.

***Lactobacillus casei* factor (LCF)** Former name for folic acid or *pteroylglutamic acid.*

Lactoflavin Riboflavin of milk; the name

given to the greenish yellow fluorescent flavin pigment of whey. A former name is lactochrome. See *Vitamin B₂*.

Lactogenic hormone See *Luteotropic hormone*.

Lactone Protein-rich food mixture in India; contains groundnut flour, skim milk powder, wheat and barley flour, vitamins, and calcium.

Lactose Also called milk sugar; a disaccharide that occurs naturally only in the milk of mammals. It is hydrolyzed by acid or enzyme action, specifically *lactase*, yielding glucose and galactose. Lactose is less sweet and less readily digested than other disaccharides. Thus some of it reaches the lower intestinal tract where *Lactobacillus* organisms change it to lactic acid and other organic acids. This acid medium aids in the absorption of many nutrients (amino acids, calcium, iron, and thiamin) and prevents the growth of putrefactive bacteria, lessening the incidence of gastrointestinal disturbances. The amount of lactose in human milk is almost twice that in cow's milk and the higher lactose/protein ratio is an added advantage of breast feeding. Excessive dietary intakes of lactose have been shown to induce cataract, impair growth, and cause demineralization of bones in animals. Too much lactose residue in the large intestines has a laxative effect and may cause diarrhea.

Lactose intolerance Lactose malabsorption is believed to be an inborn error of metabolism due to a lack of intestinal *lactase*. It is characterized by failure to grow and diarrhea in infants. In adults, diarrhea seems to disappear with prolonged intake of lactose, indicating that intestinal lactase might be an adaptive enzyme. See also *Diet, lactose-free*.

Lactum Milk formula for routine infant feeding. It is cow's milk with added corn sugar, lactose, vitamins, and minerals. (Mead Johnson.) See Proprietary foods: composition, features, and uses, Appendix P-1.

Laënnec's cirrhosis Also called portal or alcoholic cirrhosis; a form of cirrhosis that is the end result of prolonged dietary inadequacy, particularly of protein, coupled with the toxic effects of alcohol on the liver. See *Cirrhosis*.

Lambase Hypoallergenic formula for infants sensitive to milk; made with meat protein (lamb heart), corn oil, sucrose, and corn sugar with added vitamins and minerals. (Gerber.) See Proprietary foods: composition, features, and uses, Appendix P-1.

Lamina propria Connective tissue layer of a mucous membrane.

Lathyrism Neurologic disease that results from the ingestion of the seeds of plants from the genus *Lathyrus*. It is characterized by feeling of heaviness of the legs followed by weakness, jerky gait, tingling sensations in various parts of the body, and complete loss of sensation to heat and pain. See also *Osteolathyrism*.

Laubina Protein food mixture developed in Lebanon; contains wheat flour, chick-pea, sesame, skim milk, minerals, vitamins A and D, thiamin, niacin, and riboflavin.

Lauric acid A saturated fatty acid containing 12 carbon atoms; found in coconut oil, laurel oil, spermaceti, etc.

Lavage The washing out of an organ such as the stomach or bowel.

Laxative A substance that accelerates intestinal elimination. It is more specifically termed a *purgative* if it increases peristalsis. Examples are Epsom salts and castor oil.

LBF Abbreviation for *Lactobacillus bulgaricus factor*.

LBM Abbreviation for *lean body mass*.

LCT Abbreviation for *long-chain triglycerides*.

LDH Abbreviation for *lactic dehydrogenase*. See also *Serum enzymes*.

Lead Not a dietary need but of special interest because its effects are cumulative and highly toxic. Lead is naturally present in water and food in trace amounts and may be accidentally ingested from insecticides and old paint. Lead-containing solders, glazes, and enamels should not be used for cooking and storing food. See *Plumbism*.

Leaf protein Powdered product prepared from green leaves and grass that is incorporated into other foods as a rich source of protein.

Lean body mass (LBM) Active tissue mass; the part of the body weight concerned with energy metabolism. It is a measure of body composition, taken as the difference between body weight and the total mass of the adipose tissue, the extracellular fluid, and the skeleton.

Lecithin Phosphatidyl choline, a phosphatide consisting of glycerol, two molecules of fatty acids, phosphoric acid, and choline. It is widely distributed in animal cells, especially nerves. Lecithin biosynthesis depends on a dietary supply of methyl groups or choline. Lecithin exists in the cell as a dipolar ion; choline is a strong base and phosphoric acid is a moderately strong acid. This is significant in fat transport. See *Lipotropic agent* and *Phospholipid*.

Lesion An injury or cut; any loss of function of a part of the body.

Leucine Alpha-aminoisocaproic acid; an *essential amino acid* that is strongly ketogenic; acetoacetic acid is its chief catabolic product in the liver.

Leucine-induced hypoglycemia Hypoglycemia observed in certain infants after the ingestion of L-leucine. It is believed to be a hereditary defect, but the exact mechanism of its genetic transmission is not yet known. The diet restricts the ingestion of leucine to the minimum daily requirement of 150 mg/kg body weight. See *High protein, carbohydrate-restricted diet* under *Diet, protein modified* and Dietary management of selected disorders, Appendix O.

Leucovorin Synthetic folic acid. It is also called folinic acid-SF (synthetic factor). See *Pteroylglutamic acid*.

Leukemia Type of blood cancer due to proliferation of leukocytes and decreased production of red blood cells. The etiology is unknown, although ionizing radiation, the effect of certain chemicals, heredity, and hormonal abnormalities may be causative factors. Some patients with leukemia have been successfully treated with aminopterin and other folic acid antagonists.

Leukocyte (leucocyte) Also called white blood cell (WBC); the nonpigmented nucleated cell of the blood. White blood cells play an important role in the body's defense mechanism. They can destroy disease-causing organisms. The normal WBC count is about 5000 to 10,000/mm³. This is increased in acute infections and leukemia and decreased in *leukopenia*.

Leukopenia An abnormal reduction in the number of white blood cells as a result of decreased production by the bone marrow or increased destruction of the cells, usually in the spleen. The condition may be congenital or brought about by malignancy, folic acid deficiency, or some unknown causative factor (pernicious type).

Levan Also called fructosan; a *homopolysaccharide* composed of fructose units. It is derived chiefly from Jerusalem artichokes and certain grasses. *Inulin* is a levan.

Levulose Another name for *fructose* or fruit sugar to indicate that it is levorotatory.

LH Abbreviation for *luteinizing hormone*.

Licorice Black flavoring extract made from the root of a European plant. It contains glycyrrhizic acid, an agent that can cause hypertension and hypokalemia when taken in large amounts.

Liebermann-Burchard reaction Test for unsaturated sterols. It is used for the quantitative determination of cholesterol. The test sample in solution turns green when treated with chloroform, acetic anhydride, and concentrated sulfuric acid.

Lien Spleen. *Lienitis* is inflammation of the spleen. *Lienopathy* is any disorder of the spleen.

Life expectancy Number of years an adult man or woman can expect to live. There is a definite relationship between correct weight and preservation of health and, subsequently, life expectancy.

Ligament Connective tissue that is a tough fibrous band. It connects articular ends of bones and supports visceral organs.

Ligases New name for a group of enzymes that catalyze the linking of two compounds coupled with the breaking of a pyrophosphate bond. An example of a ligase is acetic thiokinase, which catalyzes the reaction:

$$\text{Acetate} + \text{CoASH} + \text{ATP} \rightarrow \text{Acetyl}$$
$$\text{CoA} + \text{AMP} + \text{P-P}$$

Light adaptation Changes occurring in the eye opposite in nature to those observed in *dark adaptation,* i.e., constriction of the pupil, diminished sensitivity of the retina, bleaching of the visual purple, and a change of pH from an alkaline to an acid reaction.

Lignin An indigestible carbohydrate. A constituent of *crude fiber* occurring in the cell wall of plants. It is resistant to hydrolysis by digestive enzymes, strong acids, and alkalies and is not attacked to any extent by intestinal microorganisms.

Lignoceric acid Fatty acid containing 24 carbon atoms that is present in cerebrosides and sphingomyelins.

Line test Biologic test for the extent of calcification, using rats as the test animals. Calcified areas of the longitudinal section of rat *tibias* are stained with silver nitrate and x-ray films are made. A wide concave epiphyseal line and coarse *trabeculae* are evident in a rachitic animal. In a normal animal the space between the *epiphysis* and shaft of the long bone is narrow. This is an accepted procedure for measuring vitamin D potency of foods.

Linoleic acid An *essential fatty acid;* a polyunsaturated fatty acid with two double bonds and 18 carbon atoms. It is found in linseed, safflower, cottonseed, and soybean oils, fish oils, and animal tissues. Human milk contains about four times more linoleic acid than cow's milk. Linoleic acid

is a dietary essential (i.e., the body cannot synthesize it) as well as a nutrient requirement (promotes growth and prevents dermatitis). The omission of linoleic acid together with two other polyunsaturated fatty acids, *linolenic* and *arachidonic* acids, from the diet of rats results in failure of growth and reproduction, dermatitis, and impaired fat utilization. There is no reported essential fatty acid syndrome in adults due to dietary deficiency. However, infants receiving milk formula lacking in polyunsaturated fatty acids develop an infantile eczema characterized by leathery skin with desquamation and oozing. Addition of trilinolein to the diet (from 5% to 7% of total calories) results in the disappearance of symptoms. The need for *essential fatty acids* will be met if linoleic acid is present in the diet at a level of at least 1% of total caloric requirement.

Linolenic acid Polyunsaturated fatty acid with three double bonds and 18 carbons that is found chiefly in linseed oil. It is considered a nutrient because of its growth-promoting effect, but it is not an antidermatitis factor. Linolenic acid is not a dietary essential since it can be synthesized in the body. See also *Linoleic acid* and *Fatty acid.*

Lipase Fat-splitting enzyme occurring in the pancreas, stomach, and certain plants. It hydrolyzes fats into fatty acids and glycerol. See Summary of digestive enzymes, Appendix J-1.

Lipemia An increased level of blood lipids. A *temporary absorptive lipemia* occurs after a fatty meal as chylomicrons discharged into the blood plasma cause a rapid rise of lipid, chiefly as triglycerides along with a small amount of protein. *Idiopathic lipemia* (unknown etiology) is frequently observed in diabetic acidosis and glycogen storage disease.

Lipid Member of a large group of organic compounds insoluble in water and soluble in fat solvents, e.g., chloroform, ether, benzene, petroleum, and carbon disulfide.

Lipids of nutritional importance are fatty acids, particularly essential fatty acids; triglycerides; phosphatides, especially lecithins; terpenes, especially carotene; and steroids such as cholesterol and the adrenocortical steroids. See Classification of lipids, Appendix C-3.

Lipid malabsorption Interference with lipid absorption brought about by bile deficiency, a lack of the pancreatic enzyme *lipase,* defective intramucosal metabolism (as in nontropical sprue and adrenal hormone insufficiency), lymphatic obstruction, and impaired lipoprotein synthesis.

Lipochromes Plant pigments that are soluble in fats and organic solvents. Examples are chlorophyll and carotenoids.

Lipogenesis 1. Synthesis of lipids or formation of body fat. 2. Specifically, the formation of fatty acids in the liver. Any dietary constituent, that supplies acetate (e.g., carbohydrate and protein metabolites) may contribute to lipogenesis. In obese persons the rate of lipogenesis may be five times greater than normal.

Lipoic acid 6,8-Dithio-*n*-octanoic acid, a cyclic disulfide. It is also called thioctic acid, protogen, pyruvate oxidation factor (POF), and *L. casei* acetate factor. It is needed for oxidative decarboxylation of alpha keto acids such as pyruvic and alpha-ketoglutaric acid. Lipoic acid functions as a hydrogen and acyl acceptor. It is an essential growth factor for various organisms. Although its function is closely associated with thiamin, lipoic acid is not considered a vitamin since it appears to be synthesized in adequate amounts in the mammalian cell. See also *Lipothiamide pyrophosphate.*

Lipoid A substance resembling fat in appearance and solubility but containing groups other than glycerol and fatty acids, which make up the true fats.

Lipolysis 1. Breakdown or degradation of lipids. 2. Specifically, the splitting of fat into glycerol and fatty acids in the liver. Glycerol enters the pathway of carbohy-

drate metabolism as glycerol-3-phosphate. The fatty acids are degraded by a series of reactions leading to the ultimate product, *acetyl CoA.* See also the *Knoop theory* and *Beta oxidation.*

Lipolytic hypothesis Theory of fat digestion and absorption that supports the view that fats are completely (or almost completely) digested in the small intestine and to some extent in the stomach into fatty acids and glycerol. See also *Partition hypothesis.*

Lipomul-Oral A corn oil emulsion providing 90 calories/15 ml. It is used as a concentrated source of calories in protein-restricted diets or after extensive surgery. (Upjohn.) See Proprietary foods: composition, features, and uses, Appendix P-1.

Lipoprotein Compound protein formed when a simple protein unites with a lipid. It has the solubility characteristics of protein; hence it is involved in lipid transport. Four types circulate in the blood: chylomicrons, alpha lipoproteins (high density lipoprotein [HDL]), prebeta lipoproteins, (very low density lipoprotein [VLDL]), and beta lipoproteins (low density lipoprotein [LDL]). See *Blood lipids* and *Hyperlipoproteinemia.*

Lipoprotein lipase Also called *clearing factor;* this lipase catalyzes the hydrolysis of fats present in chylomicrons and lipoproteins. It is found in various tissues and is important in the mobilization of fatty acids from depot fats.

Lipositol Phosphatidyl inositol. See Classification of lipids, Appendix C-3.

Lipothiamide pyrophosphate (LTPP) A conjugate of thiamin pyrophosphate and *lipoic acid* believed to be the active catalyst in the oxidative decarboxylation of alpha keto acids such as pyruvic acid.

Lipotropic agent (factor) Any substance capable of transporting or mobilizing fat and preventing or correcting the fatty liver of choline deficiency. The lipotropic agents are choline, betaine, methionine, inositol, serine, and lecithin. The exact mechanism of how these substances prevent fatty livers is not known. However, it has been suggested that neutral fats are converted to choline containing *phospholipids* to mobilize the fat and thus prevent deposition in the liver.

Liprotein Powder A high protein, high fat, low carbohydrate dietary supplement with added vitamins; used to increase calories and protein. (Upjohn.) See Proprietary foods: composition, features, and uses, Appendix P-1.

Lithiasis Formation of stones or calculi, as in cholelithiasis and pancreatic lithiasis.

Liver Also called hepatic gland; largest gland of the body, comprising about 3% of body weight, and located in the upper right quadrant of the abdomen. It is said that no other organ is concerned with so many and such varied functions as the liver so that it is fittingly called the "warehouse and chemical manufacturer" of the body. Its physiologic roles include manufacture of vital substances (bile, prothrombin, fibrinogen, heparin, and urea); regulation of bodily processes (detoxification, reticuloendothelial activity, blood volume, and blood sugar level); metabolism (carbohydrate, protein, lipid, vitamins, and minerals); and storage of nutrients and other substances (protein reserves, glycogen, iron, copper, vitamins A, D, K, and some B complex vitamins).

Liver filtrate factor Obsolete name for *pantothenic acid*.

Liver function test Test for the integrity of the liver through its functional capacity; examples include hippuric acid test (to determine the ability of the liver to synthesize hippuric acid from benzoic acid), galactose tolerance test (to determine the efficiency of the liver to convert galactose to glycogen), cephalin flocculation test (to find out the extent of protein synthesis), and Bromsulphalein test (to measure the amount of a dye excreted in a given time).

Load test Also called saturation test; a method of assessing nutritional status for a particular nutrient by measuring urinary excretion after administration of a test dose to a person on a controlled intake. It is assumed that an individual whose tissues are saturated with the nutrient will retain little and excrete most of the dose, whereas one with low nutrient reserves will retain a large amount in order to saturate tissue levels.

Lofenalac Proprietary milk formula useful in the dietary management of *phenylketonuria*. The formula is prepared by enzymatic digestion of casein followed by chemical treatment to destroy phenylalanine. It is supplemented with methionine, tryptophan, tyrosine, corn oil, sugar, minerals, and vitamins. (Mead Johnson.) See Proprietary foods: composition, features, and uses, Appendix P-1.

Lohmann reaction Transfer of high-energy phosphate from adenosine triphosphate (ATP) to creatine phosphate. The source of energy in muscle stimulation is ATP, leaving adenosine diphosphate (ADP), which in turn is resynthesized to ATP by creatine phosphate during the recovery period.

Lonalac Low sodium proprietary milk useful in *sodium-restricted diets*, particularly in infants and children. It is prepared from casein, coconut oil, lactose, minerals, and vitamins. The composition is similar to that of whole milk. (Mead Johnson.) See Proprietary foods: composition, features, and uses, Appendix P-1.

Long-chain triglycerides (LCT) Fats containing fatty acids longer than lauric acid (C_{12}). Naturally occurring fats are composed predominantly of LCT containing palmitic (C_{16}), stearic (C_{18}), oleic (C_{18} with one double bond), and linoleic (C_{18} with two double bonds) acids. LCT should be restricted in the dietary treatment of *malabsorption syndromes* and replaced with *medium-chain triglycerides* (MCT).

Low sodium milk (LSM) Milk in which about 90% of its natural sodium is removed by an ion-exchange process. Several forms of low sodium milk are produced. Thiamin, riboflavin, and calcium contents are decreased during processing. The increase of potassium is not of concern since ordinary diets contain 3000 to 5000 mg potassium/day. One quart of low sodium milk may contain as much as 2300 mg potassium and as little as 50 mg sodium (1 quart of regular milk contains 500 mg sodium).

Low sodium syndrome Disturbance characterized by the following set of symptoms: weakness, lethargy, loss of appetite, nausea and vomiting, mental confusion, acid-base disturbance, abdominal pain with general muscular cramps, renal damage, oliguria and later uremia, and possibly convulsions and shock. It is caused by prolonged periods of very low sodium intake, adrenal cortical insufficiency, and marked losses of body fluids and electrolytes as in very hot weather or excessive perspiration, severe burns, marked diarrhea, and vomiting. Prompt provision of salt (15 to 20 gm) will correct the condition.

LSM Abbreviation for *low sodium milk*.

LTH Abbreviation for *luteotropic hormone*.

LTPP Abbreviation for *lipothiamide pyrophosphate*.

Lumen Cavity or channel within a tubular organ, such as in an artery, vein, or intestine.

Lungs Pair of viscera in the thoracic cavity that forms a vital respiratory organ. The right lung has three lobes and the left two. The lobes are covered with an external serous coat called the pleural membrane. The main function of the lungs is to aerate the blood. Oxygen is brought to all parts of the body, and carbon dioxide is carried back to the lungs for expiration.

Lupus vulgaris Tuberculous disease of the skin and mucous membrane marked by the formation of brownish nodules in the corium. Vitamin D and INH are used to treat this disease.

Luteinizing hormone (LH) Also called inter-stitial cell–stimulating hormone (ICSH); one of the *gonadotropic hormones* that provokes ovulation and the formation of the corpus luteum. It stimulates the interstitial cells of the ovary and testicle.

Luteotropic hormone (LTH) Also called luteotropin, prolactin, and lactogenic hormone; a hormone secreted by the anterior lobe of the hypophysis (pituitary gland). It helps in the development of the mammary glands and also initiates milk secretion. It stimulates the corpus luteum to synthesize progesterone and estrogens.

Luxus konsumption Theory that normal people manage to keep their weight within reasonable limits by burning off any excess of food. Obese people are unable to do this.

Lyases New name for a group of enzymes that reversibly catalyze the removal of groups from substrates nonhydrolytically, leaving double bonds. An example is fumarase, which catalyzes the removal of water from malate to yield fumarate.

Lycopene The principal red pigment present in tomatoes, watermelon, and pink grapefruit. It is an isomer of carotene but has no vitamin A activity.

Lymph Fluid obtained from lymphatic ducts; one of the circulating fluids of the body. It is yellowish and alkaline in reaction. Occasionally it is pinkish due to the presence of some red blood cells. When fat globules are present it turns milky. It resembles blood plasma in appearance and composition except that lymph contains colorless cells, lymphocytes, and has a lower protein content than plasma. Its main function is to nourish and bathe cells by circulating substances from the blood into the tissues. It is believed to be important in fat absorption.

Lymph node Small bean-shaped body occurring at intervals along the lymphatic vessels. It removes foreign particles from the lymph by filtration and by *phagocytosis*.

Lymphocyte Type of white blood cell that arises in the reticular tissue of the lymph glands. The nucleus is single and surrounded by a nongranular protoplasm. The role of lymphocytes in antibody formation has been established.

Lyophilization Also called freeze drying; rapid freezing and drying under a vacuum (with controlled temperature and pressure). It is useful in biochemistry for protein fractionation and for making stable preparations of blood plasma, serum, and other tissues that are subject to decomposition.

Lysin A specific *antibody* with destructive action on cells and tissues, causing dissolution or breakdown.

Lysine An *essential amino acid;* the limiting amino acid in many cereal proteins, especially gliadin. Young rats fed a diet deficient in lysine show growth retardation and corneal vascularization. Deficiency in humans may cause nausea, vomiting, dizziness, and anemia in addition to growth failure in the young. In the tissues this basic amino acid readily converts its epsilon carbon to carbon dioxide and helps to form glutamic acid. However, it does not exchange its nitrogen with other circulating amino acids, a property unique to lysine.

Lysine intolerance Metabolic defect, probably congenital, caused by the inability to hydrolyze lysine. Symptoms include nausea, vomiting, and episodes of coma. Plasma levels of lysine, arginine, and ammonia are elevated. It is believed that the accumulation of lysine inhibits arginase action and therefore interferes with the *urea cycle.*

-lysis Combining form denoting *decomposition* or breakdown (as in glycolysis and lipolysis), *dissolution* or dissolving (as in dissolution of a blood clot), or *relief* or reduction (as in the decline of a disease or fever).

Lysolecithin A substance obtained by partial hydrolysis of lecithin with only one fatty acid liberated. It is a good detergent that aids in the emulsification of dietary lipids.

Lysophosphatides Substances that are destructive to red blood cells. They are produced from lecithin by the action of the enzyme lecithinase, which is present in the venom of poisonous snakes.

Lysosome Organelle found in the cytoplasm that contains hydrolytic enzymes capable of destroying the cell.

Lysozyme Enzyme that digests certain high molecular weight carbohydrates and some gram-positive bacteria. It is present in tears, saliva, mucous and nasal secretions, and other body fluids. It is a muramidase that catalyzes the hydrolysis of a muramic acid–containing mucoprotein found in the cell walls of many airborne cocci. This action of lysozyme protects the cornea from infection. Its activity is reduced by generalized malnutrition and particularly by vitamin A deficiency.

Lytren Oral electrolyte formula used in replacing water and electrolyte losses. (Mead Johnson.) See Proprietary foods: composition, features, and uses, Appendix P-1.

M

Macrocyte A giant red blood cell. *Macrocythemia* is an abnormal number of macrocytes in the blood. *Macrocytic anemia* is a type of anemia in which the red blood cells are unusually large.

Macronutrients Nutrients that are present in relatively high amounts in the body, constituting about 0.005% of body weight (50 ppm) or above. Protein, fat, water, and major minerals are macronutrients. See also *Nutrient classification*.

Macrophages Cells of the reticuloendothelial system; they ingest foreign particles such as bacteria and cellular debris by *phagocytosis*.

Magma 1. Suspension of finely divided material in a small amount of water. 2. Thin pastelike substance composed of organic material.

Magnesium A major mineral essential to plants and animals; a component of chlorophyll in green plants. In adults, it comprises about 0.05% of body weight, 60% of which is in bones and teeth; the rest is in soft tissues concentrated within the cells. The liver and muscles contain seven times more magnesium than the blood. As a cofactor in reactions involving adenosine triphosphate, magnesium is important in protein, fat, carbohydrate, and energy metabolism. Since it is widely distributed in nature, particularly in legumes, nuts, whole grains, and fish, an ordinary mixed diet contains an ample supply of magnesium. In conditioned magnesium deficiency, as in kwashiorkor, alcoholism, electrolyte imbalance, etc., a lack of magnesium affects the neuromuscular, cardiovascular, and renal systems. Magnesium deficiency is also seen in burns. It has been suggested that some of the psychiatric symptoms exhibited by many burned persons may be due to or aggravated by magnesium deficiency. For further details, see Summary of minerals, Appendix H.

Maidism Also called maidismus; former name for *pellagra*.

Maillard reaction Nonenzymatic browning reaction; a reaction between the free amino radical of proteins or amino acids and the free aldehyde group of carbohydrates or sugars forming brown pigments. It takes place on heating or prolonged storage of processed foods unless certain steps are taken to prevent the reaction.

Malabsorption syndrome Set of symptoms indicating defective absorption; may be functional or organic in origin. It could occur as a result of structural changes in the alimentary tract or its adjacent organs, failure of food to reach the absorptive surfaces, maldigestion, diversion of foodstuffs to intestinal organisms, or failure of the absorptive mechanism. Examples of disorders that show the malabsorption syndrome include *celiac disease, chronic pancreatitis, sprue, cystic fibrosis,* and *carbohydrate intolerance.*

Malacia Morbid softening or softness of a tissue or part as in *osteomalacia* or softening of bones.

Malassimilation Defective or incomplete assimilation, especially of nutrients, due to *malabsorption* or *maldigestion.*

Maldigestion An upset in the normal digestive processes resulting in nutritional deficiency.

Malformation Defective formation of a body part or parts.

Malignant Growing worse; resisting treatment; of cancerous growth.

Malnutrition 1. Simply stated, any disorder of nutrition; "bad" or undesirable health status due to either *lack* or *excess* of nutrient supply. 2. State of impaired biologic activity or development due to a discrepancy between the nutrient supply and the nutrient demand of cells. Malnutrition may be classified into three categories, i.e., malnutrition associated with poverty or or inadequate food supply; malnutrition associated with ignorance and indifference; and malnutrition secondary to such factors as diseases, alcoholism, drug abuse, and mental illness. See also *Nutritional deficiency* and *Deficiency disease.*

Maltase Also called alpha-glucosidase; an enzyme found in yeast and intestinal juice. It hydrolyzes *maltose* to two glucose units.

Maltose Malt sugar, a disaccharide hydrolyzed to two molecules of glucose by acid or the enzyme *maltase.* It does not occur free in the tissue, but is formed as an intermediate product of starch hydrolysis.

Mammary gland The milk-secreting gland. The breast is composed of three major parts: the lactiferous or mammary glands, the skin covering the breast, nipple, and areola, and the supporting fatty and connective tissue.

Manganese An essential trace mineral widely distributed in plant and animal cells. It is an activator of enzymes (arginase, leucine aminopeptidase, and bone phosphatase) and a cofactor in oxidative phosphorylation. It is needed in urea and hemoglobin formation, thyroxine production, and thiamin utilization. Main food sources are whole grains, legumes, leafy greens, meats, and seafoods. The human requirement is unknown, and there has been no report of manganese deficiency. However, experimentally induced manganese deficiency has been observed in animals. For further details, see Summary of minerals, Appendix H.

Manninotriose *Trisaccharide* formed by partial hydrolysis of stachyose. It is composed of one glucose and two galactose units.

Mannitol A sugar alcohol obtained from the hydrogenation of *mannose.* Commercially it is extracted from certain seaweeds. It has a sweetening power as does glucose but yields only half as many calories because it is only partially absorbed.

Mannose *Monosaccharide* containing six carbon atoms (a hexose); does not occur free in nature. It is found in legumes in the form of *mannosan,* a partially digestible polysaccharide.

Mannuronic acid A sugar acid resulting from the oxidation of the primary alcohol group of mannose to a carboxyl group. It occurs chiefly in alginic acid, a stabilizing and thickening agent.

Manometer Device for determining liquid or gaseous pressure. The *manometric technique* is commonly used in the study of tissue metabolism or cellular respiration.

MAO Abbreviation for *monoamine oxidase.*

Maple syrup urine disease (branched chain ketoaciduria) Inborn error of metabolism in which there is a block in the oxidative decarboxylation of the keto acids of the branched chain amino acids—valine, leucine, and isoleucine. Symptoms appear on the third to fifth day of life. Characteristic signs are urine that has a maple syrup odor, difficulty in feeding with jerky aspirations, cerebral disturbances, spasticity, and possibly death. The pathogenesis of the disease is related to the increased levels of valine, leucine, and isoleucine in the blood and urine. Threonine, serine, and alanine levels are reduced. Treatment consists of restricting the dietary intake of leucine, isoleucine, and valine.

Marasmus 1. Form of extreme undernutrition primarily due to a lack of calories and protein. 2. Infantile atrophy that occurs almost wholly as a sequel to acute disease, especially diarrheal diseases, and is characterized by loss of weight, loss of subcutaneous fat, and wasting of muscle tissue. See Dietary management of selected disorders, Appendix O.

Margin of safety See *Recommended dietary allowance.*

Marker Also called tracer; an indigestible material used to provide information on the amount of food or specific nutrient consumed and the extent and rate of its passage, digestibility, and utilization. Some markers are dyes, inert metals, radioactive materials, and microorganisms.

Mastitis Inflammation of the breast, particularly the *mammary glands;* a contraindication to breast feeding.

Maternal mortality rate (**MMR**) Number of women dying from causes directly related to childbearing per 10,000 live births during a calendar year.

Matrix The intercellular framework of a tissue, as of cartilage. See also *Bone* and *Organic matrix.*

Matter Anything that has mass and occupies space. The three general states of matter are solid, liquid, and gas.

Max Planck respirometer Portable apparatus based on the principle of *indirect calorimetry.* It measures the volume of expired air and simultaneously diverts a small fraction into a receptacle for subsequent analysis. See *Calorimetry.*

MCT Trade name and abbreviation for *medium-chain triglyceride.*

MDR Abbreviation for *minimum daily requirements.*

ME Abbreviation for *metabolizable energy.*

Meal Portion of food eaten at a particular time to satisfy the appetite. Meal patterns are plans or guides for the inclusion of certain foods at stated intervals during the day, usually for the main meals—breakfast, lunch, and supper.

Meals for Millions Foundation (**MMF**) International agency concerned with public health nutrition. It distributes *multipurpose food* free of charge to the poor and the sick.

Meals-on-Wheels Program started by The Lighthouse in Philadelphia in 1954. It is now available in many other communities. Volunteers and paid employees prepare meals and deliver them to the recipient's home 5 days a week. Generally a hot noon meal and a packaged evening meal are provided. The charge is based on the ability of the individual to pay for this service.

Meat Base Hypoallergenic formula for infants sensitive to milk. Made with meat protein (beef heart), sesame oil, sucrose, and added vitamins and minerals. (Gerber.) See Proprietary foods: composition, features, and uses, Appendix P-1.

Meconium The first fecal discharge of the newborn. It is a dark brownish green semisolid composed of intestinal and biliary secretions that have accumulated in the large intestine from the fourth fetal month until birth.

Medical history Record of pertinent information about an individual or patient that includes past illnesses, familial tendencies for diseases, general health status since birth, and present complaints. Routinely taken when a patient is admitted to a hospital or when one seeks medical consultation. It is a diagnostic aid in the management of a patient and a technique used in *nutrition surveys* to detect conditioning factors in nutritional inadequacy.

Medium-chain triglyceride (**MCT**) Fat composed of fatty acids shorter than lauric acid, predominantly saturated fatty acids with 8 and 10 carbon atoms. Compared with long-chain triglycerides, MCT have the following advantages: lower melting point, faster rate of hydrolysis, less need for bile acids, easier dispersion in water, smaller quantity incorporated into lipid esters, and less of a tendency to be stored in the liver. Current interest in MCT preparations is due to their usefulness in the dietary management of *malabsorption syn-*

dromes such as pancreatitis, postgastrectomy, sprue, cystic fibrosis, and chyluria.

Medulla 1. Marrow. 2. Medulla oblongata, the lowest part of the brain located at the head of the spinal cord. It controls heart rate and respiration. 3. Central portion of an organ as contrasted to its cortex. See also *Adrenal glands.*

Megaloblastic anemia Type of anemia characterized by an increased level of *megaloblasts,* which are primitive nucleated red blood cells much larger than the mature normal erythrocytes. The megaloblastic anemias of pregnancy and infancy respond readily to folic acid therapy and an adequate balanced diet.

Melanin Brown or black pigment resulting from the polymerization of the oxidation products of dopa. It is deposited in the hair, skin, and choroid of the eyes. See also *Albinism.*

Melanocyte Special cell of the skin found in the basal layer of the epidermis where *melanin* is formed. The activity of melanocytes is greater in darkskinned races and brunettes than in the white race and blondes.

Melanocyte-stimulating hormone (MSH) Also called intermedin; a hormone secreted by the neurohypophysis that increases the deposition of *melanin*. See also *Melatonin.*

Melatonin N-Acetyl-5-methoxytryptamine, a hormone of the *pineal gland* that blocks the action of melanocyte-stimulating hormone and causes lightening of the skin.

Melezitose Also spelled melizitose; a trisaccharide composed of one fructose unit and two glucose units. It occurs chiefly in poplars and conifers such as pine trees.

Melituria Former term for *diabetes mellitus.* General term indicating the presence of any sugar in the urine.

Melting point Temperature at which a solid liquefies. It is often characteristic of certain substances such as fats; useful as a means of identification and as an index of purity.

Menadione Vitamin K_3, synthetic vitamin K, which is about three times more potent biologically than the naturally occurring vitamin K. It is useful in therapy, but a dose in excess of 5 mg should be avoided since synthetic vitamin K produces toxic effects. See *Vitamin K* and Summary of vitamins, Appendix I-1.

Menaphthone Vitamin K_3 or *menadione.*

Menaquinone 2-Methyl-1,4-naphthoquinone, also known as *menadione.*

Menarche Time when *menstruation* starts.

Meningitis Inflammation of the *meninges,* the membranes covering the brain and spinal cord.

Menopause Period that marks the permanent cessation of menstruation.

Menstruation Also called menses; the periodic cycle, usually 28 to 30 days, characterized by uterine bleeding or menstrual flow. It is peculiar to women from puberty to menopause. It normally lasts from 3 to 7 days with a bloody discharge of about 125 ml; contains materials sloughed off from the uterine wall plus blood that is devoid of fibrinogen and prothrombin and hence does not clot. Many organic and psychic changes such as skin disorders, frequent urination, irritability, headache, and easy fatigability accompany menstruation. It is regulated by the following hormones: estrogen, progesterone, luteotropic hormone, luteinizing hormone, and follicle-stimulating hormone.

mEq Abbreviation for *milliequivalent.*

Mercapturic acid A complex of cysteine with naphthalene or various halogenated aromatic hydrocarbons whereby the latter compounds are detoxified and excreted in the urine.

Mercury Heavy liquid metal used in thermometers and other scientific instruments. Its salts are used in medicine as antiseptics, diuretics, fungicides, and parasiticides. The environmental concern for mercury in our food supply focuses on its toxic effect on the tissues, particularly the brain. Toxicity is due to the binding of tissue proteins and interference with cellular metabolism.

Characteristic symptoms of mercury poisoning are visual abnormalities, deafness, incoordination, proteinuria, apathy, and intellectual deterioration.

Meritene High protein dietary supplement for oral or tube feeding; made with nonfat milk, corn syrup, vegetable oil, sodium caseinate, sucrose, and added vitamins and minerals. (Doyle.) See Proprietary foods: composition, features, and uses, Appendix P-1.

Mesoinositol The preferred name is now *myoinositol.*

Mesomorph One of the anthropologic or somatic body types. The individual has a relatively predominant bony and muscular framework.

Metabolic body size Also called physiologic size; the active tissue mass of an individual. It is determined by raising the body weight in kilograms to the three-fourths power.

Metabolic chamber A room-sized chamber that permits continuous and long-term analysis of exhaled gases; used in indirect calorimetry. See *Calorimetry.*

Metabolic pool 1. Phrase descriptive of the manner in which a nutrient can change, combine with, or participate in metabolic reactions. 2. Components indistinguishable as to origin that may be employed for either synthetic or degradative processes. When the end products of digestion (e.g., amino acids, fatty acids, glycerol, and glucose) are absorbed, they enter the "metabolic pool" and intermingle with other substances or they are metabolized for various bodily functions.

Metabolic water See under *Water.*

Metabolism The sum of all the chemical changes in the body. There are two phases: *anabolism,* or constructive metabolism, which is concerned with the building up of materials and tissues; and *catabolism,* or destructive metabolism, which is the breaking down of materials and tissues. See also *Intermediary metabolism.*

Metabolizable energy (ME) The portion of gross food energy capable of transformation in the body for useful work (or net energy) and for basal metabolism. It does not include heat losses from urinary and fecal excretions.

Metalloprotein A compound protein; protein combined with a metal-containing prosthetic group. Examples are ferritin (iron-containing protein), carbonic anhydrase (zinc-containing protein), and ceruloplasmin (copper-containing protein). See Classification of proteins, Appendix C-2.

Metaprotein Denatured protein formed by the action of dilute acid or alkali on native protein, usually albumin and globulin. It behaves like a suspensoid by dissolving in dilute acid or alkali when the particles are ionized, but flocculates when its isoelectric point is reached. Metaprotein is precipitated by saturation with sodium chloride or ammonium sulfate.

Methemoglobin Also called ferrihemoglobin. See under *Hemoglobin.*

Methionine An *essential amino acid;* contains sulfur and labile methyl group. It is one of the *lipotropic agents* and participates in methylation reactions; hence it is important in protein and fat metabolism. See also *Methylating agent.*

Methylating agent Any substance that donates methyl radicals (CH_3—). Methionine is the most important source of labile methyl groups. Other donors are choline, serine, and betaine. Folic acid, vitamin B_{12}, and ascorbic acid are needed in the synthesis of methyl radicals. See also *Transmethylation.*

Methylcellulose Preparation of indigestible polysaccharide that provides bulk and satiety value. Physicians sometimes prescribe it as an aid in the dietary management of obesity.

MFS Abbreviation for *modified food starch.*

Micelle 1. Dispersed particles in a colloidal system that are held in a particulate form because of their special physicochemical properties. 2. One of the submicroscopic structural units of protoplasm.

Microbiologic assay Means of analyzing nutrients, especially vitamins and amino acids, by the use of microorganisms. A suitable microorganism is inoculated into a medium containing all the needed growth factors except the one nutrient under examination. The rate of growth is proportional to the amount of the particular nutritional factor added to the medium. The commonly used test microorganisms and the vitamins determined are as follows: *Lactobacillus fermentum 36* (thiamin), *Lactobacillus casei* (riboflavin and folic acid), *Lactobacillus arabinosus* (niacin and pantothenic acid), *Saccharomyces carlsbergensis* (vitamin B_6 and inositol), and *Lactobacillus leichmannii 313* (vitamin B_{12}).

Microbiology Branch of biology that studies living organisms invisible to the naked eye. See also *Microorganisms*.

Microcyte Red blood cell that is smaller than normal. *Microcytic anemia* is a type of anemia in which the red blood cells are smaller than normal. This is seen in iron-deficiency anemia.

Micronutrients Nutrients present in the body in amounts less than 0.005% of body weight (50 ppm). Examples are trace minerals, vitamin B_{12}, and pantothenic acid.

Microorganisms Organisms generally invisible to the naked eye; the size varies from about 100μ to about 0.1μ. The general groups of microorganisms are bacteria, protozoa, and viruses. Bacteria are the smallest form of plants that multiply by binary fission; i.e., a parent cell splits into two daughter cells. *Protozoa* are microscopic one-celled animals such as the amoeba and paramecium. *Viruses* are the smallest living unit and are not classified as plants or animals but are found in both kingdoms. Viruses that have been isolated and identified thus far are basically *nucleoproteins*.

Microscope Instrument that magnifies minute objects. There are several kinds, including simple, compound, fluorescent, ultraviolet, and electron microscopes. The development of the electron microscope, which can magnify objects up to 100,000 times (as compared to 100 times in a compound microscope), contributed tremendously to scientific progress, particularly in physiology and biochemistry.

Microsome That part of the cell that is composed of the *ribosomes* and *endoplasmic reticulum*.

Microwave Very short electromagnetic wave of high-frequency energy produced by the oscillation of an electric charge. Microwave energy is converted to heat when it is absorbed by food, as in electronic ovens.

Milk 1. Any whitish fluid resembling milk such as coconut milk. 2. Suspension of metallic oxides such as milk of magnesia. 3. Whole, fresh, clean lacteal secretion of the mammary glands. Unqualified, the term refers to whole cow's milk.

Acidified m Milk to which an acid is added to reduce curd tension and make it more digestible. Acids generally added are lactic acid, citric acid, vinegar, and acid fruit juices such as lemon, orange, or tomato juice.

Acidophilus m Milk inoculated with a culture of *Lactobacillus acidophilus*. It is used in various enteric disorders to provide a change in bacterial flora.

Artificial m Milk other than the lacteal secretion of the mammary glands. Made from a mixture of ingredients such as soybean milk and sugar; useful for those allergic to cow's milk.

Buttermilk Sour milk that is a by-product of churning sour cream to butter. Cultured buttermilk is made by using pure acid-forming cultures of lactic acid bacteria.

Certified m Milk produced under rigid sanitary conditions so that the bacterial count does not exceed 10,000/ml.

Concentrated m Milk reduced to one third of its original volume.

Dry, full-cream, or whole m Whole milk

dried under controlled conditions; has about 25% butterfat.

Dry, skim m See *Nonfat milk solids* under *Milk*.

Evaporated, full-cream m Whole milk from which about 50% to 60% of its water is removed; has no less than 9% butterfat.

Filled m Milk in which the butterfat has been replaced by vegetable oil. Coconut oil replaces milk fat in most filled milks. Some manufacturers are now using partially hydrogenated soybean and cottonseed oil to increase the percentage of polyunsaturated fatty acids.

Fortified m Milk to which vitamin D is added either by feeding irradiated yeast to a lactating cow, by direct irradiation of milk, or by adding vitamin D concentrate.

Homogenized m Milk that is mechanically treated to reduce fat globules so that they remain emulsified.

Imitation m Product resembling milk but not containing any milk constituent. It typically consists of water, sugar, vegetable fat, and a source of protein such as sodium caseinate or soybean protein.

Nonfat milk solids (NFMS) Skim milk powder; has less than 1% butterfat.

Pasteurized m Milk that has been heated sufficiently to kill pathogenic organisms. See *Pasteurization*.

Raw m Fresh, unpasteurized milk.

Recombined m Skim milk powder reconstituted to the normal fat content of whole milk by adding butterfat.

Reconstituted m Processed milk to which water is added to restore its original water content.

Skim m Milk from which most of the butterfat has been removed; may be liquid or dry.

Sweetened, condensed m Evaporated milk to which sugar is added up to 40% by weight.

Milk-alkali syndrome Occurs in persons with peptic ulcer who consume large amounts of milk and alkalies for a long period of time. The symptoms are hypercalcemia, calcium deposition in soft tissues, vomiting, gastrointestinal bleeding, and high blood pressure.

Milliequivalent (mEq) Measure of the chemical combining power of a substance per liter of solution. It is calculated by dividing the concentration in milligrams percent by the relative weight of a chemical element, radical, or compound.

Miltone Protein-rich dairy product developed in India. It is a blend of pure peanut protein, hydrolyzed starch syrup, and bovine or buffalo milk.

Mineral An inorganic element that remains as ash when food is burned. Analysis of mineral ash may show as many as 40 kinds, but only 17 are essential to human nutrition. The criteria that determine the essentiality of a mineral are as follows: a deficiency state occurs on a diet considered adequate in all respects except for the mineral under study; there is significant response (growth or alleviation of deficiency signs) when a supplement of the mineral is given; the response should be repeatedly demonstrable; and the deficiency state should correlate with a low level of the mineral in the blood or tissues. The major minerals (macrominerals) essential to man are *calcium, phosphorus, potassium, magnesium, sulfur, sodium,* and *chlorine.* The trace minerals (microminerals) needed by man are *iron, zinc, selenium, molybdenum, iodine, cobalt, copper, manganese, fluorine,* and *chromium.* See also Summary of minerals, Appendix H.

Mineral functions Minerals make up about 4% of body weight. In general, the role of minerals in the body is classified as *structural* or *regulatory*. The function of a mineral is structural when it is an integral part of the cell, tissue, or a substance, e.g., calcium, phosphorus, and magnesium in bones and teeth; sulfur in the hair, insulin, and thiamin; iron in hemoglobin; and chlorine in hydrochloric acid of gastric juice. Regulatory functions include maintenance of water and acid-base balance, muscle contractility, nerve irritability, and actions as cofactors of enzyme systems. For further details, see Summary of minerals, Appendix H.

Mineralocorticoids Adrenocortical hormones that regulate electrolyte balance. The most potent is *aldosterone*. See also *Cortisone* and Summary of endocrine glands, Appendix K.

Mineral oil Liquid petroleum preparation used as a laxative for chronic constipation. It has no caloric value, but it interferes with the absorption of fat-soluble vitamins.

Minimum daily requirements (MDR) Amounts of specific nutrients below which demonstrable deficiency states would appear. The Food and Drug Administration has established MDR for some vitamins and minerals. These are no longer used.

Miracle fruit A small, oval-shaped berry about ¾ inch long that grows mainly in Africa. It was first observed by the English in 1852 and they called it the "miraculous berry." It makes sour food taste sweet without adding caloric value. The mechanism of its action is to coat the taste buds for sweetness without affecting the other basic tastes. It is believed that the active material is a glycoprotein.

Misbranding (mislabeling) False or improper branding or labeling of food, drug, or any commodity. Food is said to be misbranded (mislabeled) if it is sold under another name; the size of the container is misleading; statements of weight or measure are not given or are wrong; the distributor or packer is not listed; artificial coloring, flavoring, and other food additives are not listed, etc.

Miscarriage Interruption of pregnancy prior to the seventh month. See also *Abortion.*

Mitochondrion Pl. mitochondria. A highly structured and complex cytoplasmic organelle. It is the powerhouse of the cell where chemical energy is converted into useful energy (adenosine triphosphate).

Mitochondria contain proteins, lipids, and a large number of systems involved in oxidation-reduction reactions.

Mitosis Process of cell division wherein two genetically identical daughter cells are produced.

MMR Abbreviation for *maternal mortality rate.*

Modified food starch (MFS) Found in commercially prepared strained and junior foods for infants. It is used to give a desirable texture and consistency and keep the components evenly distributed.

Modilac Commercial milk formula for routine infant feeding; made of skim milk, corn oil, mixed carbohydrates (lactose and corn syrup), and added vitamins and iron. (Gerber.) See Proprietary foods: composition, features, and uses, Appendix P-1.

Molality Number of moles of solute per 1000 gm of solvent; usually designated by a small "m." *One molal solution* contains 1 mole (gram molecular weight) of solute in 1000 gm of solvent.

Molarity Number of moles of solute per liter of solution; usually designated by a capital "M." *One molar solution* contains 1 mole (gram molecular weight) of solute in a liter of solution.

Molds Microscopic form of plants known as fungi that do not contain photosynthetic compounds. They form a characteristic cottonlike network of fine threads.

Molecular weight Relative weight of a substance attained by adding the weight of its constituent atoms, based on the atomic weight of carbon as the standard.

Molecule Smallest quantity into which a substance may be divided without the loss of its characteristic properties.

Molisch reaction General test for *carbohydrates.* A 5% solution of alpha-naphthol is added to the sample and sulfuric acid is poured down the side of the test tube to form a lower layer. If a carbohydrate is present, a red-violet ring appears at the junction of the two layers of liquid.

Molybdenum An essential trace material; a

component of xanthine oxidase and certain flavoproteins. It catalyzes the oxidation of purines, pterins, reduced pyridine nucleotides, and fatty acids. This mineral is widely distributed in foods and no dietary deficiency in man has been reported. For further details, see Summary of minerals, Appendix H.

Monellin Protein substance that has been isolated from West African wild red berries. It is 3000 times sweeter than an equal amount of sugar.

Monoamine oxidase (MAO) An antidepressant drug. It can cause a hypertensive reaction when taken together with tyramine-containing foods. See *Diet, tyramine-restricted.*

Monosaccharides Group of carbohydrates that are simple sugars; composed of one sugar unit that cannot be hydrolyzed into smaller units. They are classified according to the number of carbon atoms they contain as triose, tetrose, pentose, and hexose (3, 4, 5, and 6 carbon atoms, respectively). Monosaccharides of nutritional importance are glucose, ribose, fructose, and galactose. See also Classification of carbohydrates, Appendix C-1.

Monosodium glutamate (MSG) Chemical used to enhance flavor in foods. It is used extensively in Asian cookery and is thought to cause the Chinese restaurant syndrome. Large intakes can precipitate headaches, a burning sensation, facial pressure, and chest pain.

Morbidity 1. Diseased or unhealthy condition. 2. Prevalence of a disease. *Morbidity rate* is expressed as the number of reported cases of a given disease present at a given time per 100,000 population.

Mosenthal concentration test Kidney function test that measures the specific gravity and volume of urine specimens. The specific gravity of one or more 2-hour specimens is normally 1.018 or more, with a difference of not less than 0.009 between the lowest and highest readings during a 12-hour period with collections every 2 hours. The volume should be less than 725 ml for the 12-hour specimen.

Motor test meal Test diet for gastric analysis. See *Diet, motor test meal.*

Mottled enamel Condition of the teeth in which the enamel appears dull, chalky, and has white patches. In severe cases the enamel is stained yellow to brown and eventually shows pits, layers, and other depressions. This is associated with excess fluorine intake, although other conditions (genetic and other nonnutritional factors) may cause mottling.

MPF Abbreviation for *multipurpose food.*

MSG Abbreviation for *monosodium glutamate.*

MSH Abbreviation for *melanocyte-stimulating hormone.*

Mucin A glycoprotein (complex of protein and carbohydrate) that is viscous. It is secreted chiefly by the salivary glands, and it forms the basis of *mucus,* the liquid secreted by mucous glands. Mucin is soluble in water and is precipitated by alcohol and acid.

Mucoid Tightly bound polysaccharide resembling mucus, but it is different from mucus in solubility and is easily precipitated by acetic acid. If it is conjugated with protein it is called a *mucoprotein.* Examples are blood serum mucoid and ovomucoid.

Mucopolysaccharide Complex polysaccharide containing hexoses, uronic acids, and hexosamines.

Mucoprotein See *Mucoid.*

Mucosa Mucous membrane such as the lining of the gastrointestinal tract.

Mull-Soy Hypoallergenic formula made from soy protein and soy oil, with added sugar, vitamins, and minerals. (Borden.) See Proprietary foods: composition, features, and uses, Appendix P-1.

Multiple sclerosis Central nervous system disorder of unknown etiology. It develops as an acute disease and runs intermittently with exacerbations of weekly, monthly, or yearly intervals. There is destruction of the myelin sheaths of the brain and spinal cord. The symptoms are weakness, incoordination, strong jerky movements of the limbs, and scanning speech.

Multipurpose food (MPF) Mixture of ingredients especially formulated to provide cheap protein-rich food made from local vegetables such as legumes, nuts, cereals, and leaves. *Incaparina* is a multipurpose food. See Protein food mixtures, Appendix P-2.

Muscle Tissue composed of contractile fibers that makes up the muscular system and is responsible for the movement of any part of the body. It is classified as *cardiac* (heart muscle), *skeletal* (striated muscle), and *smooth* (nonstriated muscles of the gastrointestinal tract, blood vessels, and other involuntary muscles except those of the heart) muscle.

Muscle sugar See *Myoinositol*.

Muscular dystrophy Disorder of striated or skeletal muscles characterized by progressive atrophy, increased urinary creatine excretion, increased oxygen consumption, and necrosis of muscle fibers leading to paralysis. It is rare in man, and if it does occur, its onset is during childhood. A nutritional muscular dystrophy occurs in rabbits, rats, and monkeys but this is due to a vitamin E deficiency.

Mutarotation Change in optical rotation of solutions.

Mutase Enzyme that simultaneously catalyzes the oxidation and reduction of two molecules of the same substrate. For example, two molecules of acetaldehyde in the presence of one molecule of water are simultaneously oxidized and reduced by *aldehyde mutase*. The products formed are one molecule of acetic acid (the oxidized product) and one molecule of ethyl alcohol (the reduced product).

Mutation Change in the structure of DNA or a chromosome, resulting in a permanent alteration in the genetic information carried by DNA. Mutations may occur spontaneously or accidentally, but in man they are more apt to occur from changes in the cellular environment.

Myasthenia gravis Syndrome of fatigue and exhaustion of the muscular system marked by a progressive paralysis of muscles without sensory disturbance or atrophy. It may affect any muscle of the body, but especially those of the face, lips, tongue, throat, and neck.

Mycotoxin A naturally occurring poisonous substance produced by some types of molds such as *ergot* and *aflatoxin*. It has been suggested that these toxins may play a significant role in the production of cirrhosis and other liver disorders.

Myelin sheath Whitish cylindric covering of nerve fibers rich in lipids.

Myocardial infarction Also called coronary thrombosis; a syndrome due to permanent damage of a heart muscle, as in a thrombotic occlusion of a branch of an atherosclerotic coronary artery. It is accompanied by severe pain, shock, cardiac dysfunction, and often sudden death.

Myocardium Involuntary cardiac muscle tissue that makes up the walls of the heart chambers. Inflammation of the myocardium is called *myocarditis*.

Myogen Muscle protein present in the sarcoplasm and not within the muscle fibrils. It comprises about 20% of the total muscle protein.

Myoglobin Hemoglobin of muscle. It is an iron-protein complex responsible for the color of muscle meat. Oxygen is stored temporarily as oxymyoglobin; i.e., oxygen is loosely bound to the ferrous iron, giving a bright red color. *Metmyoglobin* is a brown pigment formed when ferrous iron is oxidized to the ferric state.

Myoinositol Formerly called *mesoinositol* or *muscle sugar*. This biologically active form of inositol occurs in animal tissues as *phosphoinositol*, a phospholipid concentrated in the heart, kidneys, spleen, thyroid, and testicles. Since it is present in relatively high amounts in food, it is not considered a true vitamin. It is a vitamin-like compound because of its physiologic action as a *lipotropic agent*. See also *Inositol* and *Phytic acid*.

Myosin A muscle protein found in the fibrils that constitutes about 65% of the total muscle proteins. It combines with actin to form *actomyosin,* which is responsible for the contractile and elastic properties of muscle.

Myristic acid Saturated fatty acid containing 14 carbon atoms. It is found in nutmeg, butter, coconut oil, spermaceti, etc.

Myxedema *Hypothyroidism* in adults. It is more prevalent in women than in men; usually insidious with gradual retardation of physical and mental functions. The disorder is characterized by decreased basal metabolic rate, dry, thick skin, puffy face and eyelids, enlargement of the tongue, falling out of hair and teeth, husky voice, and slurred speech. There is a general mental deterioration and decreased reproductive activity. The symptoms may be completely reversed by suitable therapy with thyroid preparations.

❧ N ❧

NAD Abbreviation for *nicotinamide adenine dinucleotide.*

NADP Abbreviation for *nicotinamide adenine dinucleotide phosphate.*

Nasogastric tube Tube that is inserted into the nose and passed into the esophagus and then the stomach. See *Diet, tube feeding.*

National Academy of Sciences/National Research Council Government group that established the Food and Nutrition Board, which is concerned with nutrition policy and the development of materials for use by professionals. It also advises national and international groups about nutrition. See also *Food and Nutrition Board.*

National Institutes of Health (NIH) Research unit of the Public Health Service in the U. S. Department of Health, Education, and Welfare. It is engaged in clinical research of diseases of public health importance, such as allergic, dental, mental, and metabolic diseases.

National Nutrition Survey In 1967 Congress requested that the Department of Health, Education, and Welfare survey malnutrition and related health programs in the United States. Kentucky, Louisiana, South Carolina, Texas, West Virginia, California, Massachusetts, Michigan, New York, and Washington were surveyed. From 1968 to 1970, data were collected regarding general demographic, dietary intake, clinical and anthropometric, dental, and biochemical considerations. See Methods of research in nutrition: nutritional surveys, Appendix M-1.

National Science Foundation (NSF) Foundation established in 1950 for the purpose of improving scientific research and education in the United States. Grants are awarded to universities and other nonprofit institutions to support research. The foundation also maintains a register of scientific personnel.

National School Lunch Act See *School Lunch Program.*

Native protein Protein in a state presumed to be identical with that present inside the living cell and possessing the unique structure required for biologic activity.

Nausea Feeling of discomfort in the stomach with a tendency to vomit; of varied causes such as overdose of drugs, food intoxication, cardiac failure, uremia, obstruction of the digestive tract, and emotional distress.

Necrosis Death of cells, tissues, or bone surrounded by healthy parts.

NEFA Abbreviation for *nonesterified fatty acid.* See under *Fatty acid.*

Neonatal mortality rate (NMR) Number of infants dying under 1 month of age per 1000 live births in 1 calendar year.

Neonate Newly born; a newborn infant.

Neoplasm New and abnormal growth such as a tumor.

Nephritis Also called Bright's disease; inflammation of the kidney; a diffuse, progressive degenerative or proliferative lesion affecting the renal parenchyma, the interstitial tissue, and the renal vascular system. The disease is called *glomerulonephritis* if the inflammation is primarily of the glomeruli.

It is called *pyelonephritis* if due to bacterial invasion from the urinary tract. Nephritis may be acute or chronic and may be caused by a number of conditions or follow such diseases as scarlet fever, tonsillitis, and influenza. See Dietary management of selected disorders, Appendix O.

Nephrolithiasis Formation of stones in the kidney or the diseased condition that leads to their formation. Kidney stones are of various types, shapes, and sizes. Causes are varied, including chronic infection of the kidney, stagnation of the urine, prolonged confinement in bed, dietary factors (e.g., excess of lime in the diet and vitamin A deficiency), and certain congenital biochemical abnormalities. A hot climate may be a contributory factor to the formation of kidney stones. See also *Diet, ash.*

Nephron The functional unit of the kidney. It consists of Bowman's capsule, renal vessels, Henle's loop, and collecting tubules.

Nephrosclerosis Also called arteriosclerotic Bright's disease; hardening of the renal arteries seen in renal hypertension and often associated with arteriosclerosis. As a rule it occurs in adults past 35 years of age and may be benign for many years. Later, albuminuria, nitrogen retention, and retinal changes appear with renal changes such as thickening of the arterioles, fibrosis of the glomeruli, and degeneration of the renal tubules, leading to renal insufficiency. Death usually results from circulatory failure.

Nephrosis Also called degenerative Bright's disease; degeneration or disintegration of the kidney without signs of inflammation. Symptoms include edema, albuminuria, decreased serum albumin, and oliguria. *Lipoid nephrosis* is a rare chronic condition frequently seen in children that is characterized clinically by proteinuria, edema, and hypercholesterolemia.

Nephrotic syndrome Set of symptoms applied to renal diseases characterized by marked edema and heavy proteinuria. As much as 30 gm of protein may be lost daily in the urine, leading to a decrease in plasma proteins, especially in the albumin fraction. See Dietary management of selected disorders, Appendix O.

Nerve Cordlike fiber that conveys impulses from one part of the body to another or from body organs to the central nervous system (brain and spinal cord). Nervous tissues make up about one fortieth of the total weight of the body. Nerves are characterized by the presence of large amounts of lipids, particularly *cerebrosides.*

Net energy value Productive energy or energy available for work.

Net protein utilization (**NPU**) Proportion of the nitrogen intake that is retained in the body.

Neural Combining form is neuro-; pertaining to nerves or nervous tissues.

Neuralgia A condition characterized by severe paroxysmal pain that extends along the course of a nerve. Many varieties are distinguished according to the cause or part affected such as facial, cardiac, gouty, anemic, or diabetic neuralgia. Neuralgia is not due to a disease of the nerve itself.

Neurasthenia Condition caused by emotional disturbance and manifested by nervous exhaustion, easy fatigue, lack of energy, and various aches and pains. Symptoms vary, being referable to the entire body in some individuals and localized in others.

Neuritis Inflammation of a nerve or nerves; usually associated with pain, anesthesia or paresthesia, paralysis, muscle degeneration, and loss of reflexes. Symptoms vary according to cause, location, and nerves involved. See also *Polyneuritis.*

Neurohypophysis The main part of the posterior lobe of the *pituitary gland.* See *Hypophysis.*

Neuron The complete nerve cell, including the *cell body,* the *dendrites* or long hairlike processes that transmit impulses into the cell body, and an *axon* that conducts impulses from the body of the cell outward.

Neurosis Any psychic or mental disorder characterized by partial disorganization of the personality but less serious than psychosis. The personality remains more or less intact without apparent structural change. Neurosis is characterized by various emotional states, including abnormal anxieties, fears, compulsions, phobias, and obsessions.

Neutralization Process that checks or counteracts the effect of another. In chemistry, a reaction in which an acid and a base unite to form water and a salt.

Neutral protamine Hagedorn (NPH) A long-acting insulin preparation developed by Hagedorn that is modified by the addition of protamine and zinc. See *Insulin preparations.*

Neutron Elementary particle of approximately the same mass as a hydrogen atom but having no electric charge.

Niacin Pyridine-3-carboxylic acid and its derivatives exhibiting the biologic activity of nicotinic acid, a member of the B complex vitamins. The term "niacin" was originally proposed to avoid association of the vitamin with nicotine of tobacco. See *Nicotinic acid.*

Niacinamide Amide form of niacin; nicotinic acid amide. See *Nicotinamide.*

Niacin equivalent Sum of the two forms in which niacin is made available to the body —as the vitamin niacin and as the amino acid tryptophan (60 mg tryptophan can be converted to 1 mg nicotinic acid).

Nibbling Small frequent feedings. With the same food intake in kind and amount, nibbling has an advantage over three regular meals: there is enzymatic adaptation due to a smaller load of food digested per unit of time, thus altering favorably the rate of substrate availability for metabolic reactions. Nibbling has been associated with increased body protein, decreased body fat, lower serum cholesterol level, decreased incidence and severity of atherosclerosis, and better management of diabetes mellitus.

Nicotinamide Preferred term for nicotinic acid amide, the amide form of nicotinic acid. It is an odorless white crystal ex-tremely soluble in water. Former name is niacinamide. See *Nicotinic acid.*

Nicotinamide adenine dinucleotide (NAD) Coenzyme I or diphosphopyridine nucleotide (DPN). See *Coenzymes I and II.*

Nicotinamide adenine dinucleotide phosphate (NADP) Coenzyme II or triphosphopyridine nucleotide (TPN). See *Coenzymes I and II.*

Nicotinic acid The preferred name for *niacin,* pyridine-3-carboxylic acid, a member of the vitamin B complex. It is soluble in water and stable to heat, acid, alkali, light, and oxygen. As *nicotinamide* (niacinamide or nicotinic acid amide), it is a constituent of nicotinamide adenine dinucleotide (NAD [DPN]) and nicotinamide adenine dinucleotide phosphate (NADP [TPN]), which act as hydrogen and electron acceptors and function in the metabolism of carbohydrate, fat, and protein, rhodopsin synthesis, and cellular respiration. Deficiency in this vitamin results in *pellagra.* Large doses of nicotinic acid can lower blood cholesterol level but also induce side effects such as flushing, burning and tingling sensation, and vasodilation. Excellent food sources include liver, kidney, and other glandular organs; lean meats; wheat germ and enriched cereals; and peanuts. It may be synthesized in the body from the amino acid tryptophan, 1 mg nicotinic acid being equivalent to 60 mg tryptophan. For further details, see Summary of vitamins, Appendix I-1.

Niemann-Pick disease Condition characterized by increased concentration of sphingomyelin in the liver, spleen, and other tissues; leukocytosis; anemia; and enlargement of the liver and spleen. This infantile disease usually ends in death within the first 2 years of life. The fundamental nature of the disturbance is not clearly understood.

Night blindness Also called nyctalopia; a condition of defective or reduced vision in the dark, especially after coming from bright light. When temporary it may be due to *vitamin A deficiency.* When permanent it may be due to diseases of the retina. See also *Dark adaptation*.

NIH Abbreviation for *National Institutes of Health*.

Ninhydrin test General test for *proteins* and *amino acids*. Pink, purple, or blue color results on interaction of ninhydrin (triketohydrindene hydrate) with amino acids, peptides, or proteins.

Nitritocobalamin Vitamin B_{12c} or alpha-(5,6-dimethylbenzimidazolyl) cobamide nitrite.

Nitrogen A chemical element essential to life; found free in the air and in combination in proteins and other organic compounds. Plants can use nitrogen from the soil, and nitrogen-fixing bacteria can use free nitrogen from the air. Animals and man, however, can utilize nitrogen only when supplied from foods. It is an important constituent of all animal and plant tissues and a unique element in *proteins*.

Nitrogen balance Measurement of the state of nitrogen equilibrium in the body. An organism is said to be in nitrogen balance or equilibrium when the nitrogen intake (from food eaten) equals the nitrogen output (in urine, feces, and perspiration). A *positive nitrogen balance* exists when nitrogen intake exceeds nitrogen output, as seen in pregnancy when the fetus is growing, during lactation when the mother is storing protein as milk, and during periods of growth and recovery from debilitating illness. A *negative nitrogen balance* exists when nitrogen intake is below output. This can be brought about by fever, surgery, burns, or shock following an accident. A negative nitrogen balance is undesirable because body protein is being broken down more rapidly than it is being built up.

Nitrogen conversion factors Values used to convert the nitrogen content of food to the protein content. The average value used is 6.25.

Nitroprusside test Color test for proteins containing cystine; they give a reddish color with sodium nitroprusside in dilute ammoniacal solution.

Nocturia Excessive urination at night.

Nonesterified fatty acid (**NEFA**) Also called free fatty acid. See under *Fatty acid*.

Nonnutritive sweetener Synthetic noncaloric product used as a substitute for sugar in foods and beverages. The most common are saccharin and cyclamate. The use of cyclamate has been banned by the FDA because of its suspected carcinogenic effects. See *Cyclamate*.

Nonprotein nitrogen (**NPN**) The total nitrogen of the blood, excluding that from protein. This may come from urea, uric acid, creatine, creatinine, etc.

Nonsaponifiable fraction Portion left after treating fats or lipids with hot alkali; does not form sodium salts or "soaps" and is soluble in ether but insoluble in water. It includes vitamin A, mineral oils, and higher alcohols such as cholesterol. See also *Saponification*.

Norepinephrine Also called noradrenaline; formerly called arterenol. A hormone secreted by the *adrenal medulla*. It is a demethylated epinephrine liberated at the end of sympathetic nerve fibers after stimulation; it may be synthesized from tyrosine. It causes an increase in blood pressure by increasing peripheral resistance, with little effect on cardiac output. Unlike epinephrine, it has little effect on carbohydrate metabolism and oxygen consumption. See also *Epinephrine*.

Norleucine An amino acid, alpha-amino-*n*-caproic acid.

Normality Number of gram-equivalent weights of solute per liter of solution; usually designated by a capital N.

Normocyte Erythrocyte that is normal in color, size, and shape.

NPH Abbreviation for *neutral protamine Hagedorn*.

NPN Abbreviation for *nonprotein nitrogen*.

NPU Abbreviation for *net protein utilization*.

NRC Abbreviation for *National Research Council*.

NSF Abbreviation for *National Science Foundation*.

Nuclease Enzyme that hydrolyzes nucleic acids. Two specific nucleases are *ribonuclease,* which acts on ribonucleic acid, and *deoxyribonuclease,* which acts on deoxyribose nucleic acid.

Nucleic acid A highly complex portion of *nucleoproteins* that yields a mixture of basic substances called *purines* and *pyrimidines,* a *ribose* or *deoxyribose* component, and *phosphoric acid* on complete hydrolysis. The two general types of nucleic acids are ribonucleic acid (RNA) and deoxyribonucleic acid (DNA).

Nucleolus Spherical particle within the nucleus composed primarily of DNA and RNA; it is involved in protein synthesis.

Nucleoplasm Fluid membrane of the nucleus; a colloidal suspension containing proteins and the nucleic acids DNA and RNA.

Nucleoprotein Compound protein that is a constituent of cell nuclei. It contains a basic protein such as histone or protamine and a nucleic acid as a prosthetic group.

Nucleoside Carbohydrate derivative (glycoside) resulting from the removal of phosphate from a nucleotide. It is a combination of a sugar (pentose or deoxypentose) and a base (purine or pyrimidine). In naturally occurring nucleosides the sugar is either D-ribose, as in ribosides (adenosine, guanosine, uridine, and cytidine) or 2-deoxy-D-ribose, as in deoxyribosides (deoxyadenosine, deoxyuridine, etc.). A *nucleosidase* is an enzyme that splits a nucleoside into its components.

Nucleosome Cell structure enclosed by the nuclear membrane. Its continuous substance is the nucleoplasm, which corresponds to the cytoplasm of the cytosome. Suspended in the nucleosome is a network of granular filaments called chromatin that is stained by basic dyes.

Nucleotide Phosphate ester of nucleoside. Examples are adenylic acid, guanylic acid, and cytidylic acid. Nucleotides of importance in metabolism are the adenosine phosphates ADP and ATP. See *Adenosine phosphates.*

Nucleus 1. The central part of an atom consisting of protons and neutrons. It is positively charged and constitutes almost all of the mass of the atom. 2. The central portion of the cell that directs cell function and contains the hereditary material of the cell. It also controls the formation of new cells for cellular growth and reproduction.

Nutrament High protein dietary supplement for oral or tube feeding; made with nonfat milk, soy oil, sodium caseinate, sucrose, vitamins, and minerals. (Drackett.) See Proprietary foods: composition, features, and uses, Appendix P-1.

Nutramigen Hypoallergenic formula for infants sensitive to milk and lactose; contains casein hydrolysate, corn oil, sucrose, arrowroot starch, vitamins, and minerals. (Mead Johnson.) See Proprietary foods: composition, features, and uses, Appendix P-1.

Nutri-1000 High fat nutritional supplement for oral or tube feeding; made with skim milk, soy and coconut oils, sucrose, vitamins, and minerals. (Syntex.) See Proprietary foods: composition, features, and uses, Appendix P-1.

Nutrient Any chemical substance needed by the body for one or more of the following functions: to provide heat or energy, to build and repair tissues, and to regulate life processes. Although nutrients are found chiefly in foods, some can be synthesized in the laboratory (e.g., vitamins) or in the body (biosynthesis). See also *Nutrition, Nutrilite,* and *Nutrament.*

Nutrient classification Nutrients are classified according to the amount present in the body, chemical composition, essentiality, and function.

    Amount present in body See *Macronutrients* and *Micronutrients.*

    Chemical composition The two categories are *inorganic* (water and minerals) and *organic* (carbohydrate, protein, fat, and vitamins). These six major groups of nutrients are composed of the following individual nutrients:

Amino acids

Essential
Isoleucine
Leucine
Lysine
Methionine
Phenylalanine
Threonine
Tryptophan
Valine

Nonessential
Alanine
Arginine
Asparagine
Aspartic acid
Cysteine
Cystine
Glutamic acid
Glutamine
Glycine
Histidine
Proline
Serine
Tyrosine

Carbohydrate
Fructose
Galactose
Glucose

Fatty acids
Arachidonic acid
Linoleic acid
Linolenic acid
Oleic acid
Palmitic acid
Stearic acid

Minerals

Major minerals
Calcium
Chlorine
Magnesium
Phosphorus
Potassium
Sodium
Sulfur

Trace minerals
Chromium
Cobalt
Copper
Fluorine
Iodine
Iron
Manganese
Molybdenum
Selenium
Zinc

Perhaps essential (?)
Arsenic
Barium
Bromine
Cadmium
Nickel
Strontium
Vanadium

Vitamins

Fat soluble
A
D
E
K

Water soluble
Ascorbic acid
Biotin
Cobalamin
Nicotinic acid
Pantothenic acid
Pteroylglutamic acid
Pyridoxine
Riboflavin
Thiamin

Vitamin-like
Choline
Inositol
Lipoic acid
Ubiquinone

Water

Essentiality All nutrients according to definition are *physiologically essential;* a nutrient that performs one function is *as important as* another nutrient that performs three functions. The coined term "nonessential nutrient" is misleading and should be appropriately revised to *"nondietary essential."* For further details and examples, see *Amino acid, Fatty acid, Dietary allowances,* and *Dietary requirement.* See also Recommended Daily Dietary Allowances, Appendix A-1.

Function Nutrients are grouped according to three general functions—*source of energy* (calorific nutrients: carbohydrate, protein, and fat); *growth and repair of tissues* (protein, minerals, vitamins, and water); and *regulation of life processes* (protein, minerals, vitamins, and water).

Nutrient content of foods Nutrients in foods are determined by *proximate analysis* and by the official methods of the *AOAC.* Data are compiled in *food composition tables,* which become the working tools of nutritionists. In using these values, certain limitations should be recognized. Starting with the raw food for analysis, variability of results in nutrient content exists even among members of the same species due to factors such as variety, climate, soil fertility, feed

161

(in the case of animal products), maturity or age, handling, transport, and length of storage. When the food is cooked or processed, many more factors such as pH, temperature, oxidation, and light alter the nutrient content.

Nutrient interrelationships Cellular metabolism is an integrated, coordinated chain of reactions, and interference with any reaction affects the whole system, which includes all nutrients. The close interrelationship of the six major groups of nutrients is best summarized as follows: *protein, fat,* and *carbohydrate* metabolites enter a common pathway to yield energy with the help of enzyme systems containing *vitamins* and *minerals* as cofactors. *Water* is the circulating medium for all reactions. Specific interrelationships can exist between two nutrients such as iron-copper, cobalamin-cobalt, water-sodium, and folic acid–vitamin C. Specific interrelationships also exist among several nutrients such as calcium–phosphorus–magnesium–vitamin D, cobalt-iron-zinc, and niacin-tryptophan-pyridoxine. See also Interrelationship of carbohydrate, protein, and fat, Appendix E.

Nutrification Addition of all necessary nutrients to a *fabricated* food to make it more completely nutritious.

Nutrilite Nutrient for microorganisms; any organic substance that is needed by a microorganism for its growth and metabolism.

Nutriment Any nourishing material. *Food* and *nutrients* are nutriments.

Nutriology Former name for the science of *nutrition.*

Nutrition Simply stated, the study of food in relation to health. As defined by the Food and Nutrition Council (AMA), nutrition is "the science of food, the nutrients and other substances therein, their action, interaction and balance in relation to health and disease, and the processes by which the organism ingests, digests, absorbs, transports, utilizes and excretes food substances." Nutrition deals with the physiologic needs of the body in terms of specific nutrients, the ways and means of supplying these nutrients through adequate diets, and the effects of failure to meet nutrient needs. In addition, nutrition is also concerned with social, economic, cultural, and psychologic implications of food and eating. The *basic concepts* in nutrition may be summarized as follows: (1) Adequate nutrition is essential for health. (2) A number of compounds and elements broadly classed as protein, fat, carbohydrate, minerals, vitamins, and water are needed daily in the food of man. (3) An adequate diet is the foundation of good nutrition, and it should consist of a wide variety of natural foods. Synthetic forms (pills, purified diets, etc.) should be employed for experimentation and therapeutic usage. (4) Many nutrients should be provided preformed in food, while a few could be synthesized within the body. (5) Nutrients are interrelated, and there must be metabolic balance in the body. (6) Body constituents are in a dynamic state of equilibrium. (7) Human requirements for certain nutrients are known quantitatively within certain limits. The search for quantitative determination for the others has been going on for over a century. (8) Effects of nutritional inadequacy are more than physical; behavioral patterns and mental performance are also affected. (9) Nutritional status of population and individuals can be measured for certain nutrients. However, for other nutrients, techniques of assessment (dietary, clinical, and biochemical) have yet to be refined. (10) Proper education, technical expertise, and the use of all resources in applied nutrition and food technology will help upgrade nutritional status of people. (11) The biologic meaning of food is attributable to the three functions of *nutrients.* To an individual or family, food is taken not only for physiologic needs but also for cultural, psychologic, social, and aesthetic values. (12) The study of nutrition as a subject or course has a broad scope and is interrelated with many allied fields—physiology, biochemistry, food technology, dietetics, public health, behavioral sciences (sociology, anthropology, and psychology), and many branches of medicine (anatomy, preventive medicine, pediatrics, etc.).

Nutrition, adolescence The adolescent period is characterized by accelerated growth rate and intense activity with physical, social, emotional, and mental changes. It is a transition period between childhood and adulthood, girls maturing earlier than boys. The nutritional needs of adolescents are unique, conditioned primarily by the building of new body tissues, the demands of increased physical activity, and to some extent the emotional changes attending maturation. In general the growing adolescent requires a high caloric intake, an abundance of good quality protein, and liberal minerals and vitamins. Because of the onset of menstruation, adolescent girls have specific nutrient needs, especially for iron, protein, and other nutrients essential for blood formation. Nutrition education is focused on the eating habits of adolescents because of the following problems that affect nutrient intake: (1) irregularity of meals—some skip breakfast; (2) poor choice of snack items—there is a tendency to eat foods with "empty calories" such as cakes, cookies, and soft drinks; and (3) some adolescent girls are so conscious of figure development that they do not eat enough. See Recommended Daily Dietary Allowances, Appendix A-1.

Nutrition, adulthood Adulthood is the period of life when one has attained full growth and maturity. The onset of this stage varies among individuals and there are no clear-cut age boundaries. However, as related to dietary needs, adulthood pertains to the years between ages 21 and 65 without stresses such as pregnancy, lactation, and convalescence. Proper nutrition needs emphasis in adulthood, since it is the longest period of the life cycle and possibly the peak productive years. Ideally one should reach adulthood with a wide range of familiarity and acceptance of different foods and must have established sound food hab-

its. An adult tends to resist changes in his food habits, hence the importance of proper training both in food selection and regularity of eating as early in life as possible. Another aim of good nutrition throughout adulthood is the maintenance of desirable body weight. It is recommended that the daily caloric allowances be reduced with increasing age. See *Nutrition, aging process*, and *Nutrition, geriatrics*. See also Recommended Daily Dietary Allowances, Appendix A-1.

Nutrition, aging process Theoretically aging is a continuous process from conception until death. However, in the young growing organism, the building-up processes exceed the breaking-down processes so that the net result is a picture of growth and development. Once the body reaches adulthood, the process is reversed. Although the rate of degenerative changes is slow during middle adulthood, it increases as the individual approaches the geriatric age. See *Nutrition, geriatrics*.

Nutrition, alcoholism Chronic *alcoholism* is a complex condition involving psychologic, social, and physiologic factors. An addict usually has faulty eating habits and an inadequate diet. *Cirrhosis of the liver* in chronic alcoholism is caused mainly by dietary neglect rather than the direct toxicity of alcohol. Protein and the vitamin B complex, particularly thiamin, are the nutrients often lacking. The metabolic explanation for induced vitamin B deficiencies is based on their involvement in enzyme systems needed to oxidize alcohol (1 gm alcohol yields 7 calories). The degradation takes place in the liver, hence the characteristic liver cirrhosis. Besides taxing the liver, excess alcohol has toxic effects on the central nervous system, heart, kidneys, and other organs of metabolism. Nutritional inadequacy is sometimes aggravated by chronic gastritis resulting from habitual drinking.

Nutrition, anemias Nutritional anemias probably constitute the most common nutritional disease in man. This statement is not difficult to believe because of the many etiologic factors that lead to anemia. All nutrients are involved directly or indirectly. *Protein* is needed for the globin portion of hemoglobin (Hb); *iron* is an integral part of heme; *copper* catalyzes the utilization of iron both in the intestinal tract and at the tissue level; *pyridoxine* helps in the formation of the pyrrole ring of Hb; *riboflavin* is important in protein synthesis; *ascorbic acid* increases the absorption of iron by keeping it in its ferrous state and catalyzes the conversion of folic acid to folinic acid; and *cobalamin* and *folinic acid* are needed for normal maturation of red blood cells and in the synthesis of methyl groups needed for heme structure. Because of interrelationships, other nutrients are indirectly involved. See also *Anemia* and *Hemopoiesis*.

Nutrition, antibiotics The increasing use of antibiotics necessitates a review of how nutrition is affected by this special group of drugs. There are several mechanisms or modes of action to explain their nutritional influence. Many antibiotics have direct effects on the gastrointestinal tract, e.g., nausea, anorexia, glossitis, stomatitis, and diarrhea. Certain antibiotics bind some nutrients; e.g., tetracycline binds bone calcium ions, chloramphenicol binds protein, and penicillin and sulfonamides bind serum albumin. Neomycin may lead to a malabsorption syndrome, whereas other antibiotics increase volume and/or frequency of stools. In general antibiotics alter microflora and inhibit bacterial synthesis of certain vitamins. See also *Nutrition, drugs*.

Nutrition, cancer Present knowledge about the relationship of nutrition and cancer is not conclusive for two main reasons: (1) the causative factors of malignant tumors are numerous and often undetermined and (2) the carcinogenic stimulus affects the organism in varying degrees, depending on factors such as the amount or dose of the stimulus, the period of exposure, and the susceptibility of the species. The observa-

tion that cancer of the stomach and the liver are the most prevalent types is of interest, since these organs are directly involved in nutrient utilization. Also certain substances found in foods are carcinogenic. Among these are the aflatoxin of moldy peanuts, cycasin in cycad meal, polyphenols in tea, excess selenium in the diet, and a toxic substance developed in overheated fats. The question of limiting or increasing a certain nutrient or specific nutrients in the diet of patients with cancer is not yet resolved. However, some trends need further study in man: e.g., a diet excessively high in phosphates may stimulate nucleic acid synthesis as well as malignant growth of tumors; restriction of essential amino acids, e.g., phenylalanine, may inhibit cancerous growth of cells; and a diet low in pyridoxine may be beneficial, since pyridoxamine tends to stimulate malignant growth.

Nutrition, childhood Childhood is the period of life between infancy and puberty, generally from ages 1 to 12 years. Nutritional needs during this period cannot be generalized because of the following factors: spurts of growth occur and growth patterns vary among children; the kind and size of food servings should be adjusted with age, development, and appetite; outside influences such as school activities and play affect eating habits; etc. Thus nutritional needs for specific ages from 1 to 12 years are considered separately. See *Nutrition, toddler; Nutrition, preschool age;* and *Nutrition, schoolchildren*.

Nutrition, dental health The time intervals involved in the development of *teeth* are important considerations in any discussion of the relationship of nutrition to tooth development. The life history of a tooth may be divided into three main eras: the period during which the crown of the tooth is forming and calcifying in the jaw; the period of maturation when the tooth is erupting into the oral cavity and its root or roots are forming; and the maintenance period while it is in full function in the oral cavity. Prenatal factors affect *deciduous teeth* (baby teeth) far more than factors after birth. At the early stage of the sixth fetal week, the tooth buds start to form and calcification begins on the sixteenth week. Eruption of baby teeth starts around the age of 7 months; the last molar tooth comes out at the age of 2 years. Calcification of the permanent teeth starts soon after birth, and eruption of the first permanent tooth appears at about 6 years of age, when the child is starting to lose baby teeth. Hence, an adequate diet is imperative as early as the first trimester of pregnancy. All nutrients directly or indirectly play an important role in dental development, as does the maintenance of dental health. Nutrients directly involved are *protein,* for the organic matrix formation; *calcium, phosphorus, magnesium,* and *vitamin D,* for deposition of the mineral compound, *apatite,* into the matrix structure; *ascorbic acid,* involved in mineral utilization and for cementum formation to connect the tooth to the bone structure and to the gum tissues; *vitamin A,* for the proper functioning of enamel-forming cells to achieve a smooth, even enamel as well as a deposit of sound dentin; and *fluorine,* to harden the enamel and prevent dental caries. Although nutrition influences dental health profoundly, other nonnutritional factors are also important, such as oral hygiene, regular visits to the dentist, and fluoridation of community water supply.

Nutrition, dermatology The *skin* is a tough but resilient covering of the body with protective, regulatory, excretory, and sensory functions. The first layer (epidermis) is the site of keratin and vitamin D synthesis; the second layer (dermis), which is rich in blood vessels, nerves, and sweat and sebaceous glands, is a storehouse for water, blood, and electrolytes. The innermost layer (subcutaneous tissue) is a storehouse for body fat and helps support the body. Protein deficiency results in dryness, scaliness,

pallid appearance, and inelasticity of the skin, often with brownish pigmentation on the face. In kwashiorkor there is extensive hypopigmentation and dryness of the skin and hair, with the characteristic "flag sign" of the hair. Lack of *essential fatty acids* results in eczematous skin lesions that are probably related to the seborrheic dermatitis of *pyridoxine* deficiency. The skin changes caused by lack of *vitamin A* include desquamation of epithelial cells, keratinization, and dry and rough gooseflesh with follicular hyperkeratosis. On the other hand, excessive carotene (provitamin A) results in jaundicelike yellow discoloration of the skin. In *riboflavin* deficiency, dermatitis is of the seborrheic type, with fine, oily scales, especially around the nose and lips. Symmetric dermatitis, i.e., dark red eruptions and desquamation appearing bilaterally, is characteristic of pellagra (*nicotinic acid* deficiency). Dry, "crackled," and scaly dermatitis is observed in *biotin* deficiency. *Ascorbic acid* deficiency results in inelastic skin with a tendency to petechial hemorrhages.

Nutrition, diet therapy Also called therapeutic nutrition; in the dietary management of diseases (diet therapy) the prescribed diet has certain nutritional effects, depending on the type of therapeutic diet and the length of time it is used. For example, the clear liquid diet is nutritionally inadequate; sodium-restricted diets reduce palatability of food; fat-restricted diets decrease absorption of fat-soluble vitamins; a high polyunsaturated fatty acid diet tends to lower serum cholesterol; a high protein intake increases the requirement for riboflavin and pyridoxine; a high carbohydrate diet tends to elevate serum triglyceride and to increase the thiamin requirement; and prolonged sodium restriction, especially at the 200 mg level, leads to the *low sodium syndrome.* For further details, see *Diet* and *Diet therapy.* See also Dietary management of selected disorders, Appendix O.

Nutrition, diseases The nutritional effects of

diseases are collectively considered as secondary factors or "conditioning factors" of nutritional inadequacy. In general a diseased condition leads to anorexia. Bed rest increases calcium and nitrogen excretion; diarrheal diseases increase motility of the intestines and the frequent bowel movements obviously cause maldigestion and malabsorption. Many diseases, particularly gastrointestinal disorders, are characterized by nausea and vomiting, affecting electrolyte and water balance. Renal diseases increase the loss of nitrogen. For other examples of the nutritional effects of diseases, see under each disease. See also *Nutritional deficiency.*

Nutrition, drugs The trends in modern chemotherapy are of interest because of the effects of certain drugs on nutrient availability or utilization. To cite the most common examples, antacids destroy thiamin; appetite-depressants such as amphetamines may irritate gastric mucosa and cause nausea and vomiting; mineral oil decreases absorption of fat-soluble vitamins; chelating agents bind many minerals and reduce their availability; cation-exchange resins also reduce available sodium, potassium, and calcium; antimetabolites for cancer therapy antagonize the physiologic role of some vitamins; barbiturates have antivitamin action against folic acid; and corticosteroids alter electrolyte, carbohydrate, and fat metabolism. See also *Nutritional deficiency* and *Nutrition, antibiotics.*

Nutrition, emergency feeding Refers to the provision of meals to persons suddenly deprived of food as a result of either man-made or natural catastrophes such as famines, floods, industrial accidents, fires, and wars. In emergency feeding the long-range objective is to sustain adequate nourishment until the victims return to their normal pattern of life. The immediate aim, however, is to provide water and warm food to maintain body temperature and to give immediate nourishment. Less emphasis is placed on dietary adequacy, especially

when the emergency is brief. Distribution of food should be orderly, and the feeding program should include the rescue workers. Special attention should be given to vulnerable groups such as infants, children, pregnant women, and those under pathologic stress. The food relief personnel or volunteers should help allay fears and anxiety, avoid panic, and maintain morale.

In emergency feeding, an allowance of 2 L of water per person per day is enough. Foods chosen should be suitable for all ages and not subject to deterioration for a few days to a week or more. Ready-to-eat food items or those that require minimum preparation or wastes are preferred. Such foods include milk solids, hard cheese, dry cereals, sugar, fats, dried legumes and nuts, canned goods, and dried foods. Many kinds of freeze-dried foods are available for stockpiling. See also *Nutrition, starvation.*

Nutrition, emotional stability Well-nourished individuals generally have a cheerful disposition and a positive attitude toward changes and can easily adjust to various situations. On the other hand, an undernourished individual tends to be nervous, tense, apathetic, dull-looking, and irritable. Examples of the relationship between nutrition and emotion include (1) women who are emotionally distressed require a higher intake of calcium (and possibly other nutrients) than happy, relaxed women; (2) the well-known depression of pellagra starts with irritability, headache, and sleeplessness in the early stages, followed by loss of memory, hallucinations, and severe depression in advanced stages; (3) persons starved for a long time are prone to excitement and hysteria; (4) fear, anger, and worry stimulate adrenaline secretion, which in turn increases the loss of nitrogen from the body; and (5) thiamin-deficient individuals show moodiness, uneasiness, and disorderly thinking. The allusion to thiamin as the "morale vitamin" originated from its ability to alleviate certain mental and emotional depressions. See also *Nutrition, mental health.*

Nutrition, eye changes See *Nutrition, ophthalmology.*

Nutrition, gastronautics See *Nutrition, space feeding.*

Nutrition, geriatrics Nutrition in the aged or persons over 65 years of age. The changes peculiar to the aging process present problems that contribute to *nutritional inadequacy.* These include poor dentition or loss of teeth, loss of appetite and acuity of taste and smell, reduced secretions of digestive enzymes, lack of neuromuscular coordination, reduced cellular metabolism, reduced circulatory and excretory functions, hormonal changes, and a tendency to develop osteoporosis, pernicious anemia, and many metabolic disorders. Aside from these physiologic changes are socioeconomic and psychologic factors that affect nutriture. Most common among the aged are boredom, inactivity, lack of interest in the environment, anxiety, faulty eating habits that resist change, and economic insecurity. Considering these changes, dietary principles that govern feeding the aged are as follows: (1) reduce caloric intake; (2) liberal intakes of protein, vitamins, and minerals; (3) liberal water intake to prevent constipation, which is common among elderly people; and (4) small frequent feedings of palatable meals that are easy to manage and digest. See Recommended Daily Dietary Allowances, Appendix A-1.

Nutrition, growth and development In a broad sense, growth and development refer to the increase in size and number of cells as well as cell maturation for functional processes of the body. Thus the study of nutrition as related to growth and development covers the whole life cycle of an individual. For nutrition principles for each period of life, see *Nutrition, pregnancy; Nutrition, infancy; Nutrition, toddler; Nutrition, preschool age; Nutrition, school-* *children; Nutrition, adolescence; Nutrition, adulthood;* and *Nutrition, geriatrics.*

Nutrition, iatrogenic Nutritional disease that results from erroneous treatment, i.e., surgery, drugs, or diet, prescribed by a physician.

Nutrition, infancy The first 12 months of life are characterized by the most rapid rate of growth and development of the entire lifetime; thus an infant's nutritional needs merit special attention. For *calories,* he should have 49 to 53 calories/pound (108 to 117 calories/kg), using the higher level for the first months of age. About two thirds of his caloric needs should come from milk and the rest from added carbohydrates and later from supplementary foods. *Protein* needs should be within 0.9 to 1 gm/pound (2 to 2.2 gm/kg). This level is higher than the protein requirement of adults and is easily supplied by adequate milk intake. *Fat* is important primarily to provide essential fatty acids to an extent of at least 1% (preferably 2%) of the total caloric needs. This is adequately supplied by human milk or whole cow's milk. *Fluid* requirement is about 2.5 ounces/pound (4.5 to 5 ounces/kg). It is the most variable of nutrient needs because of fluctuations in the infant's activities and environmental temperature. *Mineral* needs are generally met during the first 3 months of age by human milk or by the prescribed milk formula. However, after 3 months the infant's iron stores are depleted and there is need for other foods and supplementation. *Vitamins* needed by the infant are ample in his milk supply except for A, D, and C, which must be supplemented. See Recommended Daily Dietary Allowances, Appendix A-1.

The following are the main criteria of normal growth and development during infancy: (1) *steady weight gain* of 5 to 8 ounces/week that slows down toward the end of the first year to about 4 ounces/week (this means that an average infant should have doubled and tripled his birth weight at the end of 5 months and 12 months, respectively) ; (2) *normal increase in body length* is about 10 inches (50% more) at the end of the first year; (3) normal toilet and sleeping habits; (4) firm, well-formed muscles with moderate subcutaneous fat; (5) happy disposition; and (6) normal dental and motor development. See *Nutrition, dental health; Nutrition, mental health;* and *Nutrition, motor performance.*

Nutrition, infection Blood levels of vitamin A are sufficiently reduced in acute infections that xerophthalmia and keratomalacia frequently develop in children receiving diets deficient in this vitamin. Giardiasis is known to interfere with vitamin A absorption, and any intestinal infection producing malabsorption interferes with the absorption of the fat-soluble vitamins. Fat absorption is also decreased in infections. Clinical manifestations of thiamin, folic acid, vitamin B_{12}, and ascorbic acid deficiencies have all been related to a preceding infection of a vulnerable host. Increased losses of calcium and phosphorus are seen in tuberculosis. Losses of sodium, chloride, potassium, and phosphorus are seen in diarrheal diseases of infectious origin. Hookworm infections can be responsible for enough loss of blood to induce anemia. See also *Nutrition, resistance to disease.*

Nutrition, labeling The U. S. Food and Drug Administration has proposed the following regulations, which should be in effect by December 1974. Labeling of foods is voluntary except for products that are fortified or those that offer some nutrition information. The following nutrition information must be included on the label: serving size; servings per container; caloric, protein, carbohydrate, and fat content; and percentage of the United States' recommended dietary allowance of protein, vitamins, and minerals. The values for nutrient content are based on serving size. Seven vitamins and minerals must be listed: vitamin A, vitamin C, thiamin, riboflavin, niacin, calcium, and iron. If the amount is less than 2%, it may be listed as containing less than 2% rather than the specific percentage. The amounts of the other vitamins and minerals may also be listed.

Nutrition, lactation Nutrient requirements of the mother during *lactation* are increased to provide for normal secretion of milk (the recommended dietary allowances assume that an average mother produces 850 ml of breast milk a day) and for recovery from pregnancy and delivery. Thus *caloric requirement* is increased by 500 to 750 calories over the needs of the nonpregnant woman. This is approximately 90 calories/100 ml of milk secreted to provide for actual energy expenditure of the secretory function and for the caloric content of milk. Similarly, intakes for *protein, minerals,* particularly *calcium,* and *vitamins* are increased. See Recommended Daily Dietary Allowances, Appendix A-1. See also *Infant feeding* and *Lactation.*

Nutrition, mental health The relationship of nutrition and mental health is well established; i.e., proper nourishment is conducive to mental efficiency, the ability to concentrate, and ease of adjustment to environmental changes. On the other hand, nutrient inadequacy may result in permanent brain changes in size or chemical composition, thus affecting mental capacity; inborn errors of metabolism retard mental development (e.g., phenylketonuria and galactosemia); and specific nervous lesions occur as a result of nutrient deficiencies such as in *pellagra, kwashiorkor, marasmus,* and *beriberi.* For further details, see also *Nutrition, emotional stability; Nutrition, nervous system;* and *Nutrition, psychiatry.*

Nutrition, motor performance The ability of the body to coordinate its movements and to perform other physical activities has its roots in the motor development during infancy and childhood. Evidences for the significant correlation of good nutrition and motor development include kwashiorkor, beriberi, and other deficiency diseases; phenylketonuria and other inborn errors of metabolism; and *hypokinesis.* Lack of exercise and prolonged immobilization, as in bedridden patients, lead to negative nitrogen and mineral balances. The physiologic effects of moderate exercise on nurtriture and good health in general are as follows: it promotes pulmonary ventilation, circulation, and oxidation processes; it stimulates appetite, flow of digestive juices, and peristalsis; it improves muscle tonus and sleep habits; and it increases strength, mental acuity, and resistance to infection. See also *Nutrition, mental health,* and *Nutrition, nervous system.*

Nutrition, nervous system Proper nutrition is important for the integrity of nerve cells and the normal functioning of the nervous system. An obvious example is the feeling of restlessness or irritability when one is hungry. All nutrients are involved in maintaining a healthy nervous system, notably the following: *carbohydrate* (specifically glucose) is the chief energy source utilized by the brain; *protein* is needed for enzyme systems to oxidize glucose; and *B complex vitamins* are involved in carbohydrate metabolism. Certain vitamin deficiencies lead to neurologic changes varying from mild symptoms to gross anatomic nerve lesions: e.g., lack of *thiamin* results in neuromuscular incoordinations (nystagmus, hyperesthesia, ataxia, cramps, and loss of tendon reflexes) and later brain lesions and degeneration of nerve fibers and myelin sheaths with death of the parent nerve cells; *riboflavin* deficiency is characterized in the early stages by photophobia and affects nicotinic acid metabolism, in which riboflavin is indirectly involved; lack of *nicotinic acid* is associated with the psychosis of pellagra; and *pyridoxine* deficiency leads to sensory neuritis, convulsions, hyperesthesia, and loss of positional sense. See also *Nutrition, alcoholism; Nutrition, psychiatry; Nutrition, emotional stability;* and *Nutrition, mental health.*

Nutrition, ophthalmology It has long been established that the muscles, nerves, and mucous membranes of the eyes as well as the visual process are affected by nutrition. The ability to see or adapt in dim light depends in part on adequate vitamin A. Ocular changes associated with lack of *vitamin A* are xerosis, keratomalacia, Bitot's spots, night blindness, and xerophthalmia. *Riboflavin* deficiency leads to corneal vascularization, conjunctivitis, photophobia, and burning and itching of eyes. Lack of *pyridoxine* results in angular blepharitis and conjunctivitis. The *essential amino acids, vitamin C,* and *nicotinic acid* maintain the integrity of the eye lens and prevent cataracts.

Nutrition, parasitism Infestation of *parasites* in the human host, particularly in the digestive tract, is a conditioning factor of nutritional inadequacy. The common intestinal parasites are tapeworms, hookworms, pinworms, whipworms, ascarides, flukes, *Trichinella,* and *Trichuris.* The extent of their harmful effects depends on the tissues invaded, the types of secretion they produce, their rate of growth and multiplication, and the ability of the body to protect itself from these effects. The principal ways by which parasites harm the host are as follows: mechanical injury (tissue lesions and hemorrhage), inflammation, and pain; obstructions, e.g., blocking ducts; toxicity of their secretions; and robbing the host of its nutrient supply, especially proteins and vitamins. The nutritional implications of these parasitic effects do not need further elaboration. Preventive measures against parasitism include *nutrition education* (a well-nourished body can build antibodies that neutralize the toxic effects of parasites); *environmental sanitation* (e.g., proper sewage disposal, safe water and food supply, educated food handlers and consumers); and *parasitic control* (medical attention and use of chemicals or other means of interfering with the life cycle of the parasite). See also *Nutrition, resistance to disease.*

Nutrition, physical health The state of nutrition is easily reflected in a person's appearance. The physical signs of good nutrition are normal weight for height, body frame, and age; firm, moderately padded muscles; clear and slightly moist skin with good color; well-formed jaw and teeth; soft glossy hair and clear bright eyes; a well-formed trunk; good appetite and abundance of energy; endurance to physical work and resistance to disease; and in general a happy personality. See also *Nutrition, mental health* and *Nutrition, emotional stability.*

Nutrition, pregnancy A well-nourished mother during *pregnancy* is important not only for her own needs but also for the growing fetus (prenatal nutrition). Good maternal nutrition results in a lower incidence of abortion and miscarriage; fewer stillborn and premature infants and infants with congenital malformations; fewer complications during pregnancy (e.g., toxemias and anemias) and during delivery (e.g., prolonged labor, premature separation of the placenta, and hemorrhaging); healthier full-term babies; and reduced infant mortality and morbidity rates. Pregnancy imposes a physiologic stress on the mother, and the most important changes with nutritional implications are increase in basal metabolic rate (about 25% in the latter half of pregnancy); tendency to retain water; decreased gastric acidity and intestinal motility with frequent impairment of digestion and absorption in the early stage and constipation in the last trimester; simple glycosuria; hormonal changes (increased activities of progesterone, gonadotropin, estrogen, and adrenal steroid hormones); and positive nitrogen balance and increase of plasma volume with a corresponding decrease of hemoglobin concentration. With these significant changes in mind, the dietary principles try to provide for the increased maternal metabolic activities; the nutrient needs of the growing fetus; the development of reproductive tissues (uterus, placenta, etc.) and the mammary glands; and the nutrient reserves to allow for losses during delivery. In general all nutrient requirements are increased from the nonpregnant to the pregnant state. For further details, see Recommended Daily Dietary Allowances, Appendix A-1.

Noteworthy is the need of regulating weight gain during *pregnancy*. The desirable weight gain is about 20 to 25 pounds throughout the gestation period distributed as follows: normal weight of infant at birth = 7 to 7½ pounds; weight of uterus, placenta, and membrane = 3 to 3½ pounds; weight of amniotic fluids = 2 pounds; weight of mammary glands and tissues = 1 to 1½ pounds; and the remaining weight is in the form of maternal body water and increased blood volume. The total weight gain of 23 pounds (average) should be within the rate of 5, 8, and 10 pounds for the first, second, and third trimesters, respectively. In view of the rapid fetal growth and development that occur as early as the second month of pregnancy, it is recommended that *protein, mineral,* and *vitamin* intakes be increased as early as possible.

Nutrition, prematurity Premature infants have special nutritional needs because nutrient requirements are relatively high for body size and weight, yet digestive capacity is usually small; the sucking and swallowing reflexes are not well developed; respiration is irregular with a tendency to regurgitate and aspirate foods; achlorhydria is common; and fat absorption is poor, resulting in a loss of fat-soluble vitamins and calcium along with fecal fat. The dietary management of a premature infant has to be individualized, depending on his anatomic facilities and physiologic condition. His daily nourishment should provide at least 125 calories/kg and 4.5 gm protein/

kg with vitamin and mineral supplementations. He has a peculiarly high vitamin C requirement and a daily supplement of 50 mg ascorbic acid in the early weeks will prevent tyrosyluria. Some premature infants require special feeders or tube feeding. A recommended feeding regimen for a premature infant is as follows: for the *first 12 hours,* nothing is given orally; for the *second 12 hours,* a 5% glucose solution is given at 2- to 3-hour intervals, starting first with a half teaspoonful and gradually increasing by half teaspoonfuls at alternate feedings; for the *third 12 hours,* a prescribed milk formula is prepared and diluted with an equal amount of 5% glucose solution, and this mixed formula is given alternately with the pure glucose solution at 2- to 3-hour intervals, starting with half teaspoonfuls; for the *fourth 12 hours,* the mixed formula is given at 2- to 3-hour intervals, gradually increasing the amount; for the *third day* and thereafter a full concentration of the prescribed formula is given, starting with small amounts and gradually increasing as tolerated by the infant. Vitamin and mineral supplements are given by the second week. See also *Nutrition, infancy.*

Nutrition, preschool age The group of 1- to 5-year-old children constitutes a far more vulnerable group than infants. Recognizing that ages 1 to 5 years are the most formative years of child development in all aspects of his personality (physical, mental, and social), the importance of nutrition cannot be overemphasized. For a quantitative evaluation of dietary adequacy for ages 1 to 3 and 4 to 6 years, see Recommended Daily Dietary Allowances, Appendix A-1.

Nutrition, psychiatry Man associates varying emotional experiences with food, such as social acceptance or rejection, feeling of security or anxiety, pleasure or pain, satisfaction or frustration, and many other feelings. To the mentally ill these associations are often exaggerated and feeding problems are more difficult to manage. Well-known conditions with underlying psychologic disorders are obesity with uncontrollable overeating, anorexia nervosa, chronic alcoholism, and drug addiction. For successful dietary management, the dietitian must know the background of the patient (social, economic, educational, etc.), especially the underlying psychiatric defect. The feeding regimen is part of the patient's total rehabilitation program, which requires the "teamwork" approach of the physician, dietitian, nurse, social worker, hospital administrator, etc. See also *Diet therapy; Psychodietetics;* and *Nutrition, emotional stability.*

Nutrition, puberty Puberty is the period during which the reproductive organs become functionally operative and secondary sex characteristics start to develop with accompanying increased rates of growth and metabolism. Its onset varies from 10 to 15 years of age, with 12 to 13 years of age being the average. For nutritional considerations, see *Nutrition, adolescence.*

Nutrition, public health The theory and practice of nutrition as a science through organized community effort, with the family as the smallest unit under study. The overall aim of public health nutrition is to improve or maintain good health through proper nutrition. Various agencies, governmental or nongovernmental, are concerned with nutrition work at local, national, or international levels. See Agencies concerned with nutrition in the United States, Appendix L.

The years 1960 to 1970 were declared by the WHO-FAO as the decade of the "Freedom from Hunger" campaign. In the *Third World Food Survey* (FAO Report, 1963), the following findings were revealed: (1) Over half of the world's population is hungry or malnourished. This is based on food balance sheets of over 80 countries, representing about 95% of the world population. (2) Compared to the pre-World War II level, there is a slight improvement of food balance brought about mainly by developing countries, but the gap of food production between developing areas and the advanced countries has widened. (3) Deficiency diseases are still common in many areas of the world, as revealed by the retarded growth and poor physique of children, high mortality and morbidity rates, especially among children under 5 years of age, poor working efficiency, and lowered resistance to diseases. (4) Deficiency diseases are observed more frequently in countries whose fat and protein intakes are only 20% of the total calories. If 80% or more of calories are supplied by cereals, sugars, root crops, and vegetables, there is a likelihood of dietary inadequacy for most nutrients. (5) Should the world population grow according to the United Nations' projections, there is a need to increase food supply, especially animal foods, by three times the present production. As of 1970, the world population was estimated at about 3.6 billion, and by the year 2000, the world population is expected to be approximately 6.3 billion. For this reason, nutrition programs are geared toward meeting the food needs of our fast-growing population. See also *Nutritional survey* and Protein food mixtures, Appendix P-2.

Nutrition, resistance to disease Evidence suggests that there may be two ways in which nutrition can affect host resistance to disease—antibody synthesis and cellular immune response. Protein malnutrition seems to impair the production of circulating antibodies in response to certain viral and bacterial antigens. Malnutrition and the depletion of protein reserves result in atrophy of the liver, spleen, bone marrow, and lymphoid tissues, from which phagocytes and lymphocytes originate. Lysozyme activity is also reduced by generalized malnutrition. Nutritional deficiencies cause tissue changes that lower body resistance and affect wound healing and collagen formation. Deficiencies in protein, vitamin A,

ascorbic acid, and niacin are especially likely to cause tissue changes that lower resistance to disease.

Nutrition, schoolchildren Dietary principles in feeding schoolchildren are the same as those for preschoolers, but food intake differs in quantity and variety. Due to school activities, children from 6 to 12 years of age are more independent, and this includes their choice of food outside the home. Unless supervised by nutrition educators, as in the case of *school lunch programs,* feeding time and food selection could be erratic. Hurried meals, skipping breakfast, poorly selected snacks, and lack of appetite due to social and school interests are the common feeding problems faced by parents and teachers.

Nutrition, skin condition See *Nutrition, dermatology.*

Nutrition, space feeding Also called gastronautics; the preferred name is "astrophysiologic dietetics," signifying that feeding an organism beyond the earth environment is both an art and a science. Space begins about 120 miles above the earth and is devoid of air, friction, gravity, and oxygen. Thus the very nature of a trip into space imposes nutritional problems. Although water requirement remains the same, caloric needs are reduced because of weightlessness and confinement, resulting in sedentary activity. Close to 50% of total caloric intake should come from fat (this is an advantage since fat catabolism requires less oxygen); 15% of calories is provided by protein; and the rest is carbohydrates. Fecal losses are minimized by the use of low residue diets. Mineral levels for calcium, sodium, potassium, and magnesium are increased by 10% above normal needs.

Foods used should be technologically prepared to tolerate weightlessness; sudden fluctuations of pressure, temperature, light, radiation, and humidity; and other conditions during the flight. The overall aim of the feeding system is to promote maximum efficiency of the crew, whose movements are restricted even in mastication. Besides nutrient adequacy, food should be palatable, easy to manage, and not subject to deterioration. Thus the types of foods chosen are bite-sized finger foods, precooked foods, and freeze-dried foods, each packaged to serve three purposes—storage container, food utensil, and eating device. The possible use of green algae for space feeding has been explored. See *Chlorella*.

Nutrition, starvation A state of subnutrition arises from prolonged starvation caused by any of the following circumstances: lack of food as in famine, war, poverty, etc.; presence of a conditioning factor, especially disorders of the digestive tract and malabsorption syndrome; and the effect of certain toxemias that may be metabolic or infectious in origin. The outstanding changes in starved individuals are as follows: generalized atrophy or wasting of tissues with loss of body fat and increase in extracellular fluids; shrinkage of lean tissues with muscular weakness and loss of skin elasticity; disturbance of water balance as a result of loss of plasma proteins and electrolyte changes with consequent nutritional edema; digestive and renal disorders, especially nocturia and "starvation diarrhea"; lack of hormone and enzyme production, leading to decreased metabolic activities; loss of sexual function; amenorrhea in women; lowered blood pressure; mental restlessness and physical apathy; cancrum oris; and many other clinical and anatomic lesions, depending on the severity of starvation (partial or complete deprivation of food) and the length of time an individual is starved. The rehabilitation of the starved person should be gradual. Immediate needs are calories in the form of warm, easily digested, and bland foods to be given in small, frequent feedings and then gradually increased as tolerated. Recommended first foods are skimmed milk and simple carbohydrates. Some persons need special feedings with the use of a stomach tube or catheter. Medical supervision is needed for the severely starved persons. Full recovery is a slow process.

Nutrition, teen-age See *Nutrition, adolescence.*

Nutrition, therapeutic See *Nutrition, diet therapy,* and *Diet.*

Nutrition, toddler The nutritional problem of the child from 1 to 3 years of age is only an extension of his needs from infancy. The primary concern is to increase gradually the kind and amount of food and to lessen the number of feedings to three meals and in-between snacks. Significant in this period is the establishment of proper food habits at home, hence the need for nutrition education of mothers. For quantitative consideration of nutrient needs, see Recommended Daily Dietary Allowances, Appendix A-1.

Nutrition, tongue and mouth conditions Certain oral changes are associated with specific nutrient deficiencies. Two striking examples are the tongue and mouth lesions caused by a lack of riboflavin and nicotinic acid. In *ariboflavinosis,* angular stomatitis, cheilosis, and a purplish or magenta tongue are the characteristic lesions. In *pellagra,* the tongue is swollen and has a "beefy red" color; its papillae are smoothened or denuded and the tongue assumes a mushroom appearance. Mucous membranes and lips are also red and often fissured. The tongue and mouth lesions associated with lack of other B complex vitamins are as follows: a clean, pale, and smooth tongue (chronic atrophic glossitis) in pernicious anemia due to *vitamin B_{12}* deficiency; seborrheic angular dermatitis in *vitamin B_6* deficiency; edematous glossitis resulting from a lack of *folic acid;* and cancrum oris in *multiple vitamin B* deficiencies as seen in starvation.

Nutritional adaptation Maintenance of a fairly constant blood or tissue composition despite deficiencies or excesses of nutrients in the food supply. Any change in the diet that would create a condition of nutritional stress is checked by the body's ability to adapt itself to maintain constancy in nutrient composition. An increased supply of some nutrients leads to the accentuation of systems associated with wasteful excretion of the excess nutrient, increased metabolism, or the preferential use of the nutrient as a source of energy. A reduced supply of a nutrient leads to decreased activity of systems associated with its metabolism, e.g., the unusual thrift in the use of a scant supply seen in fasting. Eventually an adaptive increase or decrease in the utilization of a nutrient takes place.

Nutritional anthropometry Measurement of the physical dimensions and gross composition of the body at different age levels and degrees of nutrition. These measurements include height; weight; circumference of the arm, chest, and hip (ACH index); and the *Wetzel grid*. Nutritional anthropometry is a useful aid in the assessment of the nutritional status of a community as well as of an individual.

Nutritional deficiency (inadequacy) Condition of the body that may arise as a result of a lack of one or more nutrients in the diet (primary factor of nutritional inadequacy) and/or a breakdown of one or more of the bodily processes concerned with nutrient utilization (secondary factor of nutritional inadequacy). The underlying reasons for a dietary lack, either in quantity or quality, may in turn be due to poverty, ignorance of proper nutrition practices, faulty selection of food, lack of food supply as a result of poor agricultural practices, poor distribution of foods, lack of facilities for preservation and storage, and overpopulation. The secondary factors are sometimes referred to as conditioning factors of nutritional inadequacy (i.e., nutrient deficiencies occur even if the diet is adequate) because they interfere with ingestion, digestion, absorption, metabolism, etc., as enumerated below:

1. *Factors that interfere with ingestion:* gastrointestinal disturbances such as peptic ulcer and diarrhea, loss of teeth, anorexia, and neuropsychiatric disorders and therapy.
2. *Factors that interfere with absorption:* diarrhea, achlorhydria, biliary disease, gastrointestinal surgery, and therapy with mineral oil.
3. *Factors that interfere with utilization:* liver disease, diabetes mellitus, hypothyroidism, malignancy, alcoholism, and antimetabolite and sulfa drug therapy.
4. *Factors that increase nutritive requirement:* strenuous physical activity, fever, delirium, hyperthyroidism, growth, pregnancy, and lactation.
5. *Factors that increase excretion:* polyuria, lactation, excessive perspiration, and therapy that causes diuresis.
6. *Factors that increase nutrient destruction:* achlorhydria, lead poisoning, and alkali and sulfonamide therapy.

See also *Deficiency disease, Nutrition,* and *Nutriture.*

Nutritional status State of the body resulting from the consumption and utilization of nutrients. Clinical observations, biochemical analyses, anthropometric measurements, and dietary studies are used to determine this state. See also *Nutriture.*

Nutritional status assessment An evaluation of one's nutritional state is accomplished by one or more of the following methods: *dietary survey* (to detect a faulty diet, i.e., primary factor), *medical and clinical examination* (to detect conditioning factors), *biochemical tests* (to detect tissue levels), and *anthropometric tests* (to detect anatomic changes). These methods are used in *nutrition surveys.* Other sources of information helpful in appraising the nutritional status of groups of individuals or populations are vital and health statistics, food balance sheets, and other pertinent data compiled by government agencies, hospitals, clinics, insurance companies, etc. See also *Nutritional survey* and Methods of research in nutrition, Appendices M-1 to M-4.

Nutritional survey Study of the nutritional

status of a population group in a given area of operation. The population may be homogeneous (e.g., teen-aged girls or diabetics) or heterogeneous (e.g., hospital patients). Thus the survey may be slanted with respect to various factors such as age, sex, race, or socioeconomic, geographic, physiologic, or pathologic condition, depending on the aims of the study. In general the main objectives of the nutrition survey are to determine the extent of malnutrition and ascertain feeding problems, to provide ways and means of correcting or preventing nutritional problems, and to help in nutrition education, economic planning, and other programs for the improvement of the health status of the population or group. For methods of approach or techniques used in nutrition surveys, see *Nutritional status assessment*. See also *Nutrition, public health* and Methods of research in nutrition, Appendices M-1 to M-4.

Nutrition Foundation, Inc. A public nonprofit institution that was established in 1941 for "the advancement of nutrition knowledge and its effective application in improving the health and welfare of mankind." It is supported by food and allied industries. The foundation publishes *Nutrition Reviews,* monographs, and pamphlets for the layman. It also sponsors conferences on nutrition.

Nutritionist Person who applies the science of nutrition for the improvement of health and control of disease. He may organize and conduct training programs for paraprofessionals and members of allied professions on food and nutrition, coordinate the nutritional activities of public and private health and related agencies, plan and conduct meetings on nutrition, and participate in nutritional surveys.

Clinic n Person in a nutrition clinic who counsels patients about eating habits and nutrition practices. The dietary prescription is interpreted for the individual patient. Classes may be conducted for patients on the same dietary regimen. In addition, the clinic nutritionist may prepare nutrition education materials for the patient's use.

Consulting n Person who assists public and private health agencies in establishing nutrition programs and in-service training courses. His services may be used by institutions that do not have a house dietitian for diet planning and food service consultation.

Medical n Person who is a doctor of medicine and has professional training in nutrition. He conducts physical examinations to diagnose nutritional disorders and then prescribes therapeutic diets. He may also participate in nutrition surveys or engage in research on nutritional problems.

Public health n Person who establishes the nutritional needs of the community and then plans for a nutrition segment of the health program. He also consults with and supplies educational materials to other public health workers.

Research n Person who plans or assists in nutrition research projects.

Teaching n Person who teaches nutrition in an institution such as a college or university. He may also develop teaching aids and conduct demonstrations. The nutrition educator may conduct programs for the community and/or allied health professionals.

Nutriture State of nutrient balance between tissue supply and tissue requirement. Any factor or condition that increases tissue supply or decreases tissue requirement results in a favorable balance. The various conditions that affect the nutritive balance are classified into external and internal environment. The *external environment* includes socioeconomic factors (e.g., living conditions, income, and education), physicochemical factors (e.g., radiant energy, pressure and temperature conditions, and trauma), and dietary factors (e.g., kind and level of nutrient intake and availability). The *internal* or *bodily environment* includes digestive and metabolic factors (e.g., appetite, biosynthesis, transport, excretion, and storage) and stress factors (e.g., pregnancy, lactation, endocrine imbalance, and organic or infectious disease). Nutriture or nutrient status refers to the state of nutrition with regard to one specific nutrient, e.g., protein nutriture. The overall state of nutrition is called *nutritional status*.

Nyctalopia See *Night blindness.*

Nystagmus Also called nystaxis; involuntary rapid eye movements consisting of two varieties of motions that may be rotatory, horizontal, vertical, etc. It is seen in thiamin deficiency, certain eye diseases, and a number of neuromuscular disorders.

❦ O ❧

Obesity Also called adiposity; state of malnutrition in which the accumulation of depot fat is so excessive that functions of the body are disturbed. An individual is considered *obese* when his body weight is about 20% or more above the desirable weight. There are several causative factors (genetic, traumatic, environmental, etc.), but ultimately the overall picture is the result of caloric intake in excess of caloric output. *Simple obesity* is due to overeating, reduced physical activity, a disabling disease, decreased basal metabolism, or a combination of such factors. It is believed that most of the cases of overeating are psychologic in nature (to relieve tension, worry, and frustration or simply for security and pleasure). Some obesities are due to a metabolic disturbance that favors adiposity, such as in *hypothyroidism,* lesions of the *hypothalamus,* and gonadal or pituitary obesities. Obesity is not desirable for the following reasons: it shortens life expectancy, it may complicate pregnancy and surgery, it is a social and physical handicap, and it predisposes the person to disease (e.g., renal, cardiovascular, and gallbladder diseases, gout, diabetes, and arthritis). Management of obesity includes dietary regulation and exercise. Hormones and drugs such as amphetamines, diuretics, thyroid extracts, and methylcellulose are to be used *only* on the prescription and guidance of a *physician.* See also *Low calorie diet* under *Diet, calorie modified; Energy balance;* and *Overweight.*

Occlusion 1. State of being closed or shut. 2. Contact of the teeth when both jaws are closed. 3. Deficit in muscular tension when two afferent nerves are simultaneously stimulated.

Occult Obscure or hidden, as *occult blood,* which is not recognizable with the naked eye and can only be detected by chemical tests or the use of a microscope.

Oils Simple lipids chemically similar to *fats* but differing in that they are generally liquid at room temperature. There are several kinds, e.g., *animal* and *vegetable* oils used in cooking, medicine, and in many other ways; *volatile* or *essential* oils distilled from flowers, leaves, and other parts of plants; and *mineral* oils used for fuel.

Olac High protein milk formula with butterfat replacement (corn oil), added corn sugar, and added vitamins A, D, and E. Used for low birth weight infants unable to tolerate butterfat. (Mead Johnson.) See Proprietary foods: composition, features, and uses, Appendix P-1.

Oleic acid Monounsaturated fatty acid containing 18 carbon atoms. The double bond is in the *cis* configuration. It is one of the most abundant fatty acids in nature, occurring widely in animal and vegetable fats and oils.

Oligosaccharides Group of *carbohydrates* that yield two to ten simple sugars or monosaccharide units on hydrolysis. See Classification of carbohydrates, Appendix C-1.

Oliguria Decreased urinary output or volume.

This may occur in certain renal disturbances, cardiac conditions, and diarrhea.

Omasum The third division of the ruminant stomach.

Omophagia The practice of eating foods raw, especially flesh.

Oncotic pressure Pressure exerted by proteins that helps to regulate the distribution of fluids on both sides of a semipermeable membrane. In this manner, plasma proteins regulate water balance in the body. See also *Osmotic pressure*.

Opsin Protein in the eye that spontaneously reacts with retinaldehyde in the dark, forming rhodopsin. See *Visual process*.

Opsonin Form of antibody that can render bacteria and cells more susceptible to *phagocytosis*.

Optical activity (rotation) Ability of a substance to rotate the plane of polarized light. Solutions of many organic substances such as sugars and amino acids are optically active. A substance is described as *dextrorotatory* and is designated as a plus (+) rotation if it turns the plane of polarized light clockwise. When the plane of polarized light is turned counterclockwise, the substance is described as *levorotatory* and is designated as a minus (−) rotation.

Oral hypoglycemic agents Compounds ingested through the mouth that lower blood glucose levels and reduce glycosuria in certain types of diabetes. Preparations that have been available commercially for some time include tolbutamide (Orinase), chlorpropamide (Diabinese), phenformin (DBI), and acetohexamide (Dymelor). Newer compounds include tolazamide (five to ten times more potent that tolbutamide) and glymidine, which is about 188 times more potent than tolbutamide. Oral hypoglycemic agents are indicated for patients whose diabetes started in adulthood, who do not have complications such as acidosis, and whose disease is mild, requiring less than 40 units of insulin/day. They are *contraindicated* for patients with juvenile diabetes or growth-onset type of diabetes; for patients prone to ketosis; for

obese patients whose diabetes can be controlled by weight reduction and diet alone; for patients undergoing surgery, severe trauma, infection, or pregnancy; for patients experiencing hepatic and renal dysfunction; and in the presence of vomiting and diarrhea.

Organ Group of tissues that perform a particular function, e.g., the heart, liver, and kidney.

Organelle Structure found in cells that has a specific function, e.g., *mitochondria, ribosomes,* and *lysosomes.*

Organic chemistry Branch of chemistry dealing with carbon-containing compounds with the exception of cyanide and carbonate. Substances of animal and vegetable origin are generally organic in nature.

Organic matrix In bones and teeth the organic matrix consists largely of collagenous tissue in a gel of cementing substances.

Orinase Trade name for tolbutamide, an oral hypoglycemic agent.

Ornithine Diaminovaleric acid, an amino acid obtained from arginine by the hydrolytic removal of urea. Together with citrulline, arginine, and aspartic acid it is an intermediate product in the cyclic process of urea formation in the body. See *Urea cycle*.

Orotic acid A pyrimidine; when fed to rats it results in fatty liver.

Orthopnea Inability to breathe lying down; often associated with cardiac disease.

Oryzenin The major protein in rice belonging to the class glutelins.

Osmosis Passage of a solvent through a membrane from a dilute solution to a more concentrated one.

Osmotic pressure "Attractive" or drawing force that many substances in solution exert on water molecules (or solvent). It is the force exerted by a solute that causes the solvent to pass through the semipermeable membrane until the concentration on both sides is approximately equal. The osmotic pressure of body fluids is a result of the presence of various electrolytes and organic crystalloids. This pressure is one of the fundamental forces underlying physiologic processes such as the interchange of materials between blood or tissue cells and their surroundings, the excretion of urine, and the regulation of blood volume. However, osmotic pressure in the body is not constant. It varies as a result of metabolic processes and changes in concentrations of various constituents of the intra- and extracellular fluids.

Osseous tissue Bony tissue; *os* is the Latin word meaning bone. See *Bone*.

Ossification Process of bone formation. The *organic matrix* becomes strong and rigid as a result of calcification or deposition of minerals, chiefly calcium and phosphorus salts plus magnesium, carbonate, citrate, fluoride, and others in trace amounts. The structure resembles *hydroxyapatite* crystals, and the process is catalyzed by *vitamin D*.

Osteoarthritis Also called degenerative or hypertrophic *arthritis;* a joint disorder characterized by degeneration of the articular cartilage and bony outgrowths around the joints. It is a painful disease associated with advancing years and is often seen in overweight persons. Extra body weight puts a strain on the weight-bearing joints such as the ankles and knees.

Osteoblast A cell that produces bone.

Osteoclast A cell that destroys bone.

Osteolathyrism Syndrome characterized by skeletal abnormalities. It results from the ingestion of aminonitriles. See also *Lathyrism*.

Osteomalacia Also called adult rickets; softening of the bones resulting from a lack of vitamin D, calcium, and/or phosphorus. There is inadequate mineralization of the organic matrix of bones, resulting in skeletal deformities and fractures. It occurs in cloistered nuns not exposed to sunlight and among women who have become depleted of calcium because of repeated pregnancies. A diet high in protein, calcium, phosphorus, and vitamins A and D is a preventive measure.

Osteopetrosis Condition in which bone becomes hard and brittle or marblelike. Ex-

cessive fluoride intake has been associated with this disorder. It has been associated with a familial tendency and may be an inborn error of metabolism.

Osteophagia The eating of bone by animals caused by a phosphorus deficiency.

Osteoporosis Bone disorder characterized initially by abnormal porosity as a result of diminution in the absolute amount of bone. The remaining bone is normal in chemical composition. The primary defect is degeneration of the cellular matrix that holds the bone structure. It has been suggested that osteoporosis should be considered as a disorder resulting from a relative nutritional imbalance of calcium leading to bone resorption. Studies have shown that it is caused by a disturbance of calcium metabolism in association with hyperadrenocorticalism, hyperthyroidism, hyperparathyroidism, scurvy, various malignancies, immobilization, and rheumatoid arthritis. However, the condition is also seen in elderly bedridden patients with no demonstrable disease. It has also been found that persons drinking fluoridated water have a lower incidence of osteoporosis. Some evidence suggests that fluorine improves calcium balance by delaying the excretion of calcium.

OTC Abbreviation for *oxytetracycline*.

Ouch-Ouch disease Disease reported only in Fuchu, Japan. It resembles *osteomalacia* combined with proteinuria and glycosuria. The locally grown rice and soybeans contain large amounts of cadmium, lead, and zinc. It has been suggested that cadmium plays a role in this disease.

Ovalbumin The albumin of egg white. Although it is considered a simple *protein* because of its solubility and other physical properties, some authorities classify it with glycoproteins, since it contains small amounts of carbohydrate (less than 4% hexose).

Ovaries Pair of female sex glands lying deep in the pelvic cavity on either side of the uterus. Their main function is to produce ova and secrete sex hormones (estrogens and progesterone). See Summary of endocrine glands, Appendix K.

Overweight Term applied to a person whose weight is about 10% to 20% above the desirable weight. An athlete with well-developed muscles may be overweight but not obese. See also *Obesity* and *Weight*.

Ovoflavin Name given to *riboflavin* in egg. See also *Vitamin B₂*.

Ovulation The periodic ripening and rupture of the graafian follicles and eventual discharge of the ovum.

Ovum An egg; a female germ cell which, after fertilization, can develop into a new individual.

Oxalate Salt of oxalic acid. It forms insoluble calcium salts, rendering calcium unavailable for absorption. Oxalate may be excreted in the urine (oxaluria) or it may form urinary stones.

Oxidase Enzyme that oxidizes compounds by removing hydrogen and adding it to oxygen to form water. The new name for this enzyme is oxidoreductase. See *Oxidoreductase*.

Oxidation Any chemical reaction that involves the addition of oxygen, the removal of hydrogen, or in general a loss of electrons and an increase in valence. In biologic systems, oxidation requires energy. See *Physiologic oxidation* and *Phosphorylation*.

Oxidation-reduction (**oxidoreduction**) Oxidation involves a loss of electrons, and reduction involves a gain of electrons. Thus the electron donor or acceptor is itself oxidized or reduced during the process. Oxidation and reduction reactions occur simultaneously in cellular respiration; the reactions are reversibly catalyzed by *oxidoreductases*.

Oxidative phosphorylation See *Phosphorylation*.

Oxidoreductase Group term for enzymes that reversibly catalyze oxidation-reduction reactions. They are divided into subclasses according to the nature of the acceptor. A systematic name for such an enzyme has

the form *donor:acceptor oxidoreductase*. Thus ascorbic acid oxidase is called L-*ascorbate:O₂ oxidoreductase,* and malic dehydrogenase is called *malate:NAD oxidoreductase*. Some of the trivial names of enzymes included in this group are oxidase (if oxygen is the acceptor), dehydrogenase (if coenzymes are acceptors), and peroxidase (if hydrogen peroxide is the acceptor).

Oxybiotin Analog of biotin in which the sulfur is replaced by oxygen in the furan chain. It functions as a growth factor for some microorganisms.

Oxycalorimeter Apparatus that determines the caloric value of food by measuring the amount of oxygen consumed. It is used in *indirect calorimetry*.

Oxygen Nonmetallic element occurring free in the atmosphere as a colorless, tasteless gas. It is present in many substances combined with other elements. It constitutes 20% of the atmosphere and makes up 65% of body weight. Oxygen is essential to life for *respiration* and *physiologic oxidation*.

Oxygen debt Deficit of oxygen that arises during continuous or intense exercise when energy cannot be adequately supplied by oxidative means and lactic acid accumulates faster than it can be oxidized. When exercise is finished, the depth of respiration is increased to provide more oxygen to oxidize the excess lactic acid that has accumulated. See *Lactic acid*.

Oxyhemoglobin Oxygenated hemoglobin. See *Hemoglobin*.

Oxytetracycline (**OTC**) An antibiotic effective against a number of gram-positive and gram-negative bacteria, rickettsias, and viruses. It is marketed under the trade name Terramycin.

Oxythiamin Analog of thiamin in which a hydroxyl group is substituted for the free amino group on the pyrimidine ring. It acts like an antimetabolite and appears to displace thiamin from the tissues.

Oxytocin Also called pitocin; a hormone synthesized in the hypothalamus and transported to the posterior pituitary as a larger peptide, neurophysine. It stimulates uterine contractions and promotes lactation. The muscular walls of the intestines, gallblad- der, and urinary bladder are also stimu- lated and excited by this hormone. Pitocin is used clinically to induce labor.

❧ P ❧

PAA Abbreviation for *plasma amino acid*.

PABA Abbreviation for *para-aminobenzoic acid*.

PAG Abbreviation for *Protein Advisory Group* of the United Nations.

Pagophagia Eating of ice; common among Caucasian men and women. Ice is usually in the form of crushed ice and is swallowed before melting. The practice of eating ice has been associated with iron-deficiency anemia.

PAHO Abbreviation for *Pan American Health Organization*.

Pain A localized sensation of discomfort, distress, or agony resulting from the stimulation of specialized nerve endings.

Pair-feeding Method used in nutrition experiments whereby similar animals are paired and the food consumption of each pair of animals is measured. The amount to be fed the following day is determined by the animal consuming the least amount of food on the previous day.

Palate 1. Roof of the mouth, consisting of a hard bony forward part *(hard palate)* and a soft fleshy back part *(soft palate* or *velum)*. 2. Taste or the sense of taste.

Palmitic acid A saturated fatty acid containing 16 carbon atoms; one of the most abundant fatty acids. It is found both in animal and vegetable fats and oils.

Palmitoleic acid A monounsaturated fatty acid containing 16 carbon atoms. It is abundant in animal fats.

Palsy Paralysis in any part of the body, sometimes accompanied by involuntary tremors. It is due to lesions or injury of central nervous system areas associated with motor nerve activity. See also *Cerebral palsy*.

Panacea 1. A cure-all or remedy for all diseases. 2. An ancient name for various plants.

Pan American Health Organization (PAHO) Division of the World Health Organization that is concerned with the improvement of health through nutrition in Pan American countries. See also *World Health Organization*.

Pancreas Glandular organ extending across the upper abdomen close to the liver. It secretes into the intestinal tract the pancreatic juice, which contains enzymes that act on protein, fat, and carbohydrate. It also produces the hormones *insulin* and *glucagon* elaborated by its islets of Langerhans. See also *Pancreatic juice*.

Pancreatic insufficiency Deficiency of pancreatic secretion. It may be congenital or caused by a number of diseases such as carcinoma of the pancreas, pancreatitis, and cystic fibrosis. Symptoms include recurrent attacks of abdominal pain, alteration of bowel habits, change in character of stool, and malnutrition.

Pancreatic juice Digestive juice produced by the pancreas and secreted into the duodenum. It is alkaline (pH 7.5 to 8.0) and contains some protein and electrolytes, mainly sodium, potassium, bicarbonate, and chloride ions. It contains a number of enzymes involved in the digestion of protein, fat, and carbohydrate. For further details, see Summary of digestive enzymes, Appendix J-1.

Pancreatin Commercial preparation made from the pancreas of animals; contains the enzymes of *pancreatic juice.*

Pancreatitis Inflammation of the pancreas. *Acute pancreatitis* is characterized by severe epigastric pain, nausea, vomiting, fever, and decreased peristalsis. *Chronic pancreatitis* is characterized by a disturbance in the functioning of the pancreas, leading to inadequate production of digestive enzymes. As a result, stools become bulky and foul, with an increased excretion of protein, carbohydrate, and fat.

Pancreozymin Hormone produced by the intestinal mucosa that stimulates the pancreas to secrete enzymes. It has been shown to also stimulate insulin secretion.

Pandemic Term used to characterize a disease that is widespread throughout several countries, regions, or a great part of the world; an epidemic over a wide area.

Pantetheine *Pantothenic acid* joined to beta-mercaptoethylamine through a peptide linkage. It is the functional unit of *coenzyme A.*

Pantothenic acid Pantoyl-beta-alanine, a condensation product of beta-alanine and pantoic acid (dihydroxydimethylbutyric acid). It is found in the blood, liver, and other tissues in bound form. It is a water-soluble vitamin essential for growth, normal skin, development of the central nervous system, and adrenal cortex function. It is part of *coenzyme A* in the form of *pantetheine* and is universally distributed in all plants and animals. Human deficiency is unlikely to occur unless induced by an antagonist. Deficiency signs include decreased gastric secretion, impaired adrenal function, muscular weakness of fingers, rapid heart rate, and hyperactive deep reflexes. Best food sources are liver, kidney, yeast, egg yolk, nuts, lean meats, sweet potato, and whole-grain cereals. See also Summary of vitamins, Appendix I-1.

Pantoyltaurine Analog of *pantothenic acid,*

with the carboxyl group replaced by a sulfonic acid group. It acts as an antagonist to the vitamin.

Papain Proteolytic enzyme found in papaya; used as a meat tenderizer.

Papillae Small nipple-shaped projections such as the small elevations at the root of a developing tooth, hair, or feather.

Para-aminobenzoic acid (PABA) Formerly classified with the B complex vitamins, but present knowledge maintains that it is not a vitamin for higher animals, although it plays an indirect role as a component of *folic acid.* PABA has a growth-promoting effect on microorganisms and chickens. It stimulates lactation and prevents graying of the hair in rats. There is no known deficiency in man, but there has been some evidence that PABA increases the physiologic potency of insulin and penicillin. Best food sources are yeast, liver, bran and germ of cereals, and molasses.

Paracasein Compound produced by the action of rennin on casein. See *Rennin.*

Paracentesis Puncture of the wall of a body cavity by means of a hollow needle to draw out the fluid from within it; tapping.

Paralysis Loss or impairment of motor function as a result of a neural or muscular lesion. There are two types—*flaccid paralysis,* in which the muscles cannot resist stretch and appear soft and flabby, and *spastic paralysis,* in which the muscles are rigid with heightened deep reflexes.

Paraplegia Paralysis of the legs and lower part of the body, affecting motion and sensation. Of various causes such as nerve injury resulting from alcoholism, brain damage, and injury to the spinal cord.

Parasite Organism that lives within, on, or at the expense of another organism known as the host, from which the parasite obtains the nutrients essential for its growth, metabolism, and reproduction. *Parasitology* is the study of parasites and parasitism. See *Nutrition, parasitism.*

Parasympathetic nervous system Part of the autonomic nervous system comprising preganglionic fibers that arise from the midbrain, the medulla, or the sacral region of the spinal cord. It controls the activity below the level of consciousness, e.g., gland secretion, intestinal action, and heart function. The other part of the system is the *sympathetic nervous system.*

Parathormone (PTH) Parathyroid hormone or parathyrin, a protein consisting of a single polypeptide chain with alanine as its N-terminal amino acid. It exerts a profound effect on the metabolism of calcium and phosphorus. Administration of the hormone raises blood calcium and lowers blood phosphorus levels, increases the elimination of both minerals in the urine, causes migration of calcium from the bones if there is an insufficient supply of this element in the food, and increases the *phosphatase* activity of the serum.

Parathyroid glands Two pairs of small endocrine glands located in the posterior part of the thyroid gland, a pair in each lobe, one below the other. They are reddish or yellowish brown, egg-shaped bodies weighing a total of 0.1 to 0.2 gm in man. Their secretion is concerned chiefly with calcium and phosphorus metabolism. Insufficient secretion results in a decrease of calcium ions in the blood, which produces *tetany*. Oversecretion results in increased calcium in the blood and increased excretion of calcium and phosphate through the kidneys. As a result, there is muscular weakness and calcium phosphate stones are formed.

Parathyroid hormone See *Parathormone.*

Parenchyma 1. The essential or functional tissue of an organ as distinguished from its connective tissue, stroma, or framework. 2. A soft tissue of roundish, thin-walled cells in a plant stem or in the pulp of fruits.

Parenteral feeding (nutrition) A means of providing food by routes other than through the mouth and digestive tract, such as subcutaneous, intramuscular, or intravenous feeding. For short-term maintenance it is sufficient to give only glucose solution with electrolytes. However, some patients must be maintained for some time by the parenteral route. *Total parenteral feeding* is indicated only when oral or tube feeding is contraindicated or inadequate. Amino acids and protein hydrolysates have been employed. See also *Hyperalimentation.*

Paresis Slight or incomplete *paralysis.*

Paresthesia An abnormal sensation characterized as burning, pricking, or tingling. It is seen in beriberi and other disorders involving the nerves and spinal cord.

Parietal 1. Of or pertaining to the walls of a cavity. Parietal cells found on the margin of the peptic glands of the stomach secrete hydrochloric acid. 2. The parietal bone that forms part of the side and top of the skull.

Parkinson's disease A neurologic condition marked by muscular rigidity and tremors, abnormal gait and balance, and difficulties in chewing, speaking, and swallowing. Pyridoxine (vitamin B_6) appears to interfere with the therapeutic effect of levodopa in treating this condition.

Parorexia Abnormal craving for special foods, as opposed to *anorexia.*

Parotid glands Pair of serous glands situated near the ear that secrete saliva. *Parotitis* is inflammation of the parotid gland.

Paroxysm 1. Sudden recurrence or intensification of symptoms. 2. Spasm or convulsion such as an attack of asthma.

Partition Distribution of a dissolved substance between two immiscible solvents.

Partition hypothesis Theory about fat digestion and absorption that supports the view that fats are not completely hydrolyzed into fatty acids and glycerol. About 70% are in the form of di- and monoglycerides that are emulsified by bile salts. The resulting globules, or "particulate" fat, are absorbed by the lymph into the lacteals and lymphatics. The free fatty acids (about 30% of fat absorbed) enter the blood via the portal circulation. See also *Lipolytic hypothesis.*

Parturition Childbirth; process whereby the fetus is expelled from the uterus after the full term of gestation. In the human, gestation terminates about 280 days after the last menstrual period. The approximate date of parturition is determined by counting back 3 months from the first day of the last period and adding 7 days.

Passive transport Diffusion through a semipermeable membrane without the use of energy. See also *Active transport.*

Pasteur effect Inhibition of glycolysis to completion by oxygen, with an increase in lactic acid production. The admission of oxygen to a glycolytic system decreases anaerobic glycolysis so that more glucose is completely broken down, less lactic acid is formed, and maximum energy is derived from glucose. In the absence of oxygen, glucose is oxidized with the production of lactic acid and the entire energy content of glucose is not made available.

Pasteurization Heat treatment to kill most pathogenic microorganisms. The temperature is usually below 212° F and heat is applied by steam, hot water, dry heat, or electric currents. The conventional method is to heat at about 145° F for at least 30 minutes and then to cool rapidly to 50° F. In milk, pasteurization destroys pathogenic organisms and arrests fermentation.

Patch test Skin test for allergy administered by applying the suspected antigen on a filter paper and placing it on a certain patch of skin. The area is uncovered after 2 to 4 days and compared with an unpatched skin area.

Pathogen A microorganism capable of producing a disease. *Pathogenesis* is the development of a disease or morbid condition.

Pathology Branch of medicine that deals with the special nature of disease by studying its causes and effects and its processes and changes on the structure and performance of a tissue. A specialist in this field is a *pathologist.*

PBI Abbreviation for *protein-bound iodine.*

PCM Abbreviation for *protein calorie malnutrition.*

Pectase Enzyme that catalyzes the conversion of pectin to pectic acid.

Pectic substances Group designation for complex colloidal carbohydrate derivatives that occur in or are prepared from plants. They contain a large proportion of anhydrogalacturonic acids. The carboxyl groups may be partly esterified by methyl groups and partly or completely neutralized by one or more bases. Pectic substances include protopectin, pectin, pectinic acid, and pectic acid.

Pedialyte Oral electrolyte mixture for maintenance of body fluid and electrolyte balance in infants and children with diarrhea. (Ross.) See Proprietary foods: composition, features, and uses, Appendix P-1.

Pediatrics Branch of medicine concerned with child development and care and the treatment of diseases of children. A *pediatrician* is a specialist in this field.

Pellagra From *pelle,* meaning "skin," and *agra,* meaning "rough." A deficiency disease due to lack of niacin (nicotinic acid); characterized by dermatitis, diarrhea, dementia, and eventually death if unremedied. These pellagrous symptoms are commonly referred to as the classic 4 D's. The skin changes occur in several stages: there is thickening and pigmentation with temporary redness similar to sunburn, then atrophic thinning with dark red eruption, followed by desquamation. In its severe stage the involved parts erupt and swell with ulceration and infection. Typical pellagrous dermatosis is symmetric, clearly demarcated, and hyperpigmented. Parts of the body exposed to sunlight are commonly affected, e.g., cheeks, neck, hands, and forearms. The digestive disturbances include sore mouth with angular stomatitis, bright red or scarlet tongue with glossitis, achlorhydria, and nausea and vomiting, followed by severe diarrhea. The neurologic disturbances include insomnia, irritability, poor memory, confusion, delusions of persecution, hallucinations, and dementia. Pellagra is also seen in alcoholism, Hartnup syndrome, multiple carcinoid tumors, and in persons whose staple diet consists of jowar. Evidence indicates that an imbalance of leucine may be an important mechanism in the etiology of pellagra. In pellagrous individuals there is a reduced secretion of gastric and pancreatic digestive enzymes. This suggests that a reduced secretion of enzymes leads to poor digestion and diarrhea.

Pellagra preventive factor (PPF) White crystalline substance first isolated from yeast and rice bran. It was originally thought to be riboflavin but was later identified as nicotinamide.

Pelvis Any basinlike structure such as the pelvis or sac in the kidney and the pelvic bone in the hips.

PEM Abbreviation for *protein energy malnutrition.*

Penicillamine Chelating agent that is employed to remove excess copper from the body. It is used principally to treat patients with *Wilson's disease* and *cystinuria.* See *Chelate.*

Penicillin Antibiotic obtained from the cultures of *Penicillium notatum.* It is bacteriostatic for many microorganisms and useful in the treatment of infections caused by nearly all gram-positive bacteria.

Pentosan Also called pentan; a homopolysaccharide or a complex carbohydrate of pentose units that is widely distributed in wood, straw, gums, hulls, and corncobs. It is not digested by man, but it is hydrolyzed by acid to yield pentoses. Examples are arabans and xylans.

Pentose A 5-carbon monosaccharide. Pentoses important to nutrition are arabinose, xylose, ribose, 2-deoxyribose, xylulose, and ribulose. The first four are aldoses and do not occur free in nature; the last two are ketoses. Arabinose is obtained by hydrolyzing various gummy substances; xylose is derived from wood and straw; ribose and deoxyribose are constitutents of *nucleic*

acids; xylulose is often the sugar found in the urine in *pentosuria;* and ribulose is found only as an intermediate metabolite in the *hexose monophosphate shunt.* See also *Pentosan.*

Pentose phosphate pathway Another designation for the *hexose monophosphate shunt.*

Pentosuria Excretion of pentose in the urine. *Alimentary pentosuria* occurs temporarily in normal individuals after ingestion of large amounts of prunes, cherries, grapes, and other foods rich in pentoses (mainly arabinose and xylose). *Congenital pentosuria* is due to an inborn error of metabolism for which there is no cure at present. In this case the body cannot metabolize L-xylulose.

PEP Abbreviation for *phosphoenolpyruvate.*

Pepsin Digestive enzyme in gastric juice that converts protein to peptones and proteoses. It occurs in the stomach as an inactive precursor, *pepsinogen,* which is converted to the active pepsin by hydrochloric acid.

Peptic ulcer Ulceration on the mucous membranes of the esophagus, stomach, or duodenum. See *Ulcer.*

Peptidase Proteolytic enzyme that acts on peptide bonds.

Peptide Compound formed when two or more amino acids are linked together by the CONH linkage, called the *peptide linkage,* which is the main bond in protein structure. See also *Polypeptide* and *Protein.*

Peptization Process of making a colloidal solution more stable; conversion of a gel to a sol.

Peptone A secondary protein derivative. When protein is hydrolyzed, it is changed to proteoses, then peptones, peptides, and finally amino acids. Peptones, as distinguished from proteoses, are not precipitated by ammonium sulfate or tannic acid. *Peptonization* is the conversion of protein to peptones, using suitable proteolytic enzymes such as those found in *pancreatin* or pancreatic juice.

Peptonized milk Milk that is predigested by adding pancreatic extract and sodium bicarbonate before feeding. Curds formed in the stomach are soft and small, facilitating digestion.

PER Abbreviation for *protein efficiency ratio*.

Per capita consumption The amount of food consumed per person per day or other specified time.

Perfusion 1. Act of pouring over or through. 2. Introduction or passage of fluids through tissues and spaces.

Pericardium Membranous sac surrounding the heart. It prevents friction between the heart and the lungs and it also helps to support the heart. *Pericarditis* is inflammation of the pericardium. It may result from rheumatic fever, kidney disease, tuberculosis, or infection from neighboring parts of the heart. Symptoms include mild fever, pain and tenderness over the heart region, difficulty in breathing, and rapid pulse rate.

Periodic table Table of chemical elements arranged according to the periodic laws; i.e., the chemical and physical properties of elements are periodic functions of their atomic weight. At present there are 103 chemical elements in the periodic table.

Periodontal Occurring or situated around a tooth or periodontal membrane.

Peristalsis Normal wavy movement of the gastrointestinal tract characterized by alternate contraction and relaxation along the walls from the esophagus to the intestine, forcing the contents toward the anus. Peristaltic waves are of two kinds—*slow* progressive contraction and relaxation covering a short distance and the peristaltic *rush* that sweeps along the intestine without pause and covers a relatively long distance. *Reverse peristalsis* is an abnormal backward movement of the intestine, as seen in pyloric obstruction and diverticulitis.

Peritoneal cavity Region bordered by the parietal layer of the *peritoneum*. It contains all the abdominal organs except the kidneys.

Peritoneum Serous membrane that lines the interior of the abdominal cavity and surrounds the viscera. It is a closed sac except in the female, where it is continuous with the mucous membrane of the fallopian tube. *Peritonitis* is inflammation of the peritoneum. It is accompanied by fever, abdominal pain, vomiting, and constipation.

Perlèche Former term for *angular stomatitis*. The epithelial linings of the lips are thickened and desquamated. See also *Nutrition, tongue and mouth conditions*.

Permeability Property or state of being penetrated. *Capillary permeability* is the property of the capillary walls that allows filtration and diffusion. This is important in the exchange of substances between the blood and tissue fluids. See also *Osmosis*.

Pernicious Causing injury or death; destructive or incurable. *Pernicious anemia* is a misnomer since the advent of liver extract and vitamin B_{12} therapy. However, the term is retained traditionally to designate a clinical entity.

Pernicious anemia A chronic macrocytic anemia found mostly in middle-aged and elderly persons. The red blood cells cannot be supplied by the bone marrow as rapidly as needed because of vitamin B_{12} deficiency conditioned by the lack of intrinsic factor. This factor is a glycoprotein found normally in gastric juice and is essential for the absorption of vitamin B_{12}. Pernicious anemia is characterized by disturbances in the gastrointestinal, nervous, and blood-forming systems. The symptoms are achlorhydria, atrophy of the gastric mucosa, diarrhea, glossitis, paresthesia, ataxia, degeneration of the lateral and posterior tracts of the spinal cord, macrocytosis that is often hyperchromic, and hyperplastic bone marrow. Treatment consists of vitamin B_{12} supplementation. See also *Anemia, Hemopoiesis*, and *Vitamin B_{12}*.

Perosis Slipped tendon or hock disease seen in chickens that is primarily due to a lack of choline. It is also associated with a high intake of inorganic phosphate and calcium salts and a low intake of manganese and biotin.

Peroxidation Formation of peroxides as a result of the action of oxygen on poly-unsaturated fatty acids. Vitamin E prevents lipid peroxidation in cells.

Peroxide value 1. Measure of reactive oxygen expressed as milliequivalents of oxygen. 2. Rancidity test for fats measured by the amount of iodine released when potassium iodide reacts with rancid fat.

Perspiration Also called sweat; the secretion and exudation of fluid by the sweat glands of the skin, averaging about 700 ml/day. See also *Insensible perspiration.*

Petechiae Small, pinpoint-sized, nonraised, purplish red spots in the skin formed by subcutaneous effusion of blood. It is seen in vitamin C deficiency.

PGA Abbreviation for *pteroylglutamic acid.*

pH Symbol commonly used in expressing hydrogen ion concentration; a measure of alkalinity and acidity. It is the logarithm of the reciprocal of the hydrogen ion concentration.

Phagocyte Cell that can engulf particles or cells that are foreign or harmful to the body. Phagocytes are present in the blood, lymph, lungs, liver, and spleen.

Phagocytosis Process of ingesting a moving or foreign particle through the cell membrane. It is one of the body's defense mechanisms against bacteria and other harmful substances. In this process a portion of the cellular membrane envelops the foreign body by forming a small pocket outside the cell and then pinches it off from the surface to create an intracellular vacuole.

Pharmacology Branch of medicine that has to do with the nature, properties, effects, and uses of drugs.

Pharmacopoeia Book that describes drugs and standard preparations used in medicine. The *United States Pharmacopoeia* is revised every 5 years by a committee of experts.

Pharynx Muscular and membranous tube extending from the oral cavity to the esophagus.

Phaseolin A simple protein of the globulin type occurring in kidney beans.

Phenformin An *oral hypoglycemic agent* used for diabetics whose pancreas can still produce insulin. It is suitable for middle-aged patients with mild diabetes and is marketed under the trade name DBI.

Phenol C_6H_5OH; an aromatic derivative in which the hydroxyl group is attached directly to the benzene ring. It is a crystalline or light pink solid obtained from coal tar. It has a characteristic odor and is dangerous because of its rapid corrosive action on tissues. The liquid form is commonly called carbolic acid. It is useful as an antiseptic, disinfectant, and local anesthetic.

Phenylalanine Alpha-amino-beta-phenylpropionic acid, an *essential amino acid* rarely limiting in protein foods. It is easily converted to *tyrosine,* but the reaction is not reversible. As a precursor of tyrosine, phenylalanine is also involved in reactions where tyrosine plays a direct role, as in melanin formation. Phenylalanine participates in *transamination* and can be ketogenic as well as glycogenic. See also *Phenylketonuria.*

Phenylketonuria (**PKU**) Also called phenylpyruvic oligophrenia; an inborn error of metabolism transmitted as a simple mendelian recessive trait. The underlying biochemical defect is the failure to convert the essential amino acid *phenylalanine* into tyrosine due to the absence of the liver enzyme phenylalanine hydroxylase. Serum phenylalanine level is elevated, and phenylpyruvic acid is excreted in the urine. If not treated, it causes mental retardation; poor growth and development with reduction in stature and head size; reduced pigment production, resulting in fair skin and blond hair; eczematous dermatitis; poor muscular coordination; and the accumulation of phenylpyruvic acid in the blood, which eventually appears in the urine. The treatment requires dietary restriction of phenylalanine. See *Diet, phenylalanine-restricted.* See also Inborn errors of metabolism, Appendix G, and Dietary management of selected disorders, Appendix O.

Pheochromocytoma A vascular tumor of the adrenal medulla that causes the production of abnormal amounts of catecholamines, resulting in hypertension. Various cardiovascular and metabolic disturbances are associated with this disorder.

Phlorizin Also spelled phlorhizin or phloridzin; a bitter glycoside from the root bark of apple, cherry, plum, and pear trees. It causes glycosuria by blocking the tubular reabsorption of glucose. It is used as a test for kidney function and to examine the formation of glucose from other ingredients of the diet.

Phobia Neurotic or abnormal dread or fear.

Phosphatase Enzyme that hydrolyzes monophosphoric esters with the liberation of inorganic phosphate. It is found in practically all cells, body fluids, and tissues. Phosphatases constitute a large and complex group of enzymes, some of which appear to be highly specific.

Acid p A phosphatase active in an acid medium that is found in mammalian erythrocytes, yeast prostatic epithelium, spleen, kidney, blood plasma, liver, and pancreas. It is useful in diagnosing prostatic carcinoma metastases, Gaucher's disease, and certain diseases of the bones.

Alkaline p A phosphatase active in an alkaline medium that is found in blood plasma or serum, bone, kidney, mammary gland, spleen, lung, leukocytes, adrenal cortex, and seminiferous tubules. It is useful in diagnosing rickets, hyperparathyroidism, and liver dysfunction.

Phosphate bond energy Energy trapped in the phosphate bond of "phosphate carriers," which are of two categories—the relatively inert types or those that release 3000 calories on hydrolysis as triose phosphates and the active phosphate carriers that yield 5000 to 12,000 calories for each

energy-rich bond hydrolyzed. To the latter belong creatine phosphate and adenosine di- and triphosphate. The energy released by the energy-rich bonds is used mainly for biologic oxidation in muscular work and maintenance of cell potential. See also *Phosphorylation; Oxidation;* and *Oxidation-reduction.*

Phosphatidic acid A phosphatide that yields on total hydrolysis 1 mole each of glycerol and phosphoric acid and 2 moles of fatty acid.

Phosphocreatine Also called creatine phosphate; a constituent of the muscles that acts as a phosphate donor when hydrolyzed into creatine and phosphate. For its biologic role, see *Creatine.*

Phosphoenol pyruvate (PEP) A metabolite in the glycolytic pathway.

Phosphogluconate shunt Also called phosphogluconate oxidative pathway. See *Hexose monophosphate shunt.*

Phosphoinositide Inositol containing phosphatides. The synthesis and degradation of these compounds occur mainly in the brain. On hydrolysis, phosphoinositide yields glycerol, L-myoinositol, fatty acids, and phosphoric acid. These compounds are important in the transport processes of the cells.

Phosphokinase Enzyme that transfers the phosphate radical together with its energy to or from adenosine di- or triphosphate.

Phospholipid Also called phosphatide; substituted fat containing a phosphoric acid residue, nitrogenous compounds, and other constituents in addition to fatty acids and glycerol. Phospholipids include *lecithins, sphingomyelins, cephalins,* and *plasmalogens. Sphingomyelins* contain 4-sphingenine in place of glycerol. Phospholipids are essential components of the cell membrane. They play a role in electron transport, stimulate protein synthesis in special systems, affect cell permeability in ion transport, affect fat absorption and transport, and induce blood coagulation with the formation of thromboplastin.

Phosphoprotein Conjugated protein compounds with a phosphorus radical other than nucleic acid (nucleoproteins) or lecithin. To this group belong the ovovitellin of egg yolk and the casein of milk.

Phosphorolysis Chemical reaction wherein the elements of phosphoric acid rather than water are incorporated into the molecule of a compound. The degradation of glycogen to glucose-1-phosphate is accomplished by adding phosphoric acid.

Phosphorus Essential mineral widely distributed in nature; deficiency is not observed in man, since diets are normally adequate. Phosphorus is a constituent of a buffer system and helps to regulate the pH of blood; it gives rigidity to bones and teeth together with calcium; it regulates osmotic pressure; it is a component of nucleic acid and energy-rich compounds such as adenosine di- and triphosphate; it transports fatty acids (as phospholipids); and it is a constituent of coenzymes involved in fat and carbohydrate metabolism. For further details, see Summary of minerals, Appendix H.

Phosphorylase Enzyme that in the presence of inorganic phosphate, is able to catalyze the reversible change of glycogen into glucose phosphate (Cori ester and inorganic phosphate). It is widely distributed in animals, plants, and microorganisms.

Phosphorylation Formation of phosphate esters of sugars or their derivatives. This reaction is the initial step in the metabolism of all sugars, e.g., trioses, tetroses, pentoses, hexoses, and heptoses, as well as sugar acids and sugar alcohols. *Oxidative phosphorylation* is the formation of an energy-rich phosphate bond, adenosine triphosphate (ATP), when adenosine diphosphate (ADP) reacts with inorganic phosphate. The term "coupled oxidative phosphorylation" is the preferred term because it explains the reactions collectively, which occur in the following manner: energy obtained from the metabolism of carbohydrate, protein, and fat is trapped in a form that could be released slowly in regulated amounts as needed for the functions of the cell. The energy potential of carbon is released through decarboxylation, while the energy potential of hydrogen is released through the electron transport chain, with ATP as the "coupling agent," storing the energy released from the electron flow. The seat of coupled oxidative phosphorylation is in the *mitochondria* of cells. See also Embden-Meyerhof pathway, Hexose monophosphate shunt, Krebs cycle, and Electron transport system and coupled oxidative phosphorylation, Appendices F-1 to F-4.

Photophobia Abnormal sensitivity to light as seen in riboflavin deficiency.

Photosynthesis Process of utilizing or "fixing" carbon dioxide and water into carbohydrate in the presence of radiant energy from the sun by the chlorophyll of green plants. This photosynthetic reaction is the primary source of food in the biosphere and is referred to as *light-reaction* photosynthesis. Tracer studies have shown that photosynthesis can take place in the absence of radiant energy. This is called the *dark reaction* by which carbon dioxide fixation occurs without radiant energy but with chemical energy. Carbohydrate intermediates are synthesized by enzymatic reactions similar to the metabolic pathway of the *hexose monophosphate shunt*. See also *Carbon dioxide fixation*.

Phylloquinone 2-Methyl-3-phytyl-1,4-naphthoquinone or vitamin K_1, found in plants. See *Vitamin K*.

Physiologic fuel value See *Food, energy value*.

Physiologic oxidation Reaction taking place in cellular respiration. See *Oxidation*.

Physiologic salt solution See *Solution*.

Physiology Science that deals with the functions of living organisms.

Phytanic acid 3,7,11,15-Tetramethylhexadecanoic acid, a branched chain fatty acid. See *Refsum's syndrome*.

Phytic acid The hexaphosphoric acid ester of *inositol*, occurring in the leaves of certain plants and cereal husks. It forms insoluble or almost insoluble compounds that are eliminated in the feces. It also reduces the coefficient of utilization of minerals, particularly calcium, phosphorus, iron, and magnesium. *Phytase* is a phosphatase enzyme that splits phytin into inositol and phosphoric acid. It is present in yeast, liver, blood, malt, and seeds.

Phytohormone Also called plant hormone; substance secreted by plant cells for specific functions such as growth and cell division. There are several types, including *auxins, indolacetic acid, gibberellins,* and *kinin.*

Phytol An unsaturated aliphatic alcohol; related to xanthophyll, carotenoids, and vitamin A. It is a precursor of *phytanic acid* and is found as an ester in *chlorophyll.*

Phytosterol Also called plant sterol. See under *Sterols.*

P$_i$ Abbreviation for *inorganic phosphate.*

pI Abbreviation for *isoionic point.*

Pica An abnormal craving for unusual articles such as hair, clay, chalk, laundry starch, and dirt. Although this is rarely seen in man, it presents a nutritional problem when it occurs. The cause is not well understood. It has been observed in hysteria, mentally defective children, and some pregnant women. In experimental animals the practice appears to be a compensatory mechanism for some dietary lack.

PIDH 1-(2-Pyrimidinyl)-4-imino-1,4-dihydropyridine hydrochloride, a new oral hypoglycemic agent.

Pile Also called hemorrhoid; an enlarged vein of the anus engorged with blood.

Pineal gland (body) Also called epiphysis cerebri; a small cone-shaped body lying at the base of the brain near the pituitary gland. A tumor of the pineal body in children causes precocious puberty. In experimental animals, removal of the pineal body results in precocious sexual development.

Pinocytosis Process whereby a cell absorbs liquids. The membrane invaginates and then closes to form a liquid-filled vacuole. It is similar to phagocytosis, whereby a cell engulfs solid particles.

Pitocin See *Oxytocin.*

Pituitary gland Also called hypophysis; an *endocrine gland.* The word "pituitary" refers to mucus or phlegm, which was mistakenly thought to be the main secretion of the gland. Hypophysis ("to grow under") is the preferred name, since this gland is located under the brain. For details, see *Hypophysis.*

PKU Abbreviation for *phenylketonuria.*

Placebo An inactive substance or preparation that has no effect but is similar in appearance to a substance being tested. It is used in metabolic and controlled studies to determine the efficacy of substances.

Placenta 1. Any cakelike mass. 2. Cakelike organ within the uterus that is the means of communication between the fetus and mother through the umbilical cord. The maternal and fetal blood are separated by two thin membranes that eventually fuse. All fetal nourishment must pass through this barrier. The placenta also elaborates hormones needed for normal pregnancy. See *Gonadotropic hormones.*

Plague An acute febrile, infectious, and fatal disease. There are several types. The well-known examples are bubonic plague transmitted by rodents, hog plague, fowl plague, and bovine plague. Tuberculosis is sometimes called the white plague.

Plaque 1. Any patch or flat area. 2. A blood platelet.

Atherosclerotic p See *Atherosclerosis.*

Plasma 1. The liquid portion of the blood in which corpuscles are suspended. (When fibrinogen is separated from the plasma by blood clotting, the remaining fluid is called *serum.*) 2. The lymph without its cells. 3. The cytoplasm or protoplasm. 4. A starch glycerite used in preparing ointments.

Plasma amino acid (PAA) The amino acid levels in the plasma can be used as a measure of protein quality. It is expressed as the following ratio:

$$PAA = \frac{B - A}{Amino\ acid\ needs} \times 100$$

191

where A and B are the plasma amino acid concentrations measured immediately before and after the meal. See also *Protein quality*.

Plasmalogen A *phospholipid* containing an unsaturated ether in place of a fatty acid. On hydrolysis it yields glycerol, phosphoric acid, a nitrogen base, a fatty acid, and an unsaturated fatty aldehyde. It is widely distributed in nature, especially in cardiac and skeletal muscles, brain, egg, and liver. The biologic role is not understood except that plasmalogens are found as structural components of tissues.

Plasmin Also called fibrinolysin; proteolytic enzyme that can dissolve blood clots or fibrin by changing them to peptides. It ordinarily exists in plasma as the inactive precursor *plasminogen* (or profibrinolysin).

Platelet Also called thrombocyte. See *Blood platelet* and *Blood clotting*.

Pleurae Serous membranes such as the parietal pleura and the visceral pleura. These thin membranes envelop the lungs and line the thoracic cavity, thus completely enclosing a space called the *pleural cavity*. The pleurae are moistened with a serous secretion to facilitate movement of the lungs. *Pleurisy* is an inflammation of the pleurae and may be accompanied by exudation of serum or lymph with cellular elements.

Plexus A network or "braid," especially of nerves, veins, or lymphatic vessels.

Plumbism Chronic poisoning due to absorption of lead or its salts. Symptoms are poor appetite, stomachache, vomiting, constipation, headache, paleness, and in advanced cases convulsions and coma. See *Lead*.

Pneumothorax Increased amount of air in the pleural cavity that results in extra pressure on the lung. The air may come from the outside through a chest wound, or it may be due to a breakdown in a diseased portion of the lung, creating an opening into the pleural cavity.

Poikilocyte Erythrocyte of abnormal size and shape. *Poikilocytosis* is a condition charac-terized by the presence of poikilocytes in the blood.

Polarimetry Measurement of the rotation of polarized light in a *polarimeter* or a *polariscope*. Many substances are optically active and have the power to bend or rotate polarized light. The extent of rotation depends on the nature and the number of molecules in the substance and is expressed as the specific rotation of the substance. See *Specific rotation*.

Polarity 1. The property of having pronounced electron activity, e.g., polar groups (COO^-, NH_2, OH^-) in contrast to the nonpolar groups such as ring compounds and hydrocarbon chains. 2. The exhibition of opposite effects at the two extremities. 3. The special property of the nerve cell with regard to the flow of impulses.

Poliomyelitis Commonly called polio or infantile paralysis; an acute viral infection characterized by fever, sore throat, headache, and stiffness of the neck and back in the early stage. Later the central nervous system is affected with paralysis and subsequent atrophy of certain muscles, ending in permanent contraction and deformity. There are several types—the *spinal paralytic* type is the classic form of acute anterior polio, the *bulbar* type is a serious form affecting the medulla oblongata and marked by difficulty in swallowing, and the *cerebral* type involves the brain cells, leading to paralysis of the skeletal muscles.

Polycythemia Increased number of red blood cells. This has been observed in animals consuming an excess of cobalt.

Polydipsia Excessive thirst due to loss of body fluids, especially in the urine, as seen in *diabetes mellitus*.

Polymer Compound, usually of high molecular weight, formed by the combination of simpler molecules. *Polymerization* is the process of forming a compound by combining simpler molecules.

Polymorphism Occurrence of different crystal forms of the same chemical substance. Fat exhibits polymorphism; hence its melting point occurs over a temperature range.

Polyneuritis Condition that involves the inflammation of many nerves. It occurs in thiamin deficiency.

Polyneuropathy Multiple noninflammatory degeneration of nerves. *Nutritional polyneuropathy* is caused by a lack of nutrients, particularly the B complex vitamins. It is characterized by bilateral lesions of the legs with cramps, ataxia, foot drop, loss of vibratory and positional senses, and paresthesia. It is seen in beriberi, chronic alcoholism, starvation, and toxemias of pregnancy.

Polypeptide A long chain of amino acids (usually about 100 units) linked by the *peptide linkage*. Polypeptides are smaller than proteins but larger than proteoses.

Polyphagia 1. Swallowing abnormally large amounts of food at a meal. 2. Excessive appetite as in diabetes mellitus.

Polysaccharide Also called glycan; a carbohydrate containing ten or more monosaccharide units. Polysaccharides are classified according to digestibility (digestible, partially digestible, and indigestible) or according to the type of products resulting from their hydrolysis (homo- or heteropolysaccharide). Those of nutritional significance are glycogen, starch, and cellulose. See *Homopolysaccharide* and *Heteropolysaccharide*. See also Classification of carbohydrates, Appendix C-1.

Polysome (polyribosome) A polymer of *ribosomes,* which are the site of protein biosynthesis.

Polyunsaturated fatty acids (PUFA) Fatty acids that have more than one unsaturated linkage in the chain. See *Fatty acids.*

Polyuria Excessive secretion and discharge of urine as seen in *diabetes mellitus.*

Ponderal index Measure of obesity based on height in inches divided by the cube root of weight in pounds. For example, a ponderal index of less than 12.4 is indicative of obesity in adolescent girls.

Pons 1. Bridge of tissue connecting two parts

of an organ. 2. Whitish tissue situated at the base of the brain consisting of fibers and nuclei that receive impulses from the cerebral cortex and send fibers to the contralateral side of the cerebellum.

Porphyrin Derivative of the fundamental substance *porphin* that contains four pyrrole-like units linked by four CH groups or methene bridges to form a large ring structure. Porphyrins form metal chelates with a variety of ions, including magnesium, iron, zinc, cobalt, and copper. This type of structure is found in hemoglobin, cytochrome, and chlorophyll. *Porphyria* is a condition in which excessive amounts of porphyrins are excreted.

Portacaval shunt Formation of an anastomosis between the portal vein and the vena cava. Digested nutrients enter the general circulation rather than the portal vein, which goes directly to the liver. This is done when there is limited liver function, portal hypertension, and hemorrhage.

Portagen Nutritionally complete dietary product that contains 95% of the fat as *medium-chain triglycerides* and 5% as safflower oil to provide linoleic acid. It is used when fat is not well digested or absorbed. (Mead Johnson.) See Proprietary foods: composition, features, and uses, Appendix P-1.

Portal vein The superior mesenteric and the splenic vein merge to form the portal vein, which enters the liver. The capillaries of the villi in the small intestine empty into the portal vein. In this way the absorbed nutrients are carried to the liver.

Postprandial blood sugar Amount of sugar in blood immediately after a meal. It will be elevated from the fasting level due to the absorption of digested sugars from the intestine.

Potassium Mineral that is the chief cation in the intracellular fluids. It plays the same role as sodium in the extracellular fluids. Although dietary deficiency is unlikely to occur, it may result from prolonged diarrhea, abnormal kidney function, diabetic acidosis, and renal disease. Symptoms of deficiency are weakness, nervous irritability, mental disorientation, and cardiac irregularities. *Hyperkalemia* refers to an elevated level of potassium in the blood. See Summary of minerals, Appendix H.

PPF Abbreviation for *pellagra preventive factor.*

Precipitin Antibody that causes bacterial antigens to precipitate out as a mass.

Precision-LR Nutritionally complete low residue food for oral and tube feeding; made with egg white solids, maltodextrin, sugar, vegetable oil, and added vitamins and minerals. (Doyle.) See Proprietary foods: composition, features, and uses, Appendix P-1.

Precursor A forerunner; something that precedes another factor; e.g., carotene is a precursor of vitamin A. See also *Provitamin.*

Prediabetes The period when one can detect an early abnormality that precedes diabetes mellitus and is not dependent on insufficient insulin activity. It is a phase during which the body is coping successfully with diabetogenic forces. The period of prediabetes may be a span of a few years in childhood to several years in patients in whom diabetes mellitus did not develop until middle or later life.

Preeclampsia A *toxemia* of pregnancy characterized by hypertension, albuminuria, and edema of the lower extremities. See *Toxemia* and *Eclampsia.*

Preformed Ready for use by the body in contrast to *precursor.*

Pregestimil Protein hydrolysate formula containing glucose, MCT oil, vitamins, and minerals for infants with malabsorption problems. (Mead Johnson.) See Proprietary foods: composition, features, and uses, Appendix P-1.

Pregnancy Also called gestation; the condition of having a developing embryo or fetus in the body after the union of an ovum and a spermatozoan. In women the period of pregnancy is about 266 to 280 days. It is divided into three main phases,

i.e., *implantation,* the first 2 weeks of gestation during which the fertilized ovum becomes embedded in the wall of the uterus and the placenta develops; *organogenesis,* the next 6 weeks during which the developing fetal tissue undergoes differentiation; and *growth,* the remaining 7 months of pregnancy, characterized by rapid cell division and development. See also *Nutrition, pregnancy,* and *Parturition.*

Premature infant A liveborn infant weighing less than 2500 gm (5½ pounds) at birth or born before the thirty-sixth week of the gestational period. There are many causes of premature births, some of which are unknown. Undoubtedly maternal malnutrition is a significant cause.

Pressor nerve Afferent nerve that on stimulation causes an increase in blood pressure by a reflex constriction of the blood vessels.

Pressure Force per unit area. See *Osmotic pressure* and *Oncotic pressure.*

Probana High protein formula with banana powder and lactic acid for infants with diarrhea, cystic fibrosis, and celiac syndrome. (Mead Johnson.) See Proprietary foods: composition, features, and uses, Appendix P-1.

Proconvertin Also called serum prothrombin conversion accelerator (SPCA), cothromboplastin, and autoprothrombin I; a name synonymous with *factor VII* (stable factor); required for the conversion of prothrombin to thrombin. See *Blood clotting.*

Proenzyme *Zymogen* or proferment.

Progesterone Hormone produced by the *corpus luteum.* Its main function is to prepare the uterus for the reception and development of the fertilized ovum.

Prognosis Prediction of the probable course of a disease and the chances of recovery as indicated by the nature and symptoms of the condition.

Proinsulin Compound believed to be a precursor in the biosynthesis of insulin. The mechanism involves a proteolytic process that results in the liberation of insulin from "proinsulin."

Project Head Start Program started in 1965

by the Office of Economic Opportunity to help disadvantaged preschool children from poverty areas attain their potential in growth and physical and mental development before entering school. Nutrition is an important part of this project. Meals and snacks are provided at the Head Start centers. In addition, meal planning and preparation classes are held for the parents of these children.

Prolactin See *Luteotropic hormone.*

Prolamine Simple protein insoluble in water, neutral solvents, and absolute alcohol but soluble in 70% to 80% alcohol. Examples are *zein* (corn) and *gliadin* (wheat). See Classification of proteins, Appendix C-2.

Proline A heterocyclic nonessential amino acid. See *Amino acid.*

Prolo Protein food mixture developed in the United Kingdom; made of soya flour, DL-methionine, minerals, vitamin A, thiamin, riboflavin, and niacin. See Protein food mixtures, Appendix P-2.

Pronutro Protein food mixture developed in South Africa; made of maize, skim milk powder, peanut, soybean, fish protein concentrate, yeast, wheat germ, sugar, iodized salt, vitamin A, thiamin, riboflavin, and niacin. See Protein food mixtures, Appendix P-2.

Properdin Protein found in normal serum in trace amounts. It has an antibacterial action and protects the body against certain bacterial, viral, or even protozoan diseases.

Prophylaxis Prevention of disease. A prophylactic is a remedy or agent that helps protect from disease.

Propionic acid CH_3CH_2COOH; an acid found in chyme and sweat. It is one of the products of alcoholic and propionic fermentation. Its calcium and sodium salts are used as fungicides.

Proprietary foods Commercially prepared foods under the patent, trademark, or brand of a company. They are prepared to conform to certain standards and are properly labeled. For common examples, see Proprietary foods: composition, features, and uses, Appendix P-1.

Proprietary milk Special preparation that may or may not be made from cow's milk to meet specific needs of infants. For examples, see Proprietary foods: composition, features, and uses, Appendix P-1.

Prosobee Milk-free formula made with soy protein isolate, soy oil, corn sugar, and sucrose with added iron, vitamins, and minerals. (Mead Johnson.) See Proprietary foods: composition, features, and uses, Appendix P-1.

Prostaglandins New family of hormones composed of 14 fatty acids with 20 carbons, of which carbons 8 to 12 are involved in a five-membered ring. The polyunsaturated fatty acids serve as precursors for these compounds. They perform a variety of functions in the body—blood pressure depressants, smooth muscle stimulants, and antagonists to several other hormones.

Prosthetic group Nonprotein molecule that confers characteristic properties on the complex protein. The binding to protein is very firm, as in the heme of hemoglobin. See also *Coenzyme* and *Cofactor.*

Protamine A simple protein soluble in water or in ammonium hydroxide but not coagulated by heat. This basic polypeptide contains a relatively small number of amino acids. Examples are salmine (in salmon) and sturine (in sturgeon). See also Classification of proteins, Appendix C-2.

Protease Enzyme that hydrolyzes protein into smaller fragments, e.g., proteoses, peptones, peptides, and amino acids.

Protease inhibitor A substance that has the ability to inhibit the proteolytic activity of certain enzymes. It is found throughout the plant kingdom, particularly among the legumes. *Trypsin inhibitor* is found in soybeans, lima beans, and mung beans. *Chymotrypsin inhibitor* is found in cereal grains and potato. Protease inhibitors are destroyed by heating.

Protective foods Milk, eggs, meats, vegetables, and fruits. These groups were called "protective" by McCollum because they are good sources of many nutrients that prevent deficiency diseases in contrast to foods that supply *"empty calories."*

Protein Organic compound essential to all living organisms. It is a polymer of *amino acids* linked together by peptide bonds. This forms the primary structure. Hydrogen bonds and disulfide, ester, and salt bridges also contribute to the structure. A protein molecule always contains carbon, hydrogen, oxygen, and nitrogen, and occasionally phosphorus, sulfur, copper, and iron. The nitrogen content distinguishes protein from fat and carbohydrate. Protein in solution is colloidal because of its high molecular weight (6000 to several millions). Protein is easily denatured, acts as an electrolyte, forms zwitterions, hydrates with water, and precipitates at its isoelectric point. For further details, see Classification of proteins and Utilization of proteins, Appendices C-2 and D-2. See also *Amino acids, Denaturation,* and *Native protein.*

Protein Advisory Group (PAG) Group of the United Nations that is concerned with high protein foods, protein concentrates, and protein food mixtures. This group publishes the *PAG Bulletin,* which reviews international actions to improve world protein nutriture.

Protein-bound iodine (PBI) Thyroxine-binding globulin. This is the form in which the thyroid hormone, bound to a plasma protein, is transported in the blood. The normal concentration is about $5\mu/100$ ml of plasma or serum. It increases to about $8\mu/100$ ml in hyperthyroidism and falls below $3\mu/100$ ml in hypothyroidism. The PBI determination provides a good index of thyroid function and is useful in measuring basal metabolism.

Protein calorie malnutrition (PCM) Also called protein energy malnutrition; generic term to cover any protein calorie deficiency state. Some occur as a definite clinical syndrome such as kwashiorkor and marasmus, whereas others are manifestations of multiple nutritional deficiencies, as seen in starvation or secondary to certain diseases. Particularly affected are infants and children. Early symptoms are loss of appetite, lassitude, easy fatigability, loss of weight, retarded growth, decreased resistance to disease, and hypoproteinemia. Later manifestations include anemia, nutritional edema, and slow mental and motor development. See *Kwashiorkor; Marasmus;* and *Nutrition, starvation.*

Protein classification The chemistry and physiology of proteins are so complex that a single scheme of classification is not sufficient. Proteins are classified according to *composition and chemical properties* (simple, conjugated or compound, and derived proteins), *quality* (complete, partially complete, and incomplete proteins), *structure* (fibrous or globular proteins), and *solubility* (in water, acid, or alcohol). See *Protein quality, Protein structure,* and Classification of proteins, Appendix C-2.

Protein efficiency ratio (PER) Biologic method of evaluating *protein quality* in terms of weight gain per amount of protein consumed by a growing animal. Feeding, usually for a month, is ad libitum. Casein is often used as a control protein. PER is calculated as follows:

$$PER = \frac{\text{Weight gain (gm)}}{\text{Protein consumed (gm)}}$$

Protein energy malnutrition (PEM) See *Protein calorie malnutrition.*

Protein functions The biologic role of protein is so unique that it merits its name, which originated from a Greek word, *proteios,* meaning "to take first place." An important function of protein is in tissue synthesis. It is a *structural component* of all living cells and is found in muscles, nerves, bone, teeth, skin, hair, nails, blood, and glands. Almost all body fluids contain protein, with the exception of urine, sweat, and bile. All enzymes and some hormones are composed of protein. As a *source of energy,* protein yields 4 calories/gm; this function should be spared by fat and carbohydrate so that protein is used for building and repairing tissues. Protein is a *regulator* of blood pH, osmotic pressure, and water balance. It forms *antibodies* and aids in building resistance to infections. Other specific functions of protein are attributable to certain amino acids such as *tryptophan* for vitamin synthesis, *methionine* as a lipotropic agent, and *phenylalanine* and *tyrosine* for melanin formation. See also *Nutrient* and *Nutrient classification.*

Protein hydrolysate A predigested protein that contains a mixture of amino acids and peptides. It is useful for oral or parenteral feeding of patients with poor or impaired digestion, as seen in pancreatic diseases, postoperative cases, and severe burns.

Protein measurement The quantity of protein can be estimated by a number of techniques, including colorimetry, microbiologic assay, isotope dilution, countercurrent distribution, enzymatic method, and chromatography. For practical purposes the *Kjeldahl method* is most commonly used, since proteins contain an average of 16% nitrogen. Thus %N × 6.25 = %Protein. See also *Proximate analysis.*

Protein quality An attribute of a protein that depends on the kinds and amounts of *amino acids* present relative to body needs. No two food proteins are alike in their efficiency for tissue synthesis. In general plant proteins are lacking or "limiting" in the essential amino acids—lysine, methionine, threonine, and tryptophan. Animal proteins are of high quality or are said to be complete proteins. A *complete* protein contains all the essential amino acids in amounts sufficient for growth and life maintenance, e.g., casein and egg albumin. A *partially complete* protein can maintain life but cannot support growth, e.g., gliadin. An *incomplete* protein cannot support life or growth, e.g., zein and gelatin. The last two classes of protein can be used effectively for anabolic processes by combining with small amounts of complete proteins, by adding the limiting amino acid in synthetic

form, or by mixing several plant proteins to obtain a complete assortment of amino acids in the amounts needed for tissue synthesis. The last method has been the object of extensive research, notably by the FAO and WHO. Many methods of assessing protein quality have been proposed—biologic, microbiologic, enzymatic, or chromatographic methods. For the techniques commonly used, see *Balance study, Biologic value, Microbiologic assay, Plasma amino acid, Protein efficiency ratio,* and *Chemical score.* See also *Protein supplementary value* and *Protein sparing action.*

Protein requirement Protein needs vary among individuals according to age, body size, physiologic condition (growth, pregnancy, and lactation), state of health, type of protein in the diet, and adequacy of caloric intake. For practical purposes the protein *requirement* and *allowance* for normal adults are 0.35 gm/kg and 0.8 gm/kg, respectively (based on desirable body weight and assuming that the caloric supply is adequate). It is recommended that a considerable portion of protein in the diet be derived from animal sources. For specific needs of various age groups, see Recommended Daily Dietary Allowances, Appendix A-1. A practical guide for meeting daily protein needs is provided by the basic food groups. See Four basic food groups, Appendix B-1.

Protein reserve The body does not store protein in the same way or to the same extent that it stores fat and carbohydrate. To a limited extent all organs and tissues store protein, which is more appropriately termed "labile tissue protein." The latter designation signifies that the protein reserve is in a dynamic state, being constantly broken down or resynthesized and is at equilibrium with the metabolic pool of amino acids. Muscle protein is not as readily available as is protein stored in the liver, kidney, and other organs. The determination of plasma amino acids or the regeneration of other blood constituents and protein in the liver is indicative of the extent of protein storage or depletion.

Protein score See *Chemical score.*

Protein-sparing action The ability of a substance to save protein from being catabolized to supply energy so that it is used for its unique function of anabolism or tissue synthesis. Fats and carbohydrates are protein sparers.

Protein structure The structure of protein consists of four levels: *primary* (right number and sequence of amino acids joined by peptide bonds), *secondary* (hydrogen bonding between carbonyl and imido radicals), *tertiary* (folding and coiling of the polypeptide chain due to salt, ester, and disulfide bonds), and *quaternary* (extent of polymerization of a protein). According to the shape of the protein molecule, the two general classes are fibrous and globular proteins. *Fibrous protein* is composed of long filamentous chains joined laterally by tertiary or cross linkages; it is relatively stable and insoluble. Examples are myosin, keratin, and collagen. *Globular protein* is elliptical and shows considerable coiling and folding. Examples are enzymes, antigens, and globulins. See also *Protein synthesis.*

Protein supplementary value The effect of a protein to provide or add the "limiting" or missing amino acid of another protein so that the combination approximates a *complete protein.* For example, the combination of rice or corn with nuts and legumes. See *Multipurpose food* and *Protein quality.*

Protein synthesis Building of protein as opposed to catabolism and proteolysis. A specific protein is synthesized according to the genetic code as governed by the deoxyribonucleic acid (DNA) for a particular cell. The DNA in the nucleus uncoils, and a complementary strand of messenger ribonucleic acid (mRNA) is formed. It carries the genetic message from DNA to the *ribosome,* the site of protein biosynthesis. Transfer RNA picks up an amino acid that has been activated by adenosine tri-

phosphate in the cytoplasm and brings it to a specific site on the mRNA. The amino acids are added one at a time by means of a peptide bond until the complete protein is synthesized. Protein synthesis follows the *all-or-none law:* all amino acids (both essential and nonessential) needed according to the genetic code must be present at the same time at the site of protein synthesis. The absence of a single amino acid will prevent synthesis. See also *Nucleic acid.*

Proteinuria Appearance of protein in the urine as a result of faulty reabsorption of protein by a damaged tubule or leakage of an excessive amount of protein through a damaged or inflamed glomerulus, as in glomerulonephritis.

Protenum Proprietary milk formula useful as a high protein, low fat supplement. (Mead Johnson.) See Proprietary foods: composition, features, and uses, Appendix P-1.

Proteolysis Enzymatic or hydrolytic conversion of protein into simpler substances such as polypeptides, proteoses, peptones, and amino acids. See Summary of digestive enzymes, Appendix J-1.

Proteose Protein derivative intermediate between a polypeptide and a peptone. It is soluble in water and not coagulated by heat. It precipitates in salt solution. *Protease* hydrolyzes proteoses.

Prothrombin Protein in blood plasma needed for *blood clotting.* Prothrombin time is the length of time it takes the plasma to clot. This is useful for measuring the prothrombin level and reflects the intake of *vitamin K.*

Protinal High protein supplement low in fat, sodium, and potassium. It contains refined soya and corn, sugar, nonfat dry milk, vegetable oil, and calcium. (National.) See Proprietary foods: composition, features, and uses, Appendix P-1.

Protogen See *Lipoic acid.*

Protone Protein-rich mixture developed in the United Kingdom and used in the Congo; made of maize, skim milk powder, yeast, vitamins, and minerals. See Protein food mixtures, Appendix P-2.

Protoplasm The organized colloidal material considered as the essential substance of living cells. It is the seat of vital functions, i.e., nutrition, movement, growth, reproduction, etc. Protoplasm is composed of water, organic substances (especially protein), and inorganic salts.

Provitamin A vitamin *precursor;* e.g., carotene is the provitamin of vitamin A. A provitamin is chemically related to the preformed vitamin, but it has no vitamin activity unless it is converted to the biologically active form.

Proximate analysis Also called Weende scheme; named after the Weende Experimental Station in Germany, which established the analytic methods in 1865. A method of analyzing food and biologic materials according to their molecular components, such as water, ash or minerals, protein, fat, and carbohydrate by difference. The first four are determined as follows: the sample is dried and the difference in weight before and after drying represents *moisture content* or water; a subsample of the dried material is extracted with ether and the ether extract represents *crude fat;* another subsample is analyzed for nitrogen content using the *Kjeldahl method* and the percent nitrogen multipled by the factor 6.25 represents *crude protein;* the third subsample is boiled for 30 minutes in dilute sulfuric acid, filtered, and the residue boiled in dilute sodium hydroxide. The insoluble residue is made of crude fiber and ash; when ignited, the remaining residue is *ash,* representing minerals, and the loss or difference in weight is taken as *crude fiber* or indigestible carbohydrate. The proximate analysis of food is the basis of food composition tables. It is the starting point for analyzing individual nutrients. See *Carbohydrate by difference.*

Pruritus Intense itchiness. Examples are *pruritus ani* (anus), a symptom in certain intestinal parasitism, and *pruritus vulvae* (female external genitalia), as seen in diabetes mellitus.

Psoriasis Skin disease of many varieties. It is characterized mainly by scaly red patches on the extensor surfaces of the body. A taurine-restricted diet is recommended for patients with psoriasis. See *Diet, taurine-restricted.*

P/S ratio Ratio of polyunsaturated to saturated fatty acids. See *Fatty acid.*

Psychiatry Branch of medicine that deals with disorders of the mind (psyche). See *Nutrition, mental health,* and *Nutrition, psychiatry.*

Psychodietetics The interrelationship between psychology and nutrition. It deals with the study of the meanings of food, the attitudes and habits of people, the interaction of diet and behavior, and the emotional aspects of eating. See *Nutrition, emotional stability,* and *Nutrition, psychiatry.*

Psychology Study of the science of the mind and mental operations.

Pteroylglutamic acid (PGA) Name designated to replace folic acid (folacin). A member of the B complex vitamins that contains glutamic acid, para-aminobenzoic acid (PABA), and a substituted pterin. The combination of pterin and PABA is called *pteroic acid.* PGA occurs in a number of active forms conjugated with two to six glutamic acid molecules. The physiologically active form is the reduction product tetrahydrofolic acid. See also *Folic acid* and Summary of vitamins, Appendix I-1.

PTH Abbreviation for *parathormone.*

Ptomaine Amino compound resulting from microbial decomposition of dead animal matter. It should *not* be confused with bacterial products causing food poisoning.

Ptyalin Obsolete name for *salivary amylase,* an enzyme in the saliva that converts starch to maltose. See Summary of digestive enzymes, Appendix J-1.

Puberty Age at which reproductive organs become mature functionally and secondary sex characteristics develop. See *Nutrition, adolescence*.

Public health Science and art of preventing diseases, promoting health, and prolonging life through organized community efforts. See *Nutrition, public health*.

Puerperium Period between parturition and the time the mother's womb or uterus returns to normal, usually about 6 weeks.

PUFA Abbreviation for *polyunsaturated fatty acids*.

Pulse 1. Expansion and contraction of an artery that is felt on the temporal, carotid, or femoral arteries. Pulse rate is the number of pulsations of an artery per minute. For men it is normally about 70 to 72 and for women it is 78 to 82. 2. Another term for legumes such as peas, beans, and lentils.

Purine $C_5H_4N_4$; a nitrogenous ring structure widely distributed in nature, especially in *nucleic acids*. Examples are *adenine* (6-aminopurine), *guanine* (2-amino-6-oxypurine), *hypoxanthine* (6-oxypurine) *xanthine* (2,6-dioxypurine), and *uric acid* (2,6,8-trioxypurine).

Purpura Latin, meaning "purple." A condition characterized by purplish spots or *petechiae* over any part of the body. There are many types and causes.

Putrefaction Enzymatic or microbial decomposition of protein under anaerobic conditions, resulting in the production of incompletely oxidized substances. Many of these products are foul smelling, such as hydrogen sulfide, ammonia, and mercaptans.

Pyelitis Inflammation of the kidney pelvis. It may be due to calculi, cysts, and local bacterial infections. It occurs more frequently in children, particularly girls.

Pyelonephritis Inflammation of both the kidney and its pelvis. It is caused by bacterial invasion from the urinary tract, bloodstream, or periureteral lymphatics. See also *Nephritis*.

Pyknic Type of body composition characterized by a short and stocky build.

Pyloric Pertaining to the opening between the stomach and duodenum. *Pyloric stenosis* is a narrowing of the pyloric orifice (pylorus).

Pyorrhea 1. Purulent discharge. 2. Periodontal disease marked by purulent gum margins with bleeding and necrosis. This is later accompanied by loosening of the teeth.

Pyran Cyclic compound with one oxygen and five carbon atoms. *Pyranose* is a structural configuration of a sugar in which the oxygen ring links carbon atoms 1 and 5 for aldoses and atoms 2 and 6 for ketoses.

Pyrexia Fever or a febrile condition.

Pyridoxal See *Pyridoxine*.

Pyridoxal phosphate (**PALP**) Also called codecarboxylase; the biologically active form of *pyridoxine*. PALP functions as a coenzyme for nearly all reactions of amino acid metabolism, such as transamination, racemization, decarboxylation, desulfhydration, and deamination. It is needed for the conversion of tryptophan to niacin and serotonin. As a coenzyme of phosphorylase, it is important for carbohydrate metabolism, particularly the breakdown of glycogen to glucose. It is also indirectly involved in fatty acid metabolism, particularly in the conversion of linoleic to arachidonic acid; sterol synthesis, particularly cholesterol; and antibody formation. See also *Pyridoxine*.

Pyridoxamine See *Pyridoxine*.

Pyridoxamine phosphate (**PAMP**) Coenzyme of vitamin B_6 that participates only in transamination reactions.

Pyridoxic acid Metabolite of *pyridoxine* that is excreted in the urine. It can be used to assess vitamin B_6 nutriture.

Pyridoxine Name for the alcohol form of vitamin B_6; the accepted group designation for compounds possessing vitamin B_6 activity. The aldehyde form is *pyridoxal* and the amino derivative is *pyridoxamine*. See *Vitamin B_6* and *Pyridoxal phosphate*.

Pyridoxol *Pyridoxine*. This term is no longer used.

Pyrimidine $C_4H_4N_2$; a six-membered ring

compound with the two nitrogen atoms separated by a carbon atom. Pyrimidine bases are found in nucleic acids. Examples are *cytosine* (2-oxy-4-aminopyrimidine), *thymine* (2,4-dioxy-5-methylpyrimidine), and *uracil* (2,4-dioxypyrimidine). See also *Nucleic acid.*

Pyrithiamin Pyridine analog of *thiamin* that is antagonistic to the vitamin.

Pyrophosphate $P_2O_7^{-4}$; a salt of pyrophosphoric acid.

Pyruvate oxidation factor See *Lipoic acid.*

Pyruvic acid $CH_3COCOOH$ or ketopropionic acid; an important compound in the intermediary metabolism of carbohydrate, protein, and fat. It is the key substance or starting point of many reactions, including the following: (1) complete oxidation to carbon dioxide and water, providing energy via the Krebs cycle; (2) oxidative decarboxylation, supplying acetyl CoA, the starting point for lipid metabolism; (3) reversible reduction to lactic acid, i.e., the Pasteur effect; (4) transamination to alanine, an amino acid; and (5) glycogenesis or the storage of glycogen in the liver and other tissues. In mammalian cells, the first two reactions are the major pathways taken by pyruvate. For further details, see the metabolic charts in Appendices D-1 to D-4, E, and F-1 to F-4.

Pyuria Presence of pus in the urine. This may be a clinical sign of renal disease.

Q

Q_{O_2} Oxygen consumption per milligram of tissue (dry weight); the amount of oxygen is expressed in terms of microliters at standard pressure and temperature. It is a measure of the rate of respiration of different tissues.

Q enzyme Factor isolated from potatoes that catalyzes the formation of branching linkages of the alpha-1,6 type in starches.

Q substance Term applied to a giant molecule complex of cholesterol with proteins and lipids that may be associated with the development of atherosclerosis.

Quackery The actions, claims, or methods of a quack. A *quack* is an untrained person who practices with deception. *Food quackery,* like food faddism, leads people to believe that a particular food has miraculous properties to cure diseases. It makes use of vague, meaningless terms such as "health foods" and "cure-alls" that have scientific overtones and emotional appeal to gullible people.

Quadrivalent Having the ability to replace four atoms of hydrogen in a compound.

Qualitative analysis Determination of the nature of substances without regard to the amount present.

Quantitative analysis Determination of the actual amounts of substances. In chemistry, analysis is commonly done by gravimetric or volumetric method.

Quercetin A flavone derivative found in onion skin, tea, red rose, and the bark of the American oak.

Quinhydrone electrode Electrode used for the determination of pH. It consists of an inert metal immersed in a solution saturated with quinhydrone. The potential developed on the metal is proportional to the hydrogen ion concentration of the solution.

Quinic acid An acid that is incompletely oxidized in the body; it forms hippuric acid and is excreted in the urine. Found in large amounts in plums, prunes, and cranberries.

Quinine An alkaloid of cinchona bark; used as an antipyretic in malaria, typhoid fever, and other fevers or as a tonic to relieve fatigue.

Quinolinic acid One of the intermediary products formed in the metabolism of tryptophan. The level of its excretion in the urine is a measure of the extent of tryptophan utilization in the body.

Quinone 1. A substance obtained by the oxidation of quinic acid. 2. Any benzene derivative in which two hydrogen atoms are replaced by two oxygen atoms. Vitamin K is a quinone derivative.

R

Racemic mixture Composed of equal parts of dextrorotatory and levorotatory forms of optical isomers and therefore optically inactive. *Racemization* is the conversion of an optically active substance into its racemic form.

Rachitic Pertaining to or affected with rickets. *Rachitic rosary* is a descriptive term used for the costochondral beading (appearance of nodules or beadlike swelling) on the ribs at the junction with the cartilage often seen in children with rickets. See also *Rickets.*

Rachitogenic Capable of producing *rickets,* as a diet low in calcium or vitamin D.

Radiation 1. Divergence from a central point, as radiation of light. 2. Emission of electromagnetic waves such as those of light or particulate rays, e.g., alpha, beta, and gamma rays.

Radical Group of elements joined in a set formation that acts as a unit in a series of compounds without dissociating in chemical reactions. Examples are ammonium (NH_4) and phenyl (C_6H_5) radicals.

Radioactive Giving off radiant energy. *Radioactivity* is the property of certain elements, e.g., radium, to spontaneously emit radiation detected as alpha or beta particles or gamma rays. The phenomenon is produced naturally during the radioactive decay of radioactive isotopes or may be produced artificially by bombardment of heavy elements with high-velocity particles, as in a cyclotron (a high-voltage accel-

erating machine). See also *Radioactive isotope* under *Isotopes.*

Radioactive decay Loss of *radioactivity,* which is commonly expressed in terms of the *half-life* of the radioactive element, an interval designated as the time required for the initial number of radioactive atoms to be reduced by one-half. The decay time is an intrinsic property of a radioactive substance and is independent of temperature, pressure, presence of catalysts, or other factors that commonly influence chemical reactions.

Radioautography Photograph of the distribution of a radioactive substance in a tissue section of an organism; used in detecting tumors or endocrine gland dysfunction.

Radioisotope A radioactive *isotope.* Used as a tracer or labeled substance incorporated in a compound to follow the course of the latter in a series of reactions; also used in the diagnosis and treatment of certain types of tumors, cancers, and thyroid gland disorders. See Applications of isotopes in biology and medicine, Appendix N.

Radiology Branch of medicine that deals with x-rays, radioactive substances, and other ionizing radiations and their use in the diagnosis and treatment of diseases. A specialist in this field is a *radiologist.*

Raffinose Naturally occurring trisaccharide composed of a unit each of glucose, galactose, and fructose. It is found in sugar beets, roots and underground stems, cottonseed meal, and molasses. It is only partially digestible and not well utilized by man but can be hydrolyzed by enzymes of the gastrointestinal bacteria of herbivorous animals.

Rancidity Chemical change in fats and oils that results in the formation of compounds with a disagreeable odor and taste. Rancidity may be caused by *hydrolysis* of fat into free fatty acids and glycerol or mono- and diglycerides. This is hastened by warm temperature and the presence of moisture and lipolytic enzymes. Rancidity may also be a result of *oxidation* at the double bonds of unsaturated glycerides, forming various ketones and aldehydes with an unpleasant odor and taste.

RBC Abbreviation for *red blood cell*. See *Erythrocyte*.

RBP Abbreviation for *retinol-binding protein*.

RDA Abbreviation for *recommended dietary allowances*. See *Recommended dietary allowances* and Recommended Daily Dietary Allowances, Appendix A-1.

RE Abbreviation for *retinol equivalent*.

Recall Method used to assess an individual's dietary intake. The patient recounts what he has eaten during the previous 24 hours or some other specific time period. For other methods, see *Dietary study methodology*.

Receptor Peripheral nerve ending in the skin and special sense organs.

Recommended dietary allowances (RDA) Suggested or recommended amounts of various nutrients for use in planning diets. The term *"allowance"* is used to avoid the implication that these are absolute standards and to emphasize that the levels of nutrient intake recommended are based on *judgments* that should be reevaluated periodically as new information becomes available. Dietary allowances are designed to maintain good nutrition in *healthy* persons and are based on the *average* body sizes of adult men and women at different levels of activity, pregnant and lactating women, and children and adolescent boys and girls grouped according to age. It should be noted that dietary allowances are higher than *dietary requirements* in order to afford a 10% to 50% *margin of safety* above normal physiologic requirements. The amount added differs for each nutrient because of the differences in the body's ability to store the nutrient, the range of observed requirements, the precision of assessing requirements, and the possible hazards of excessive intake of certain nutrients. This additional amount is also intended to cover nutrient losses that might occur during the storage, preparation, cooking, and service of food, to provide for possible incomplete availability or absorption of certain nutrients, to serve as a buffer against additional needs for certain nutrients in periods of stress, and to allow for a wide range of variation in the nutrient requirement of the population at large.

Rectum Distal portion of the large intestine, from the sigmoid flexure to the anal canal. It is about 13.5 cm long.

Red blood cell (RBC) See *Erythrocyte*.

Redox potential The electric potential developed when an inert electrode is placed in a solution containing the oxidation-reduction states of a substance. The potential varies in proportion to the logarithm of the ratio of oxidant to reductant.

Redox system Simultaneous and reversible system of oxidation-reduction reaction. See *Oxidation-reduction*.

Reduction Gain of electrons or decrease in positive valence; in general any process in which electrons are supplied to an atom. A reducing agent or an electron donor is called a *reductant*.

Reference man Standard originally used by the FAO Committee on Caloric Requirements and now adopted by the Food and Nutrition Board in the recommended dietary allowances. He is described as a man 22 years old, weighing 70 kg, living in a moderate climate with a mean temperature of 20° C, wearing light clothing, and engaged in light physical activity. His estimated caloric allowance is 2700 kcal. This baseline can be used to adjust caloric allowances of individuals in different circumstances. See Recommended Daily Dietary Allowances, Appendix A-1.

Reference woman She is 22 years old, weighs 58 kg, lives in a moderate climate with a mean temperature of 20° C, wears light clothing, and is engaged in light physical activity. Her estimated caloric allowance is 2000 kcal. See *Reference man.*

Reflux esophagitis Condition characterized by heartburn that is felt substernally and is often accompanied by regurgitation of fluid in the mouth. It may occur after meals but is typically associated with a change in posture (e.g., bending, lifting, or straining) that produces a rise in intra-abdominal pressure.

Refsum's syndrome Rare neurologic disease in which *phytanic acid* cannot be catabolized so it accumulates in cerebrospinal fluid, liver, kidney, and blood. Since phytanic acid comes from exogenous sources, the treatment involves restriction of foods containing phytanic acid and its precursors. See *Diet, phytanic acid–restricted.*

Refuse Discarded and inedible parts of food; waste matter.

Regimen A systematic course or plan, including food and medication, to maintain or improve health. For specific dietary regimen, see *Diet.*

Regional ileitis Chronic, nonspecific inflammatory process involving the lower portion of the *ileum,* although other parts of the intestine may be affected.

Regurgitation 1. Backflow of food from the stomach to the mouth without the effort of vomiting. 2. Return of blood through a heart valve that is defective.

Reichert-Meissl number The milliliters of 0.1N alkali required to neutralize the volatile acid obtained from 5 gm of fat that has been saponified, acidified to liberate the fatty acids, and then steam distilled. Butterfat, which is high in short-chain fatty acids, has a Reichert-Meissl number of 26 to 33 as compared to lard, which has a number of only about 0.6.

Relapse Return of symptoms after a disease seems to have been cured. The relapse-response-relapse method is one of the criteria for determining the essentiality of a substance. For example, deficiency signs of a specific nutrient disappear when the nutrient is administered; withdrawal of the nutrient leads to recurrence of the signs, and therapeutic supplementation will again alleviate the deficiency signs. Thus the proof of essentiality is a series of alternate relapse-response-relapse reactions to the nutrient.

Relaxin Water-soluble polypeptide hormone with a molecular weight of about 9000. It is found in the ovary, testis, blood, and placenta of various mammals, including human placental tissue. It causes relaxation of the pelvic ligaments and softening of the connective tissue of the pubic symphysis; it probably acts in combination with estrogen and progesterone.

Remission The disappearance of symptoms of a disease or the time that it takes for this to occur.

Renal Pertaining to the *kidney.*

Renal acidosis Reduction or lack of alkali reserve caused by the inability of the kidney to conserve base while excreting acid. See *Acidosis.*

Renal diabetes Type of diabetes characterized by the presence of sugar in the urine even with a normal or below normal blood sugar level. The condition is not associated with a disturbance in carbohydrate metabolism. It is ascribed either to a low renal threshold for sugar or a defective reabsorption process in the kidney tubules, allowing glucose to find its way into the urine. This condition is more appropriately called *renal glycosuria.*

Renal hypertension Elevation in blood pressure as a result of reduction in the flow of blood to the kidney, as in ischemia. The ischemic kidney liberates into the blood an enzyme, *renin,* that splits angiotensin I (formerly called hypertensin or angiotonin) from angiotensinogen, an alpha globulin formed in the liver. An enzyme present in the plasma acts on angiotensin I to form angiotensin II, which is a powerful pressor agent. However, the kidney tissues in general contain a dipeptidase enzyme, angiotensinase (formerly called hypertensinase or angiotonase), that destroys angiotensin II.

Renal threshold Concentration of a substance in plasma above which the substance appears in the urine. Various substances in plasma, e.g., glucose, do not appear in the urine until their plasma concentrations rise to certain values. Such substances are referred to as *threshold substances.* The glucose renal threshold in the adult varies between 140 and 170 mg/ 100 ml of plasma.

Renin Proteolytic enzyme formed in the kidney and released into the blood by *ischemia* of the kidney. It liberates angiotensin I from its inactive precursor, angiotensinogen. See *Renal hypertension.*

Rennet Enzyme preparation containing pepsin and rennin obtained from the stomach lining of a calf or lamb. Used in making cheese and junket.

Rennin Enzyme present in gastric juice that is primarily responsible for the coagulation of milk (casein). It is capable of clotting about 10 million times its weight of milk at 37° C in 10 minutes. The process of clotting involves a change in the casein molecules to *paracasein,* which then forms calcium paracaseinate, or the milk clot.

REP Abbreviation for *roentgen equivalent physical.* A roentgen unit used to measure beta radiation. Defined as the amount of ionizing radiation capable of producing 1.615×10^{12} ion pairs/gm of tissue or that will withstand an absorption in tissue of 93 ergs/gm.

RES Abbreviation for *reticuloendothelial system.*

Residue The remainder; portion remaining after a part has been removed. In nutrition, it refers to the amount of bulk remaining in the intestinal tract following digestion. It is composed of undigested and unabsorbed food as well as metabolic and bacterial products. See also *Diet, residue modified.*

Respiration Commonly used to mean "external" respiration or *breathing,* which consists of two acts: *inspiration* or taking in atmospheric air (i.e., consumption of oxygen) and *expiration* or expulsion of modified air (i.e., elimination of carbon dioxide). "Internal" respiration refers to the exchange of gases at the cellular level between the systemic blood and the tissues. See *Physiologic oxidation.*

Respiration calorimeter See *Respirometer.*

Respiratory carriers Group of electron carriers, including coenzymes I and II (NAD and NADP), the flavoproteins (FMN and FAD), coenzyme Q, and the cytochrome systems (cytochrome a_1, a_3, b, and c). They convey electrons from the dehydrogenated substrates to oxygen, harnessing free energy in the course of the reaction for the synthesis of adenosine triphosphate, a form of energy utilized in the endergonic processes of a living cell. See *Electron transport chain.*

Respiratory enzymes Enzymes found in the *mitochondria* that catalyze a series of reactions involved in the cellular oxidation of substrates, resulting in their complete oxidation to carbon dioxide and water. Electrons removed from the substrates are passed on to a highly ordered array of *electron* or *respiratory carriers* and thence to oxygen, forming water. The principal types of respiratory enzymes are the *oxidases* and *dehydrogenases.*

Respiratory quotient **(RQ)** Ratio of the volume of carbon dioxide eliminated to the volume of oxygen used. According to Avogadro's law, one molecule of carbon dioxide has the same volume as one molecule of oxygen. Thus complete oxidation of carbohydrate will give a respiratory quotient of 1. Oxidation of fat and oxidation of protein give approximate respiratory quotients of 0.7 and 0.8, respectively. Since the three foodstuffs are metabolized simultaneously, the respiratory quotient is always a resultant of the three. It is about 0.85 on an ordinary mixed diet.

Respiratory tract Air passage from the nostrils to the air sacs in the lungs.

Respirometer Also called respiration calorimeter; an apparatus designed to measure the extent of respiration in man, which is regarded as a function of two factors: food ingestion and metabolism. Many respirometers have been designed based either on the principle of direct or that of indirect *calorimetry.* Examples are the Atwater-Rosa-Benedict respiration calorimeter and the Kofranyi-Michaelis respirometer.

Resuscitation Prevention of death by asphyxia through artificial respiration, as in the case of a person unconscious as a result of near drowning.

Reticulin One of the structural elements of skeletal muscle, together with elastin and collagen. It is thought to be a precursor of a degraded form of *collagen.*

Reticulocyte Immature erythrocyte with a delicate interior network or reticulum that stains with basic dyes. Normally present in the blood in small numbers (0.5% to 1.5% of total erythrocytes), its presence in greater number (reticulocytosis) indicates stimulation of erythropoiesis, as seen in response to liver treatment in pernicious anemia.

Reticuloendothelial system (RES) Group of cells (except for leukocytes) with phagocytic properties. They are distributed throughout the body, particularly in the spleen, bone marrow, liver, and lymph nodes. These cells have the property of engulfing and digesting foreign particles or cells harmful to the body. The reticuloendothelial system also removes red blood cells on their destruction. Protein and iron are recovered for formation of new erythrocytes, and the heme portion is converted to *bile pigments.* See also *Hemopoiesis.*

Reticulum 1. Second division of the ruminant stomach. 2. A fine network.

Retina Photosensitive portion of the eye; the innermost of the three coats of the eyeball and the terminal expansion of the optic nerve. It consists of several layers, including the pigmented epithelium, photoreceptors (rods and cones), associated cells, and ganglion cells. The retina receives light sensation and transforms it into nervous impulses via the optic nerve, which transmits the impulses to the brain for translation into a visual experience.

Retinal See *Retinaldehyde.*

Retinaldehyde Name now designated for vitamin A_1 aldehyde, retinal, or retinene.

Retinene See *Retinaldehyde.*

Retinitis Inflammation of the retina. Caused by a number of conditions such as diabetes, leukemia, kidney diseases, and syphilis. Results in some form of interference with vision.

Retinoic acid Name for vitamin A_1 acid. It does not occur in nature but has been prepared synthetically by oxidizing the alcohol group to a carboxyl group. This compound has no activity in the visual process. It has two thirds the potency of vitamin A, using the growth rate of young rats as a measure.

Retinol Name for vitamin A_1 alcohol. Its corresponding aldehyde and acid are called *retinaldehyde* and *retinoic acid,* respectively. Retinol and retinaldehyde can be reversibly oxidized and reduced, but retinoic acid cannot be converted back to the other two. Retinol circulates in plasma bound to a specific transport protein as retinol-binding protein. See *Vitamin A.*

Retinol equivalent (RE) Unit used to express vitamin A activity. One RE equals 1μ retinol, 6μ beta-carotene, and 12μ of other provitamin A carotenoids.

Rhamnose 6-Deoxy-L-mannose, a deoxyhexose in which the terminal —CH$_2$OH group is replaced by —CH$_3$. Occurs in glycoside combination in many plants, particularly vegetable gums.

Rheumatic fever Acute or chronic inflammatory process that comes as a sequel to hemolytic streptococci infection. It occurs most frequently in children and tends to recur. The inflammatory process may spread to many organs and, when pronounced, conditions such as myocarditis and arthritis occur. *Acute rheumatic fever* is characterized by a sudden onset with high fever and swelling and pain of the joints. Heart damage is particularly common.

Rheumatism Generally indicates diseases of the connective tissue, especially joints and muscles, accompanied by physical incapacity and discomfort. It includes such diseases as acute rheumatic fever, osteoarthritis, rheumatoid arthritis, gout, and bursitis.

Rheumatoid arthritis Also called arthritis deformans and atrophic arthritis; a painful, chronic condition common among young women over the age of 30 years and characterized by swelling, stiffness, and eventual deformity of the joints. Its cause is not known, although the condition is often associated with cold and damp weather and a variety of stress factors such as infection and psychologic shock. See *Arthritis*.

Rh factor Element in the blood so called because it was first found in the blood cells of the rhesus monkey. "Rh *positive*" and "Rh *negative*" are terms that indicate the presence or absence of this element in the blood. When the father is Rh positive and the mother is Rh negative, the Rh-positive factor is transmitted to the developing fetus within the mother's womb. This stimulates the mother to produce antibodies against the Rh factor; these are transmitted to the blood of the developing fetus and destroy its red blood cells. This may result in abortion or stillbirth; if born alive, the infant may die of jaundice or anemia. See *Erythroblastosis fetalis*.

Rhodopsin Also called porphyropsin; formerly called *visual purple*. It is a light-sensitive pigment responsible for the ability to see in dim light and is found in the rods of the retina. On exposure to light, it is bleached through a series of products, forming at the end opsin and retinaldehyde (formerly called retinal). See *Visual process*.

Riboflavin Also called vitamin B$_2$; a heat-stable, orange-yellow crystalline compound with a bitter taste; highly sensitive to light and easily soluble in water. It has been isolated from milk (lactoflavin), eggs (ovoflavin), and liver (hepatoflavin) and has been identified with Warburg's yellow enzyme. Riboflavin is associated with the health of the skin and eyes. As an essential component of the flavoprotein coenzymes flavin mononucleotide and flavin adenine dinucleotide, it participates in biologic oxidations as a hydrogen acceptor in aerobic dehydrogenases. Deficiency in the vitamin results in *ariboflavinosis,* which is characterized by burning and itching of the eyes, photophobia, corneal vascularization, cheilosis, and glossitis with a characteristic magenta color of the tongue. Manifestations of riboflavin deficiency in animals vary with the species. Richest food sources are yeast, milk, eggs, organ meats, and lean meat, especially pork. For further details, see Summary of vitamins, Appendix I-1.

Ribonuclease Enzyme present in the pancreas and other organs capable of hydrolyzing ribonucleic acid to its constituent parts. It is a globular protein with a single peptide chain containing 124 amino acid residues; it has a molecular weight of 14,000.

Ribonucleic acid (RNA) Also called ribose nucleic acid; one of the two main types of *nucleic acid,* with ribose as the pentose constituent. It is present in the cell cytoplasm and nucleolus and plays an important role in protein synthesis. Three distinct types of RNA are involved in *protein synthesis,* each type different in size, shape, origin, and function.

Messenger RNA (mRNA) Also called template RNA or informational RNA; conceived to be a complementary copy of DNA, thus containing the genetic "information" for protein synthesis. mRNA functions at the site of protein synthesis and carries the genetic message from DNA to the *ribosome,* the site of protein synthesis. It has a molecular weight that varies from 30,000 to 50,000 and represents only a small percentage of RNA in the cell.

Ribosomal RNA (rRNA) Ribonucleic acid in the ribosome, which is believed to direct the arrangement of the amino acids of proteins into their proper sequence within the polypeptide chain. It consists of long chains of nucleotides containing more than 1500 purine and pyrimidine nitrogenous bases.

Transfer RNA (tRNA) Also called soluble RNA or acceptor RNA; short-chain RNA molecule with a low molecular weight of 20,000 to 30,000. It occurs free in the cytoplasmic fluid and transfers the activated amino acid to a specific site on the ribosomal RNA template, resulting in an alignment of amino acids in a particular sequence to form the primary structure of a protein.

Ribose Pentose sugar of significant physiologic importance. It is a constituent part of ribonucleic acid, the coenzymes nicotinamide adenine dinucleotide and nicotinamide adenine dinucleotide phosphate, and adenosine triphosphate. Any glycoside containing ribose as the sugar component is called a *riboside.*

Ribosome Site of protein synthesis within the cells; contains 80% to 90% of the ribonucleic acid within the cell. As seen by electron microscopy, it appears as a delicate network of membranous tubules attached to numerous dense spherical granules with diameters of 100 to 150 Å.

Rice Grain of *Oryza sativa.*

Brown r Rice with the outer husk removed; has the bran layer still intact and is rich in vitamins and minerals but is oily.

Converted r Also called parboiled rice; rice soaked in water and boiled for a short time before removing the husk; contains more of the natural rice nutrients than hulled or brown rice. Parboiling causes the nutrients to be redistributed within the grain, moving from the outer layers toward the center.

Enriched r Rice enriched with vitamins and minerals.

Glutinous r Waxy or sweet rice; a variety of rice in which starch is composed wholly of *amylopectin.* On cooking, it disintegrates and the grains adhere in a sticky mass.

Parboiled r See *Converted rice* under *Rice.*

Polished r White rice or milled rice. Polishing removes the surface layer, commonly called the "bran layer," which is brownish and oily but rich in vitamins and minerals. White rice is palatable because of the absence of oil.

Premix r Ordinary rice coated with a highly concentrated solution of thiamin, niacin, and iron and protected by an edible coating that is insoluble in cold water.

Unpolished r Whole-grain rice without the hull and embryo or germ and only part of the bran layer removed; contains more nutrients than polished rice. Since the oil is in the bran layer, unpolished rice does not keep well and becomes rancid.

Whole-grain r Hulled grain with the embryo and bran layer still intact; contains the natural nutrients in the grain but is rich in rice oil, which accounts for its brownish color, unpalatable taste, and increased susceptibility to fat rancidity.

Ricinoleic acid A monohydroxy monounsaturated fatty acid containing 18 carbon atoms; found in castor oil.

Rickets Called "English disease" in Great Britain; it is a nutritional deficiency disease occurring in infancy and early childhood. It is caused by a disturbance in calcium-phosphorus metabolism and/or a lack of vitamin D. It is essentially a disease of defective bone formation, manifesting itself in many ways: e.g., delayed closure of the fontanelles; softening of the skull and bulging of the forehead; poor muscle tone, resulting in a "pot-belly" appearance of the abdomen; soft fragile bones, leading to bowing of the legs; enlargement of the wrists, knees, and ankle joints; costochondral beading at the junction of the rib joints, forming the "rachitic rosary"; and projection of the sternum, giving the appearance of a "pigeon breast."

Adult r See *Osteomalacia.*

Conditioned r Rickets occurring as a secondary result of other diseases that "condition" the calcium deficiency. This may be caused by impaired absorption of fat and hence of the fat-soluble vitamin D, which is necessary for normal absorption and utilization of calcium. Celiac disease is a typical example of a malabsorption syndrome that may cause conditioned rickets.

Late r Rickets appearing first in infancy which, instead of healing, continues throughout childhood and even into adulthood. Exact cause is not known but is possibly associated with the malabsorption syndrome, Fanconi's syndrome, or renal acidosis.

Renal r Rickets resulting from kidney failure, as in chronic glomerulonephritis, causing the retention of nitrogen, various acid metabolites, and phosphorus. Retention of the latter produces a secondary hyperparathyroidism with consequent withdrawal of calcium from the bones. Retention of acids produces acidosis; the acids eventually are neutralized and excreted by the kidney with consequent loss of bases, including calcium. See also *Fanconi's syndrome.*

Resistant r Rickets that fails to respond to ordinary therapeutic doses of vitamin D; probably caused by factors that "condition" rickets. A hereditary factor appears to be involved.

Rigor mortis The stiffening and rigidity of muscles that occur after death. Cessation of circulation in the muscles causes tissue metabolism to be anaerobic, with formation of lactic acid and a fall in pH. This causes swelling and precipitation of muscle colloids, leading to hardening of muscles.

RNA Abbreviation for *ribonucleic acid.* Abbreviations for the three types of RNA are mRNA, rRNA, and tRNA for messenger RNA, ribosomal RNA, and transfer RNA, respectively.

Rochelle salt Potassium sodium tartrate, a substance used to combine with the copper in Fehling's test for reducing sugars.

Roentgenogram A roentgen-ray photograph; an x-ray film.

Rose hip The brightly colored fruit of the rose. It is a good source of vitamin C.

Roughage Indigestible carbohydrate material in plants; it passes through the intestines unchanged, but absorbs and holds water, thus acting as a laxative. Usually composed for the most part of cellulose. Commonly used to mean indigestible fiber. See also *Fiber* and *Diet, fiber modified.*

RQ Abbreviation for *respiratory quotient.*

Rubner's law Rubner formulated a "law" to the effect that the different foodstuffs may replace each other in the diet for energy as well as for heat production in proportion to their caloric value.

Rumen First compartment of the stomach of the ruminant, where food is temporarily stored while undergoing fermentation prior to regurgitation and remastication.

Ruminant Animal having a stomach with four cavities: abomasum, omasum, reticulum, and rumen.

Rutin A crystalline alcohol from tomato stems, tobacco, rye leaves, and buckwheat plants. It has the properties of vitamin P and has been used to reduce capillary fragility.

❧ S ❧

Saccharidase Enzyme that splits di- and tri-saccharides to monosaccharides.

Saccharin Artificial sweetener about 700 times sweeter than cane sugar. It has no caloric value.

Saccharimeter Also called saccharometer; a floating device used to determine the specific gravity of sugar solutions.

Saci Caramel-flavored soybean beverage. It has 3% protein, contains added vitamins, and is stable without refrigeration.

Safflower oil Edible oil from the seeds of the safflower plant *Carthamus tinctorius*. It is a good source of polyunsaturated fatty acids.

Saliva Secretion of the *salivary glands* in the mouth. It serves to moisten and hold particles of food together, thus aiding in chewing and swallowing. It contains an enzyme, *salivary amylase,* that helps in the digestion of starch. Salivary secretion also has some bacteriostatic properties.

Salivary amylase Former name is ptyalin. It is the principal enzyme of human saliva, acting on starches with oligosaccharides and maltose as end products. It requires chloride ion and an optimum pH of 6.6 to 6.8 for its action. Digestion in the mouth is not appreciable, since food stays in contact with the enzyme for just a short time. Salivary amylase is easily inactivated at a pH of 4.0 or less, and its action ceases when food enters the stomach.

Salivary glands Three pairs of glands that secrete *saliva* by reflex response: the *parotid, submaxillary,* and *sublingual* glands.

Salmonella A genus of gram-negative bacteria, some species of which are intestinal pathogens. *Salmonella* infection, or *salmonellosis,* is characterized by abdominal cramps, vomiting, chills, fever, and prostration. The usual medium of infection is through eating contaminated foods, particularly meats, poultry, milk and milk products, bakery goods, egg dishes, and sandwich fillings. *Salmonella* grows well in moist foods of low acidity. It is readily destroyed by heat but not by freezing.

Salt 1. Common table salt or sodium chloride ($NaCl$). 2. Class of compounds formed when the hydrogen atom of an acid radical is replaced by a metal or metal-like radical, as in neutralization reactions.

Salt bridge One of the protein linkages; formed between a carboxyl group of one polypeptide chain and an amino group or similar cationic group of another chain.

Salting in Solubilizing effect of salt; usually attributed to the effect of salt on proteins. By partially neutralizing the surface charges of the protein, salt diminishes the attraction between the molecules, making the protein more soluble.

Salting out Decrease in the solubility of a substance or precipitation of colloids in greater salt concentrations.

Saponification Formation of sodium or potassium salts ("soaps") when fat or lipid is boiled with alkali. The portion of total lipid that forms soap and is soluble in water but insoluble in ether is called *saponifiable fraction.* The remaining portion

211

that does not form soap and is insoluble in water but is soluble in ether is the *non-saponifiable fraction.*

Saponification number Amount of potassium hydroxide (in milligrams) required to neutralize the free or uncombined fatty acids in 1 gm of fat. The saponification number is useful in determining the mean molecular weight of fatty acids present in a fat or lipid.

Saponins Group of glycosides occurring in a wide variety of plants, particularly legumes. Saponins are good emulsifiers, can form soapy lathers with water, and can hemolyze red blood cells even at extreme dilutions.

Saprophyte Organism that thrives on dead organic matter, as dead tissue.

Saridele Vegetable protein mixture in Indonesia; contains dry soybean meal and sesame, sugar, calcium carbonate, thiamin, vitamin B_{12}, and vitamin C.

Satiety Feeling of fullness or gratification of appetite.

Saturation 1. Property of having all the chemical affinities satisfied. 2. Point beyond which a solution can no longer dissolve a given substance.

Saturation test See *Load test.*

Schistosomiasis Infestation with *Schistosoma,* a genus of trematode parasites commonly called the blood flukes. They affect chiefly the liver, spleen, and lungs. The condition is characterized by ascites, bronchial disorder, cachexia, fever, and urticaria.

School Breakfast Program Established in 1966 as part of the *Child Nutrition Act.* In some schools, breakfast is served to children who are poor or have traveled a long distance from home.

School Lunch Program A practical nutrition program designed to train schoolchildren in proper food habits and to improve their dietary intake of nutrients. The National School Lunch Act became a law in 1946, and the program is under the supervision of the U. S. Department of Agriculture. A participating school is given financial and technical assistance to enable it to serve nutritious, hot lunches on a nonprofit basis. Two types of lunches are available free of charge to indigent children: *type A* lunch, which is planned to furnish one third of the day's nutrient requirements, and *type B* lunch, which is planned to supplement the food brought from home.

Scintillation counter Particle detector that emits light when a charged particle passes through it. The apparatus is widely used in industry and research. It is particularly useful in tracer techniques or metabolic studies using radioactive isotopes.

Scleroprotein Group of simple proteins that are insoluble in water and neutral solvents and resistant to digestive enzymes. They include the *collagen* of skin, tendons, and bones and the elastic proteins known as *elastin* and *keratin.* Scleroproteins have a protective and supportive function in bones, cartilages, ligaments, tendons, and other tough parts of the animal body. For more details, see Classification of proteins, Appendix C-2.

Sclerosis Hardening of a part of the body due to the growth of tough, fibrous tissues. The term is more commonly used to describe a disorder of the nervous system characterized by hardening of the tissues as a result of hyperplasia.

Scoliosis Abnormal lateral curvature of the spinal column.

Scotopia Vision in very dim light; twilight vision.

SCP Abbreviation for *single-cell protein.*

Scurvy Deficiency disease caused by a lack of *vitamin C* (ascorbic acid). The characteristic symptoms are loss of appetite, restlessness, spongy gums that tend to bleed, and pinpoint-sized skin hemorrhage (petechiae). Retarded growth, delayed dentition, bone deformities, general soreness to touch, and swollen joints and thighs also accompany this condition in infants and children.

SDA Abbreviation for *specific dynamic action.*

Sebaceous 1. Secreting an oily, lubricating substance, as the sebaceous glands of the skin. 2. Pertaining to sebum or suet.

Seborrheic dermatitis Skin lesion characterized by greasy scaling, especially on the nasolabial folds and around the eyes and ears. Hard sebaceous plugs also form over the bridge of the nose. The condition may be a result of various factors such as oily skin, hormonal imbalance, emotional disturbance, and nutritional deficiency (as in riboflavin and pyridoxine deficiencies).

Secretin Hormone secreted by the intestinal mucosa when gastric acid or chyme reaches the intestine. It is carried by the bloodstream to the pancreas and stimulates it to secrete the pancreatic juice.

Sedimentation The deposition of precipitates or the settling out by gravity of the solid particles in a suspension. This is an analytic procedure for separating solids of different particle size. The rate at which a molecule will settle to the bottom of a tube in a centrifugal field depends on the size and density of the molecule as well as the viscosity of the solvent.

Sedimentation rate Also called sed rate; the speed with which the red blood cells settle to the bottom of a glass tube. The sedimentation rate varies under certain circumstances and in some diseases. The rate is increased in cancer, tissue injury, and infectious and inflammatory diseases. The rate is decreased in allergic states and in certain types of shock and anemia.

Sedoheptulose A 7-carbon ketose sugar; an intermediary metabolite in the *hexose monophosphate shunt*. It is a transitory compound in the cyclic regeneration of D-ribulose for carbon dioxide fixation in plant photosynthesis.

Segmentation 1. Division into parts, as the cleavage of a cell to form new organisms. 2. Alternate contraction and relaxation of circular muscle fibers in the distal colon to push intestinal contents toward the rectum.

Seizure 1. A sudden attack or recurrence of a disease. 2. An epileptic attack.

Selenium Trace mineral essential to plants and animals, including man, but quite toxic at certain levels, depending on the dose tolerance of the organism. It can replace vitamin E or supplement its action in promoting growth and fertility and certain metabolic reactions dependent on the antioxidant property of vitamin E. Selenium is present in both plant and animal tissues, often occurring with sulfur. A deficiency state in man has not been observed. For further details, see Summary of minerals, Appendix H.

Semen 1. Thick whitish secretion of the reproductive organs in the male. 2. Any seed or seedlike fruit.

Senescence Process or condition of growing old.

Septicemia Condition caused by the presence of pathogenic bacteria and their toxins in the blood. It is accompanied by chills, excessive perspiration, intermittent fever, and weakness.

Sequestrant A substance that can combine with a metal ion or acid radical to make it inactive. Sequestrants are used in the food industry to inactivate interfering substances. Commonly used are ethylenediaminetetraacetic acid (EDTA), citrates, tartrates, phosphates, and calcium salts.

Serine Alpha-amino-beta-hydroxypropionic acid, a *nonessential amino acid* first obtained from the silk protein sericin. It is converted to glycine and one carbon (C_1) fragment with *tetrahydrofolic acid* as the acceptor. The C_1 fragment becomes the source of methyl groups needed in the biosynthesis of many compounds.

Serotonin 5-Hydroxytryptamine, a *tryptophan* derivative. It is found in the serum and a number of tissues, including the gastrointestinal tract, blood platelets, brain, and nerve tissues. Serotonin is a powerful vasoconstrictor and plays a role in brain and nerve function, gastric secretion, and intestinal peristalsis.

Serum Clear liquid left after protein has been clotted; refers both to blood and milk serum. The serum from milk is called *whey*. Blood serum is plasma *without* its fibrinogen. See also *Plasma*.

Serum enzymes Enzymes, present in blood plasma (serum), that result from the breakdown of tissue and blood cells. Examples are *SGPT* (serum glutamic pyruvic transaminase), *SGOT* (serum glutamic oxalacetic transaminase), and *LDH* (lactic dehydrogenase). Measurement of the activity of these enzymes provides useful diagnostic and clinical information.

Sex hormones Androgens (male sex hormones) and estrogens (female sex hormones) that are responsible for the development of secondary sex characteristics. See *Androgen* and *Estrogen*.

SGOT Serum glutamic oxalacetic transaminase, now called aspartate aminotransferase. This *serum enzyme* is widely distributed in all body tissues (except bone), but its levels are highest in the heart muscle, skeletal muscle, liver, kidney, and brain. The normal level ranges from 5 to 40 units. Activity is high in myocardial infarction, infectious hepatitis, extrahepatic biliary obstruction, and liver damage from toxic agents. It is moderately increased in rheumatic fever and in disorders involving necrosis of the heart, liver, or muscle.

SGPT Serum glutamic pyruvic transaminase, now called alanine aminotransferase. A *serum enzyme* found in higher concentration than SGOT in the liver. It is also found in heart muscle but in lower concentration than SGOT. This concentration difference between the two enzymes provides a more accurate diagnosis of myocardial infarction and liver disease.

Shigellosis Bacillary dysentery caused by a genus of rod-shaped bacteria *(Shigella)* that grow readily in foods. The organism is transmitted to food by contamination with feces or as a result of unsanitary handling by a carrier. The boiling of food or pasteurization of milk kills the organism.

Shock Condition characterized by pallor, clammy perspiration, low blood pressure, feeble rapid pulse, restlessness, confusion, and sometimes unconsciousness. The precipitating causes are many and varied, e.g., severe injury, loss of blood, burns, fright, pain, and surgery.

Sialic acid Acetyl derivative of an amino sugar acid; present in saliva, glycoproteins, lipids, and polysaccharides.

Sickle cell anemia Type of anemia hereditary in nature. Red blood cells take a "sickle moon" shape caused by a looping effect between two amino acids, resulting in the formation of slender strands of hemoglobin that tend to elongate the cell. This type of anemia is common among Negroes.

Siderophilin Also called *transferrin;* an iron-carbonate-protein complex; the form in which iron is transported in the blood plasma.

Siderosis The presence of excess iron in the body. This may occur under several circumstances such as excessive destruction of red blood cells as in hemolytic conditions, following multiple blood transfusion or excessive intake of iron, and accompanying failure to regulate iron absorption and metabolism.

Similac Commercial milk formula for routine feeding of infants; made of skim milk with added lactose, corn and coconut oils, iron, and vitamins. *Similac PM 60/40* is a mixture of electrodialyzed whey and nonfat milk, corn and coconut oils, lactose, minerals, and vitamins. The protein in the formula is 60% lactalbumin and 40% casein. (Ross.) See Proprietary foods: composition, features, and uses, Appendix P-1.

Simmonds' disease Also called hypopituitary cachexia; a condition caused by a wasting away of the *adenohypophysis*. It results in premature aging, severe weight loss, mental disturbance, low basal metabolic rate, and low body temperature.

Single-cell protein (SCP) Protein produced by the growth of single-cell organisms such as algae, bacteria, yeast, and fungi.

Sinus Any space or cavity in an organ, tissue, or bone; usually refers to the paranasal sinuses of the face. *Sinusitis* is inflammation of the mucous membranes lining the paranasal sinuses.

Sitos Greek, meaning "food." *Sitology* is the science of food.

Sitosterol Plant sterol similar to cholesterol but having an extra methyl group. Large doses can lower blood cholesterol and beta-lipoprotein levels. High intakes, however, produce toxic effects such as anorexia, diarrhea, and cramps.

Skatole The substance that gives the characteristic foul odor to feces. It is a product of tryptophan deamination in the intestines.

Skeletal system The bony framework of the body that gives support and structure. The human *skeleton* is composed of two parts: the *axial part* or bones of the trunk, which include the skull, vertebral column, ribs, and sternum, and the *appendicular part,* or bones of the extremities. The tendons attach the muscles to the skeleton. This aids in locomotion.

Skin Also called integument; the outermost covering of the body consisting of a double-layered, tough, resilient epithelium averaging 1.7 square meters of surface area. The outer layer, or *epidermis* (cuticle or scarf skin), produces the pigment *melanin.* The inner layer, or *dermis,* is the true skin, sometimes called the corium. It is highly vascular and well supplied with nerve endings, sweat and sebaceous glands, and hair follicles. The skin protects the underlying tissues from mechanical injury, helps regulate body temperature, synthesizes vitamin D, and is sensitive to sensations of pain, touch, and temperature. The general condition of the skin is taken as an index of health and state of nutri-

tion (e.g., pallor of anemia, petechiae of vitamin C deficiency, follicular keratosis of vitamin A deficiency, and pellagrous dermatitis of niacin deficiency).

Skinfold measurement Also called pinch test; measurement of the thickness of a fold of skin at selected body sites where adipose tissue is normally deposited, as in the outer arm, abdomen, outer thigh, and pectoral region. The skinfold is measured with a *caliper* and gives an estimate of the degree of fatness of an individual.

SM Vegetable protein mixture used in Ethiopia; made of teff, peas, chick-peas, lentils, and skim milk powder. See Protein food mixtures, Appendix P-2.

S-M-A Synthetic milk adapted; a proprietary milk formula for infant feeding. *S-M-A Formula S-26* is a mixture of partially demineralized whey and nonfat milk, vegetable oils (corn, coconut, and soy oil), oleo, lactose, vitamins, and minerals. (Wyeth.) See Proprietary foods: composition, features, and uses, Appendix P-1.

Smoke point Temperature at which heated fat gives off a thin bluish smoke, indicating fat decomposition. It ranges from 160° to 260° C, depending on the type of fat or oil.

Sobee Proprietary hypoallergenic formula made from soybeans; used in allergy to cow's milk and in lactose intolerance. (Mead Johnson.) See Proprietary foods: composition, features, and uses, Appendix P-1.

Sodium A major *mineral* essential to life; the chief cation in the extracellular body fluids. It regulates water and acid-base balance, osmotic pressure, and absorption of nutrients across membranes. Sodium is also necessary for muscle contraction and nerve sensitivity. Dietary lack is unlikely to occur because it is easily supplied by table salt (NaCl) and many foods. Sodium depletion in the body may occur as a result of conditioning factors such as excessive vomiting, burns, diarrhea, and

215

other disorders marked by loss of body fluids. Sodium deficiency is characterized by muscular cramps, weakness, oliguria, and possibly vascular collapse and coma in severe deficiency. For more details, see Summary of minerals, Appendix H. See also *Low sodium syndrome* and *Diet, sodium-restricted*.

Sol Liquid *gel:* a colloidal system with water or liquid as the dispersing medium.

Solanine Toxic glycoside found in potato, especially in the sprouts. It contains glucose, galactose, rhamnose, and the alkaloid solanidine.

Solution Uniform liquid mixture of two or more substances in homogeneous molecular dispersion. The *solute* is the dissolved substance and the *solvent* is the dissolving medium.

Concentrated s Solution containing relatively more solute than is normally dissolved in the medium or solvent.

Hypertonic s Solution with an osmotic pressure greater than that within the cell. Water moves from the cell to the solution, causing the cell to shrink.

Hypotonic s Solution with an osmotic pressure lower than that within the cell. Water passes from the solution into the cell, causing the cell to burst.

Isosmotic s Solution that contains the same number of particles per unit volume.

Isotonic s Solution with the same osmotic pressure as body fluids, such as *physiologic salt solution*.

Physiologic salt s *Isotonic solution* of sodium chloride; distilled water that contains 0.9% sodium chloride.

Saturated s Solution that holds the maximum amount of solute at a given temperature, beyond which additional solute will not dissolve. The saturation point of a solution becomes higher as the temperature is increased, as in heating.

Supersaturated s Solution that contains more solute than would normally dissolve at a given temperature so that some of the solutes crystallize and remain undissolved.

Somagen Dietary food supplement high in protein and the B complex vitamins; made of nonfat milk with yeast, liver concentrate, vitamins, and calcium. (Upjohn.) See Proprietary foods: composition, features, and uses, Appendix P-1.

Somatic Pertaining to the body framework as distinguished from the viscera.

Somatotropin (somatotropic hormone) Growth hormone secreted by the anterior lobe of the *pituitary gland.* Its main action is to stimulate the growth of the epiphyseal cartilages of long bones. It also increases nitrogen retention, facilitates the transfer of amino acids from extracellular to intracellular compartments of the body, influences carbohydrate metabolism by its insulin-like effect, and causes lowering of fat content in the body.

Sorbic acid A mycostatic agent; an additive used to inhibit mold and yeast growth.

Sorbitol A 6-carbon sugar alcohol formed by the reduction of glucose or fructose. It is used to sweeten dietetic foods, since it can apparently be metabolized without insulin. However, sorbitol has the same caloric value as glucose. Sorbitol is slowly absorbed and delays the onset of hunger. It can be converted to utilizable carbohydrate in the form of glucose. Excessive use may cause gastrointestinal distress and diarrhea.

Soxhlet Apparatus for extracting solids, particularly fats. It is commonly used in the *proximate analysis* of foods.

Soyalac Milk-free formula made of soy protein, soy oil, corn sugar, sucrose, and added vitamins and minerals. Used in lactose intolerance and milk allergy. (Loma.) See Proprietary foods: composition, features, and uses, Appendix P-1.

Special Milk Program Under the School Lunch Act, milk can be provided to children not taking part in the lunch program or as a snack. This is paid for by the U. S. Department of Agriculture.

Specific dynamic action (SDA) Increase in metabolism as a result of extra heat production when food is digested, absorbed, and metabolized. It varies with the type and amount of food eaten. The SDA of protein is about 30%; fat, 13%; and carbohydrate, 4% to 5%. For a mixed diet the SDA is estimated to be 10% of the calories needed for basal metabolism and activity.

Specific fuel factor (value) Coefficient of digestibility and particular caloric contribution of foods coming from similar sources. For example, the coefficient of digestibility of proteins in milk, egg, and meat is 97%, whereas that of cornmeal protein is only 60%. Thus the caloric value per gram of protein would be much less for corn protein than for the proteins in milk, egg, and meat. Specific fuel factors (values) for estimating calories from various foods have been established.

Specific gravity Weight of a substance compared with that of an equal volume of another substance taken as a standard (water for liquids and solids, hydrogen for gases). The specific gravity of water is 1 (i.e., 1 gm/ml); it is less than 1 for fats.

Specificity The peculiar ability of an enzyme to catalyze a single reaction or a limited range of reactions. Specificity is the main distinction between enzymes and inorganic catalysts, which are nonspecific.

Specific rotation Extent or degree of rotation of a plane of polarized light by an optically active substance such as sugar.

Spectrophotometer Optical instrument that measures the amount of light absorbed at a particular wavelength.

Sphincter Ringlike muscle that closes a body orifice.

Sphingomyelin Complex *phospholipid* composed of 4-sphingenine (a basic amino alcohol), fatty acids, phosphoric acid, and choline. It is a part of cell structures and is found primarily in brain and nervous tissue as a constituent of the myelin sheath.

Sphygmomanometer Instrument for measuring arterial blood pressure.

Spinal column The spine or backbone. Also called vertebral column because it is made up of 33 bones called *vertebrae* joined longitudinally one on top of the other. It contains the *spinal cord* and provides support and structure to the trunk.

Spinal cord Long nervous tissue inside the *spinal column;* about 44 cm long, extending from the medulla below the skull to the second lumbar vertebra. The spinal cord contains nerve centers that control a number of reflex actions. It also conveys impulses to and from the brain.

Spirits Distilled alcoholic drinks, e.g., whiskey and rum.

Spirometer Also called respirometer; an apparatus that measures air taken into and from the lungs. It is used in indirect calorimetry. See *Respirometer* and *Calorimetry.*

Spleen Ductless organ situated in the upper part of the abdomen just below the diaphragm and to the left of and behind the stomach. It is composed of a mass of sinuses with various openings. The spleen is an organ of the *reticuloendothelial system.* It also serves as a reservoir for the storage of blood and is capable of increasing and decreasing its volume to maintain normal red blood cell levels in active circulation.

Sporadic Occurring occasionally or in scattered instances, as a disease.

Spore Inactive form of bacterium or its resting state. It is thick walled and strongly resistant to high temperature; under appropriate conditions it can germinate and become active again.

Sprue Afebrile disease characterized by fatty diarrhea, malabsorption, weight loss, and anemia. There are two types: nontropical and tropical sprue.

Nontropical s Form of celiac syndrome in adults resulting from sensitivity to gluten in wheat, rye, and oat cereals. It occurs sporadically in Europe, South America, and the United States. Unlike tropical sprue, it is not associated with a poor diet and responds dramatically to a gluten-free diet. See *Celiac disease.*

Tropical s Type of sprue common in certain tropical areas (East Indies, Southeast Asia, Ceylon, and Puerto Rico). The characteristic symptoms are anorexia, glossitis, abdominal distention, diarrhea characterized by bulky, frothy, and foul stools containing unabsorbed fats, macrocytic anemia, reduced adrenal cortex activity, and increased pigmentation on the trunk and extremities. The exact cause of the disease is not known. The syndrome responds dramatically to folic acid and antibiotic therapy.

Squalene Unsaturated hydrocarbon formed by four molecules of acetic acid. It is an intermediate step in the synthesis of cholesterol.

Stachyose Tetrasaccharide containing glucose, fructose, and two molecules of galactose. It is found in tubers, peas, lima beans, and beets.

Staphylococcus A genus of bacterium that includes the species *Staphylococcus aureus,* which produces a toxin that causes food poisoning. *Staphylococcus* poisoning affects the gastrointestinal tract, causing abdominal cramps, severe nausea, and vomiting. The organism is commonly transmitted by food handlers with droplet infection, boils, and infected cuts. Improper storage and refrigeration of foods also encourage bacterial growth and toxin formation.

Starch Storage form of carbohydrates in plants. It is a polysaccharide composed of many glucose units linked in a straight line (amylose) or with branches (amylopectin). Starch is the principal source of energy and the basic staple of the daily diet. Chief food sources are cereals and cereal products, root crops such as potatoes and yams, tapioca, legumes, and starchy vegetables.

Starvation Prolonged unsatisfied hunger or deprivation of food; a condition of dying or suffering resulting from lack of food.

Stasis Stagnation or stoppage of the flow of blood or body fluids in any part of the body.

Steapsin Former name for *pancreatic lipase,* the fat-splitting enzyme in the pancreatic juice.

Stearic acid Long-chain saturated fatty acid with 18 carbon atoms. It is present in most animal and vegetable fats as the triglyceride *stearin.*

Steatorrhea Presence of fat in stool. It may be caused by defective fat absorption, lack of bile, or lack of lipase. Fatty stools are seen in celiac disease and other malabsorption syndromes.

Stenosis Narrowing or stricture of a duct or canal, as in pyloric stenosis.

Stercobilin Also called urobilin; one of the brown pigments of the feces. See *Urobilin.*

Stereoisomers Substances having the same molecular formula and structure but differing in configuration (i.e., arrangement of atoms in space). They are of two types: optical isomers and geometric isomers.

Sterilization Destruction of all living cells by heat, chemicals, light, x-rays, or electron beams. In infant feeding the two techniques of sterilizing the formula and bottles are aseptic and terminal sterilization. See *Aseptic sterilization* and *Terminal sterilization.*

Sternum Also called breastbone; the flat, narrow bone in the median line of the body in front of the chest.

Steroids Large group of cylic lipid compounds. Included in this group are the *sterols, sex hormones, adrenocortical hormones, bile acids, vitamin D, saponins,* and *sterol glycosides.*

Sterols Class of *steroids* that are complex monohydroxy alcohols universally found in both plants and animals. Mycosterols are found in yeasts and fungi; the most important is *ergosterol,* a precursor of vitamin D. Phytosterols, or plant sterols, include *sitosterol,* which is found in oils of higher plants, especially wheat germ oil. Cholesterol is the most familiar sterol present only in animal sources. See *Cholesterol.*

STH Abbreviation for *somatotropic hormone.* See *Somatotropin.*

Stigma Distinguishing mark or peculiarity associated with a particular disease or disorder. For stigmas suggestive of nutritional deficiencies, see Methods of research in nutrition: clinical tests, Appendix M-3.

Stilbestrol Former spelling is stilbesterol. A synthetic organic substance with estrogenic properties. It is widely used for fattening poultry and for stimulating the growth of cattle.

Stoma Any minute pore, orifice, or opening on a free surface.

Stomach Gaster or gastric gland; the most dilated part of the alimentary canal situated below the diaphragm. It is composed of three parts: the *cardia,* or the upper part; the *fundus,* which secretes digestive juices and stores food temporarily; and the *antrum,* which provides powerful mixing movements. Three types of cells in the stomach secrete the gastric juice. They are *mucous cells,* which secrete mucin; *parietal cells,* which secrete hydrochloric acid; and *zymogenic* or *chief cells,* which secrete the enzymes pepsin, rennin, and lipase.

Stomatitis Inflammation of the oral mucosa or soft tissues of the mouth such as the lips, palate, tongue, gums, and floor of the mouth. See *Nutrition, tongue and mouth conditions.*

Stomato- Combining form pertaining to the mouth.

Strepogenin Also called streptogenin; a peptidelike fraction believed to be essential for the growth of mice and certain microorganisms such as hemolytic streptococci and lactobacilli. It is present in the liver and in enzymatic hydrolysates of casein and other purified proteins.

Streptococcus Any of various spherical bacteria occurring in chains. It includes a species that causes septic sore throat and scarlet fever. The organism can be transmitted through food contaminated from nasal and oral discharges, contaminated air, or objects handled by infected persons.

Stress 1. Time of extreme pressure or a trying period. 2. Any stimulus that disrupts the homeostasis of the organism. Stress factors that alter nutrient needs are *physiologic stresses,* as in growth, pregnancy, and lactation; *pathologic stresses* such as fever, infection, and disease; *physical stresses* such as heavy labor, strenuous exercise, and severe environmental conditions; and *psychologic stresses* such as anorexia nervosa and psychic overeating.

Stroke 1. A sudden and severe attack of a disease. 2. Common term for *apoplexy,* a symptom complex caused by hemorrhage of the brain or thrombosis of the cerebral vessels.

Stroma Tissue that forms the ground substance or matrix of an organ; the supporting framework of an organ.

Strontium Mineral found in the body but not yet established as essential to man. Strontium has the ability to replace calcium in bone formation. Of major concern is the possibility of ingesting radioactive strontium 90 by drinking milk from cows fed grass and hay that have absorbed the element from the soil or the atmosphere as radioactive fallout from nuclear testing.

Stupor State in which the mind and senses are dulled; partial consciousness.

Sublingual Beneath the tongue, as the sublingual glands.

Submaxillary Beneath the lower maxilla or mandible, as the submaxillary glands.

Substrate Organic substance acted on by an enzyme.

Sucaryl Trade name for *cyclamate,* an artificial sweetening agent. See *Cyclamate.*

Succinic acid One of the intermediate products in the *Krebs cycle,* the final common pathway of energy metabolism.

Succus entericus The intestinal juice. It is slightly alkaline and contains mucin, amylase, lipase, peptidases, disaccharidases, and other enzymes. Its composition and volume varies throughout the intestines.

Sucrose Table sugar; made from cane or beet sugar. It is a *disaccharide* consisting of glucose and fructose. Sucrose is easily hydrolyzed by acid or the enzyme invertase to form *invert sugar*. Intestinal *sucrase* readily splits sucrose into glucose and fructose.

Sugar 1. Any sweet, soluble, crystalline organic compound belonging to carbohydrates. 2. Specifically refers to sucrose extracted from sugar cane and sugar beet.

Sulfur (sulphur) An essential major mineral present in all cells of the body. It is a constituent of several organic compounds, e.g., insulin, glutathione, thiamin, biotin, and the amino acids cystine, cysteine, and methionine. Sulfur occurs in most food proteins, and the need for this mineral is met when protein supply is adequate. For further details, see Summary of minerals, Appendix H.

Superamine Formulated protein-rich food developed by FAO, WHO, and UNICEF in conjunction with the Algerian government. It is composed of hard wheat, chickpeas, lentils, skim milk powder, sugar, and vitamin D. See Protein food mixtures, Appendix P-2.

Supplementary feeding The giving of food in addition to the regular meals to increase or supplement nutrient intake.

Suprarenal glands The *adrenal glands*. The term "suprarenal" means lying above the kidneys.

Supro Protein food mixture used in East Africa; made of maize and barley flour, *Torula* yeast, skim milk powder, salt, and condiments. See Protein food mixtures, Appendix P-2.

Surface tension Inward force acting on the surface of a liquid as a result of the attraction of the molecules below the surface. This force tends to keep a liquid in a shape (usually a sphere) that minimizes its volume, thus reducing surface area.

Suspension Solution containing very tiny solid dispersed particles.

Suspensoid Colloidal solution in which the dispersed particles are solid, as distinguished from an emulsoid where the dispersed particles are also liquid.

Sustacal High protein nutritional supplement for oral or tube feeding. Made with skim milk, sugar, soy fat, sodium caseinate, corn syrup, vitamins, and minerals. (Mead Johnson.) See Proprietary foods: composition, features, and uses, Appendix P-1.

Sustagen Proprietary food concentrate used as a nutritional supplement. It is a mixture of whole and skim milk, casein, maltose, dextrins, vitamins, and minerals. (Mead Johnson.) See Proprietary foods: composition, features, and uses, Appendix P-1.

Sweetening agent A substance that gives a sweet taste; may be *natural*, e.g., sugar, glycine, and glycerol, or *synthetic*, e.g., the nonnutritive or artificial sweeteners. Sucrose is the most common and is used as the standard (100%) for comparing the sweetness of other agents. The relative sweetnesses of natural agents are as follows: fructose, 173%; glucose, 74%; maltose, 33%; lactose, 16%; glycerol, 60%; sorbitol, 60%; and glycine, 70%. The sweetening powers of the nonnutritive sweeteners are 550, 250, and 30 times sweeter than sucrose, respectively, for saccharin, dulcin, and Sucaryl.

Symbiosis The living together of two different organisms. The relationship may be helpful to both (mutualism), beneficial to one without any harm to the other (commensalism), beneficial to one but harmful to the other (parasitism), harmful to one without effect on the other (amensalism), or harmful to both organisms (synnecrosis).

Sympathetic nervous system One of two parts of the autonomic nervous system. Its actions are opposite those of the parasympathetic nervous system. For example, heart action is accelerated by the sympathetic but decelerated by the parasympathetic system; intestinal peristalsis is decreased by the sympathetic system and increased by the parasympathetic system. See also *Parasympathetic nervous system*.

Symptom The manifestation or expression

of a disease as the patient experiences it in contrast to *sign,* or the manifestation of a disease as the examiner perceives it. Headache is a symptom; rapid pulse is a sign.

Syndrome Set of symptoms and signs that occur together to characterize a particular disease or condition.

Syneresis Opposite of imbibition; the "weeping" of a gel, or the squeezing out of its liquid.

Synergism Joint action of agents so that their combined effect is greater than the algebraic sum of their individual effects. Malnutrition lowers resistance to infection and infectious diseases tend to magnify an existing malnutrition. The simultaneous presence of malnutrition and infection results in an interaction with an enlarged effect that is more serious than would be expected if malnutrition or infection acted separately.

Synovial fluid Clear lubricating fluid secreted by the synovial membrane of a joint.

Synthesis Combination of two or more substances to form a new material. *Biosynthesis* is the process of building up a chemical compound in the body or within an organism.

System Functional unit composed of parts (usually a set of organs and tissues) working together for a definite physiologic role. The nine systems in the body are the muscular, skeletal, digestive, circulatory, endocrine, reproductive, nervous, respiratory, and excretory systems. *Systemic* means pertaining to or affecting the body as a whole, as in systemic disease.

Systole Period when the heart is contracting.

T

T₃ Abbreviation for *triiodothyronine* or thyronine, a thyroid hormone. See *Thyroid gland*.

T₄ Abbreviation for *tetraiodothyronine* or thyroxine. See *Thyroid gland* and *Thyroxine*.

Tachycardia Rapid heartbeat. The term is usually applied to a pulse rate above 100/minute; the rapid stimulus of heart action is associated with several causes, varieties, and sites in the heart.

Tachysterol An isomer of ergosterol produced by irradiation, as is calciferol. It has no antirachitic activity unless reduced to dihydrotachysterol.

Taenia Type of worm that is flat, long, sectional, and ribbonlike; ordinarily known as tapeworm. It is a food-borne parasite of several species, of which the most common are *Taenia solium* (pork tapeworm), *Taenia saginata* (beef tapeworm), and *Diphyllobothrium latum* (fish tapeworm). Taenia infection can be prevented by thorough cooking of meats and fishes, proper sewage and garbage disposal, and good personal hygiene.

Tangier disease Familial high-density lipoprotein deficiency, an inherited disorder of lipid metabolism. Characterized by storage of large amounts of cholesterol esters in foam cells, enlargement of the tonsils, and an orange color of the pharyngeal and rectal mucosa. It is probably caused by a defect in the synthesis of high-density lipoprotein.

Tannin 1. Tannic acid. 2. Any of the astringent plant acids that can precipitate collagen and darken in the presence of ferric salts.

Taurine Aminoethylsulfonic acid, a substance that occurs in bile combined with cholic acid as *taurocholic acid*. This bile acid is synthesized in the liver from cysteine sulfinic acid. Taurine excretion in the urine results from excessive intake of protein foods rich in sulfur-containing amino acids. See *Diet, taurine-restricted*.

Tautomerism Form of stereoisomerism in which the compounds formed are mutually interconvertible under normal conditions. The mixture formed is thus in a state of dynamic equilibrium.

Tears Clear watery secretion of the lacrimal glands in the eyes. It is isotonic when freshly secreted, but becomes hypertonic when the fluid passes over the cornea as a result of evaporation. Tears lubricate eye surfaces, improve optical properties by filling corneal surface irregularities, and protect the eyes from injury.

Tendon Fibrous connective tissue that attaches muscles to bones and other structures. It is similar to *ligament* but it does not possess elasticity.

Tenesmus Ineffectual straining; usually applied to painful straining during defecation or urination without any excretion of feces or urine.

Ten-State Nutrition Survey See *National Nutrition Survey* and Methods of research in nutrition: nutritional surveys, Appendix M-1.

Teratology Study of congenital malformations, monstrosities, and other serious deviations from the normal.

Terminal sterilization As applied in infant feeding, a technique of sterilizing the milk formula and bottles together or at the same time. See also *Aseptic sterilization*.

Terpene Unsaturated hydrocarbon having the empirical formula $C_{10}H_{16}$. It is soluble in alcohol and organic solvents but insoluble in water. Terpenes are formed by the condensation of C_5H_8 isoprene units and occur in most essential oils and oleoresins of plants.

Terramycin Trade name for the antibiotic *oxytetracycline*.

Testis (testicle) The male gonad; an egg-shaped gland containing the spermatozoa and male sex hormones. The testes in human males are paired and located in the scrotum. See *Androgen*.

Testosterone The principal male sex hormone produced by the testes; the most potent of the biologically active androgens. It is necessary for the normal development of the male reproductive organs and such secondary sex characteristics as deep voice, body hair growth, and manly skeletal and muscular development.

Tetanus Tense and sustained contracted state of a muscle or muscles. The term more commonly refers to an acute infectious disease called lockjaw that is caused by toxins produced by *Clostridium tetani* present in rusty nails and areas contaminated by animal manure. The condition is characterized by tonic spasm of the voluntary muscles, exaggerated reflex actions, and convulsions; it is usually fatal.

Tetany Syndrome characterized by intermittent bilateral spasms, muscle twitchings, cramps, and sharp flexion of the wrist and ankle joints. Causative factors include alkalosis or excessive ingestion of alkaline salts, parathyroid hypofunction,

abnormal calcium metabolism, and vitamin D deficiency.

Tetracycline Generic name for the parent structure of certain antibiotics such as *chlortetracycline* (Aureomycin) and *oxytetracycline* (Terramycin).

Tetrahydrofolic acid (THFA) Designated term for the compound tetrahydropteroylglutamic acid $(PGAH_4)$ or tetrahydrofolacin; the most active form of *folic acid*. It acts as the carrier of 1-carbon fragments that are important for the synthesis of *purines* and *pyrimidines* and for methylation reactions.

Textured protein Fabricated food product made from vegetable protein sources such as peanuts, sesame seeds, soybeans, and wheat and suitably flavored, colored, and textured to simulate commonly used foods such as bacon, beef, and chicken.

Thalamus Mass of gray matter at the base of the brain; the middle and larger portion of the brain. It is the sensory nerve relay center and consists of fibers from all parts of the cerebral cortex; it connects these fibers to the spinal cord.

Theine Alkaloidal stimulant in tea chemically identical to caffeine.

Theobromine Alkaloidal stimulant in cocoa beans; also occurs in tea leaves and cola nuts. It is closely related to caffeine and used as a diuretic, an arterial dilator, and a myocardial stimulant.

THFA Abbreviation for *tetrahydrofolic acid*.

Thiamin (thiamine) Vitamin B_1, a member of the B complex vitamins. It is a component of the coenzyme *thiamin pyrophosphate,* which is important in carbohydrate metabolism, regulates muscle tone of the gastrointestinal tract, maintains normal nervous system activity, and prevents *beriberi.* Early signs of thiamin deficiency include loss of appetite, irritability, depression, gastrointestinal disturbances, and easy fatigability. Severe thiamin deficiency is clinically recognized as beriberi. The chief food sources are yeast, lean pork, liver and other glandular organs, whole-grain and enriched cereals, legumes, and nuts. For further details, see Summary of vitamins, Appendix I-1.

Thiaminase Enzyme found in many species of fish and certain bacteria. It catalyzes the hydrolysis of thiamin to pyramin and a thiazole derivative. It destroys the vitamin, causing a thiamin deficiency state.

Thiamin pyrophosphate (TPP) Also called cocarboxylase; the thiamin-containing coenzyme that participates in the oxidative decarboxylation of alpha keto acids and in the formation of alpha ketols.

Thiochrome 1. The yellow coloring matter of yeast. 2. A thiamin derivative formed in vitro by the action of mild oxidizing agents.

Thioctic acid Another name for lipoic acid. See *Lipoic acid*.

Thio-oxazolidone See *Goitrogens*.

Thiouracil Antithyroid pyrimidine derivative that interferes with the formation of thyroxine; used in the treatment of thyrotoxicosis.

Thiourea Also called thiocarbamide; an antithyroid substance used in the treatment of thyrotoxicosis. It inhibits the production of thyroxine by interfering with the incorporation of inorganic iodine to the organic form.

Thoracic Pertaining to the chest or *thorax*. The human thorax is composed of 12 ribs, 10 of which are joined to the breastbone or *sternum* in front and to the vertebral column at the back. The remaining two ribs are short and "float" in front just above the diaphragm. The *thoracic cavity* contains the heart, lungs, and mediastinal structures.

Threonine Alpha-amino-beta-hydroxybutyric acid, an *essential amino acid* that participates in many of the reactions involving glycine, which is important in purine synthesis and methylation reactions. Its metabolism is similar to that of serine, and both act as phosphate carriers in phosphoproteins.

Thrombin Enzyme that hastens the conversion of fibrinogen to fibrin, forming the blood clot. It exists in shed blood as an inactive precursor, *prothrombin,* which is changed to active thrombin by the action of thromboplastin and calcium ions. See *Blood clotting.*

Thrombocyte Also called blood platelet; one of the three formed elements of the blood. See *Blood.*

Thrombokinase Enzyme found in plasma globulin and crude tissue extracts. It catalyzes the conversion of prothrombin to thrombin and is perhaps identical to *thromboplastin.*

Thromboplastin Specific enzyme that accelerates the conversion of prothrombin to thrombin; a cephalin-protein complex.

Thrombosis Formation of an intravascular clot, or thrombus. It is likely to occur when there is slowing, stasis, or eddying of the blood current as a result of circulatory or cardiac disorders or secondary to certain infections. If a thrombus or any part of it is dislodged, it may be carried through the bloodstream as an *embolus.*

Thrush Also called parasitic stomatitis; a fungal disease marked by the formation of whitish spots in the mouth, especially on the buccal mucous membranes and tongue. In infants these spots should be differentiated from temporary white spots formed by milk.

Thymine 5-Methyl uracil, a pyrimidine base occurring in nucleic acids. It was first isolated from the thymus gland.

Thymus Ductless glandlike body located behind the sternum at the base of the throat and upper mediastinum, just above the heart. It is developed early in fetal life, increases in size and weight shortly after birth, then retrogresses by fatty metamorphosis after puberty. The thymus gland is believed to influence the maturation and proliferation of lymphoid cells involved in cell-mediated immunity and general host resistance. Other possible functions include its roles in malignant growth, reproduction, and calcium and phosphorus metabolism.

Thyrocalcitonin Thyroid hormone having

significant effect on the calcium content of blood and bone. It is secreted in response to elevated plasma calcium level and acts principally on bone, causing inhibition of bone resorption. Thyrocalcitonin is a polypeptide composed of 32 amino acids.

Thyroglobulin Gelatinous iodine-containing protein synthesized by the thyroid gland. Hydrolysis of thyroglobulin yields *thyroxine* and other iodinated amino acids. See *Thyroid gland.*

Thyroid gland Butterfly-shaped endocrine gland consisting of two major lobes connected by a central isthmus. It is located in the neck, just below the larynx. The thyroid gland has the unique ability to remove and concentrate blood iodide. This activity is influenced largely by the *thyrotropic hormone* and other chemical substances such as thiouracil, thiourea, thiocyanates, sulfonamides, and goitrogens. The chief function of the thyroid gland is to elaborate the thyroid hormones thyroxine, mono- and diiodotyrosine, and di- and triiodothyronine. Thyroxine and triiodothyronine are the most active biologically. The thyroid hormones regulate metabolism by stimulating oxygen consumption. For the effects of hypo- and hyperfunction of the thyroid gland, see *Cretinism, Goiter, Hyperthyroidism, Hypothyroidism, Myxedema,* and *Thyrotoxicosis.* See also Summary of endocrine glands, Appendix K.

Thyronine Triiodothyronine. See *Thyroid gland.*

Thyrotoxicosis Hyperactivity of the thyroid gland resulting from excessive secretion of thyroxine, tumor formation, or toxins that have entered the thyroid gland. See *Goiter* and *Hyperthyroidism.*

Thyrotropic hormone Thyroid-stimulating hormone (TSH) or thyrotropin; a hormone secreted by the anterior lobe of the pituitary gland. It stimulates the thyroid gland to oxidize iodide to iodine and to release the thyroid hormones into the circulation.

Thyroxine Also called tetraiodothyronine; the principal hormone of the thyroid gland. It is secreted into the blood bound to plasma protein (as protein-bound iodine) for transport to the tissues. Thyroxine regulates the rate of oxygen consumption in the cells. It is also involved in growth and differentiation of the tissues.

Tissue Aggregate of similar cells and their intercellular substances. The different kinds of tissues are *epithelial* tissue, which covers and lines surfaces; *muscular* tissue, e.g., the smooth, skeletal, and cardiac muscles; *nervous* tissue such as neurons and nerve fibers; *vascular* tissue, as the circulatory vessels; *connective* tissue such as collagen and elastin; and *adipose* tissue for storage of body fat.

Tocopherols Group designation for all methyl tocols; complex alcohols of the chromanol type. Several tocopherols have been isolated, but only four forms have vitamin E activity (alpha-, beta-, gamma-, and delta-tocopherol). Alpha-tocopherol is the most potent biologically, and delta-tocopherol is the most active antioxidant. Tocopherols occur naturally in certain plant oils, particularly in wheat germ, or they can be produced synthetically.

Tolbutamide Oral hyoglycemic agent used in the treatment of diabetes mellitus. See *Oral hypoglycemic agents* and *University Group Diabetes Program.*

Tolbutamide test Blood sugar determination before and 20 minutes after the intravenous administration of a solution containing 1 gm tolbutamide. A fall in blood sugar level by more than 89% in 20 minutes is diagnostic of diabetes mellitus.

Tolerance 1. Limit to which substances can be ingested, absorbed, and metabolized without any deleterious physiologic effect. 2. Maximum limit established by the Food and Drug Administration to which additives may be incorporated in food.

Tongue Movable muscular organ in the mouth that aids in mastication, swallowing, speech, and taste perception. It is covered by a mucous membrane and has numerous papillae, the minute nipplelike projections containing the taste buds. Color changes and lesions in the tongue are indicative of certain disorders, including nutritional deficiencies. See *Nutrition, tongue and mouth conditions.*

Tonic 1. Producing normal tonus or tone. 2. Characterized by continuous contraction, as tonic spasms. 3. Drug or agent that improves the normal tonus of an organ or of the musculature in general.

Tooth One of the calcified structures supported by the gums of both jaws. It is important for biting and chewing, supports the facial contour, and helps in articulation of sounds (speech). Several nutrients are essential for proper tooth formation and calcification. Protein influences matrix formation in the enamel and dentin of the developing tooth. The presence of vitamin A affects the formation of the enamel matrix and the maintenance of the epithelium of the periodontal tissue. Vitamin C influences the formation of the collagen matrix in dentin, cementum, and periodontal membrane. Vitamin D, calcium, and other minerals are needed for the calcification of enamel, dentin, and cementum. Deficiencies and excesses of several minerals (fluoride, calcium, phosphorus, etc.) affect the composition of the calcified tissues.

Tophus Pl. tophi. Mineral deposit in the joints, ear, or bone, as sodium urate in gout.

TOPS Abbreviation for *Take Off Pounds Sensibly.* A noncommercial self-help group concerned with the management and problems of obesity.

Toxemia 1. Condition in which blood contains toxic or poisonous substances either produced by the body or elaborated by microorganisms. 2. Collective term for toxemias of pregnancy. See *Eclampsia* and *Preeclampsia.*

TPN Abbreviation for *triphosphopyridine nucleotide* or coenzyme II.

TPP Abbreviation for *thiamin pyrophosphate.*

Trabecula Connective tissue or fibrous band that extends from the capsule into the interior of an organ. It also refers to the small needle-shaped component of bones called spicule.

Trace minerals Elements needed by the body in minute amounts. See *Mineral* and *Micronutrients.*

Tracer technique Research method that uses a radioactive element to follow the fate of a substance or its reactions. Compounds containing tracer elements are said to be "tagged" or "labeled."

Trachea Also called windpipe; the cartilaginous and membranous tube of the respiratory system, extending from the larynx to the bronchi.

Trans Latin, meaning "on the other side." A prefix used to designate geometric isomers with a double bond between two carbon atoms. The isomer is called *trans* when a given atom or radical is in the opposite location; it is called *cis* when positioned on the side of the carbon axis.

Transamination Transfer of an amino group from one compound to another, with *pyridoxal phosphate* acting as the intermediate amino carrier. The reaction is catalyzed by the enzyme *transaminase.* By this process the body is able to use urea and synthesize the nonessential amino acids.

Transcobalamin The transport protein of vitamin B_{12}.

Transferases Class of enzymes that catalyze the transfer of groups or radicals. Examples are transaminases, kinases, and transacetylases. See Summary of enzymes, Appendix J-2.

Transferrin Also called siderophilin; a glycoprotein in the blood plasma that transports iron to the liver and spleen for storage, to the bone marrow for hemoglobin synthesis, or to the other tissues for their use.

Transfusion Transfer of blood, plasma,

plasma substitute, or any injectable solution directly into the bloodstream.

Transketolase Enzyme found in blood, cells, liver, and other tissues that is necessary for the synthesis of the 5-carbon sugars found in DNA and RNA. It requires thiamin pyrophosphate as a coenzyme.

Transmanganin Protein carrier that transports manganese in the blood. See *Manganese*.

Transmethylation Transfer of a methyl radical (—CH₃ group) from one compound to another. This reaction is important in intermediary metabolism, particularly in fat, sulfur, and creatine metabolism. Vitamin B₁₂ and folic acid are both involved in the synthesis of methyl groups. Methionine is considered the primary methyl donor in transmethylation reactions. Choline and betaine are also methyl donors.

Transmutation Process by which the atoms of one element may spontaneously change into atoms of another element. An example is the radioactive decay of uranium.

Tricarboxylic acid (TCA) cycle Krebs cycle or citric acid cycle; the final common pathway of energy metabolism for carbohydrate, protein, and fat. See *Krebs cycle*.

Trichinosis Food-borne parasitic infection caused by *Trichinella spiralis*. The condition is characterized by acute food poisoning; painful and inflamed muscles, particularly muscles of respiration, speech, mastication, and swallowing; fever; edema; and toxemia. The organism is transmitted through eating raw or partially cooked infected pork.

Triglyceride Fat in which the glycerol molecule has three fatty acids attached to it.

Trigonelline An inactive form of *niacin* that is found in seeds and nuts. Roasting coffee beans activates this substance.

Triiodothyronine A thyroid hormone. See *Thyroid gland*.

Triose A sugar that contains three carbon atoms. It is an intermediate product of metabolism and does not occur naturally. *Glyceraldehyde* is a triose.

Triphosphopyridine nucleotide (TPN) Also called coenzyme II. See *Coenzymes I and II*.

Trisaccharide An oligosaccharide containing three monosaccharide units. Examples are *raffinose* (has fructose, glucose, and galactose) and *melezitose* (has two molecules of glucose and one molecule of fructose).

Tritium The hydrogen isotope with a mass of three. It is radioactive and has a half-life of 31 years. Tritium is used in tracer studies and body water determination.

Tropic (trophic) Combining form meaning to influence, change, or stimulate. A tropic hormone is one that causes another gland to function.

Trunk 1. The torso or body without head and limbs. 2. The main stem of a lymphatic or blood vessel or of a nerve.

Trypsin Proteolytic enzyme of the pancreas secreted as the inactive precursor *trypsinogen*. It is an endopeptidase and catalyzes the hydrolysis of peptide linkages containing the carboxyl group of lysine and arginine, yielding polypeptides with C-terminal lysine and arginine groups.

Trypsin inhibitor A substance capable of reducing the activity of the proteolytic enzymes in the digestive juices; can also slow down the absorption of some amino acids, either by reducing the utilization of nitrogenous material in food or by raising the needs of the organism for certain amino acids. It is found in raw egg white, soybeans, peanuts, peas, beans, and lentils.

Tryptophan Alpha-amino-beta-indolylpropionic acid, an *essential amino acid* for man and animals. It is frequently a limiting amino acid for tissue synthesis. Tryptophan is the only amino acid with an indole nucleus; it can be converted to nicotinic acid, serotonin, and melatonin.

TSH Abbreviation for *thyroid-stimulating hormone*. See *Thyrotropic hormone*.

Tube feeding See *Diet, tube feeding*.

Tularemia Food-borne disease caused by the

organism *Pasteurella tularensis*. It is popularly known as rabbit fever because it is frequently transferred to rabbit hunters from wild rabbits that have the infected ticks, lice, and fleas that carry the organism. The disease is also transmitted to man through the bite of an infected animal or insect. It is characterized by recurrent fever, headache, prostration, and focal ulcers at the site of infection.

Tumor Growth of a mass of new tissues independent of surrounding tissues; the growth has no physiologic role. It may be malignant or benign.

Tyndall effect Scattering of a beam of light when it passes through a colloidal dispersion. The amount of scattering depends on the size and concentration of the dispersed particles. The effect is useful in estimating the molecular weight of protein molecules.

Typhoid fever Food-borne infection caused by *Salmonella typhosa*. It occurs endemically wherever sanitation is poor and the water supply is likely to be contaminated with sewage. The organism is transmitted through polluted water and food, especially milk, shellfish, and raw vegetables.

Tyramine Base found in putrefied animal tissue, ergot, certain cheeses and wines, and other foods. It can cause severe hypertensive reaction when taken with monoamine oxidase inhibitory drugs. See *Diet, tyramine-restricted*.

Tyrosinase Copper-containing enzyme that oxidizes tyrosine and other phenolic compounds, forming brown to black pigments. Lack of this enzyme results in *albinism*.

Tyrosine Alpha-amino-beta-hydroxyphenylpropionic acid, a nonessential amino acid that has some sparing action on the essential amino acid phenylalanine. It participates in transamination reactions and is the starting material for the synthesis of melanin, thyroxine, and epinephrine.

Tyrosinosis Hereditary disorder characterized by high plasma levels of tyrosine, renal tubular defects, liver damage, and increased excretion of para-hydroxyphenyllactic acid and para-hydroxyphenylpyruvic acid in the urine. It results from a lack of the enzyme *para-hydroxyphenylpyruvic acid oxidase*. A diet low in tyrosine and phenylalanine has been recommended. Tyrosine can be formed from phenylalanine. See Inborn errors of metabolism, Appendix G.

U

Ubichromenol Compound similar in structure to vitamin E. It has vitamin activity.

Ubiquinone General term for a group of related quinones with variable numbers of isoprene residues. Ubiquinone is found in the mitochondria and serves as an electron transport agent. See *Coenzyme Q*.

UDPG Abbreviation for *uridine diphosphate glucose*.

UGDP Abbreviation for *University Group Diabetes Program*.

Ulcer An eroded lesion or an excavated sore. A *peptic ulcer* is any ulcer in the gastrointestinal tract that is a result, at least in part, of the digestive action of gastric juice. Thus *esophageal ulcer* is found in the lower portion of the esophagus; *gastric ulcer* affects the mucosa of the stomach, generally in the lesser curvature near the pylorus; *duodenal ulcer* is usually found in the first 4 cm of the anterior wall of the duodenum near the pylorus; and *marginal ulcer* is near the mouth or junction between the stomach and the jejunum and is a result of *gastroenterostomy*. The exact cause of peptic ulcer is unknown, although a number of factors contribute to its formation. These include hyperacidity, lowered cellular resistance, insufficient secretion of mucus, local trauma or injury, and nervous and emotional factors. Epigastric pain is the most *outstanding* symptom; it is often described as burning, piercing, or boring and is characterized by its chronicity, periodicity, rhythm, and location. For dietary management, see *Diet, bland,* and *Diet, progressive bland*.

Ultracentrifuge Centrifuge with a very high speed of rotation that can separate and sediment small particles in a colloidal suspension. It is used for the determination of proteins and viruses of different particle sizes.

Ultrafiltration Filtration under pressure through an appropriate membrane, such as clay or porcelain, with minute pores. It is used to separate colloidal particles from the dispersion medium.

Ultramicroscope Microscope with powerful side illumination capable of making visible minute particles such as virus and colloidal particles that cannot be seen with an ordinary microscope.

Ultraviolet rays Rays of light of shorter wavelength than that of visible light.

Umbilicus The navel; the scar at the site of attachment of the umbilical cord in the fetus. The *umbilical cord* is the connection between the navel of the fetus and the placenta of the uterus.

Underweight Term applied to individuals whose body weights are more than 10% below the established standard for individuals of the same age, sex, and height.

UNESCO Abbreviation for *United Nations Educational, Scientific, and Cultural Organization*. An organization that aims to eliminate illiteracy and to help people, through education, to use science and to

229

understand cultural forces for the improvement of their lives.

UNICEF Abbreviation for *United Nations International Children's Emergency Fund*. An organization that aims to help children all over the world by eradication of disease, improvement of health, and provision of emergency relief rations by milk distribution and school feeding and through the establishment of maternal and child health-care centers.

United States Department of Agriculture (USDA) Department of the federal government consisting of a Human Nutrition Research Division, experiment stations, and extension services, all of which are concerned with nutrition. These divisions carry out research and program services such as the Food Stamp Program and publish data on the nutritive value of common foods and information on the eating patterns of persons residing in the United States.

United States Department of Health, Education, and Welfare (HEW) Department of the federal government that has several agencies that deal with nutrition, such as the Maternal and Child Health Service, the Office of Education, the Food and Drug Administration, and the National Institutes of Health and its Public Health Services agency.

United States Pharmacopeia (USP) The standard weight reference of nutrients in the United States. The USP standards for ascorbic acid, calcium pantothenate, choline chloride, nicotinamide, nicotinic acid, pyridoxine hydrochloride, riboflavin, thiamin hydrochloride, eight essential amino acids, and vitamins A and D are available to the public. When an international standard exists, the USP standard is compared and brought as closely as possible into agreement. A USP unit is therefore equal to an international unit.

University Group Diabetes Program (UGDP) Program started in 1961 and consisting of 12 university clinics and a coordinating center. Their objectives were to evaluate the effect of hypoglycemic agents on the development of vascular disease in diabetes, to collect information on the natural history of diabetes and the relationship of blood glucose levels to vascular disease, and to develop methods for other long-term clinical trials. The investigators found a higher incidence of cardiovascular disease in diabetics treated with tolbutamide. They also found that the combination of diet and tolbutamide is no more effective than diet alone in the treatment of diabetes.

Uracil One of the pyrimidine bases of *nucleic acids*.

Urate A salt of *uric acid*. An increased amount of urates in the urine is called *uraturia*.

Urea NH_2CONH_2; the diamide of carbonic acid. It is the major end product of human nitrogen (protein) metabolism and the chief nitrogenous constituent of the urine. Urea formation occurs chiefly in the liver.

Urea clearance test Test that measures the quantity of blood "cleared" of urea per minute to determine renal function.

Urea cycle The overall reactions of the urea cycle proceed as follows: the combination of CO_2, NH_3, and adenosine triphosphate forms carbamyl phosphate, which combines with ornithine to form citrulline, which combines with aspartic acid to form argininosuccinic acid; then the cleavage of argininosuccinic acid forms arginine and fumaric acid and finally the hydrolytic cleavage of arginine yields urea and ornithine.

Urease (urase) Specific enzyme that decomposes urea, forming ammonia and carbon dioxide. It is obtained from the jack bean and watermelon seeds. Urease was the first enzyme to be crystallized.

Uremia Retention of urinary constituents in the blood. It is a toxic condition and the terminal manifestation of renal failure. The clinical features include nausea and vomiting, anorexia, dizziness, convulsions, and coma.

Ureter Long narrow tube that conveys the urine from the pelvis of the kidney to the bladder. See also *Kidney*.

Ureterolith A stone in the ureter. The formation of a stone or calculus in the ureter is called *ureterolithiasis,* and the surgical removal of a stone in the ureter is called *ureterolithotomy.* See also *Urinary calculi*.

Urethra Membranous canal that conveys the urine from the neck of the urinary bladder to the external opening. It also serves to convey the spermatozoa in the male. *Urethritis* is inflammation of the urethra.

Uric acid The end product of purine metabolism in man and protein metabolism in birds and some reptiles. In man, uric acid is excreted in the urine in the free state and as the urates of sodium, potassium, and ammonium. It is formed in part from purines taken in the food (exogenous uric acid) and in part from body purines as a result of the breakdown of nucleic acids (endogenous uric acid). Abnormal metabolism of uric acid is characteristic of *gout*.

Uricase Enzyme that catalyzes the aerobic oxidation of uric acid to *allantoin*. It is present in the liver of most mammals except man.

Uridine Nucleoside that consists of uracil and ribose. This is obtained by the removal of phosphate from uridylic acid.

Uridine diphosphate glucose (**UDPG**) The glucose ester of uridine diphosphate formed from glucose-1-phosphate in the presence of a pyrophosphorylase. It is the prosthetic group of the enzyme responsible for the conversion of galactose to glucose.

Uridylic acid Nucleotide containing ribose, phosphoric acid, and the pyrimidine uracil. The nucleotides of uridine monophosphate, uridine diphosphate, and uridine triphosphate function as coenzymes in a wide variety of reactions.

Urinalysis Physical, chemical, and microscopic analysis of the urine. This includes a description of color, the determination of pH, the quantitation of specific gravity, and the observation of the presence or absence of abnormal constituents such as proteins (albumin), sugar, ketone bodies, casts, pus, and blood cells. See Normal constituents of urine, Appendix R.

Urinary calculi Insoluble constituents in the urine that precipitate in the urinary passages; these contain urates, cystine and calcium oxalates, phosphates, and carbonates. Urinary calculi formation is the result of a number of factors, including hyperfunction of the parathyroid glands; vitamin A deficiency; systemic infections; inadequate fluid intake; metabolic disturbances; prolonged bed rest; and obstruction in the renal flow, producing stasis of the urine. See Dietary management of selected disorders, Appendix O.

Urinary ketosteroids Steroid compounds in the urine that may be derived from bile acids, estrogens, and other endocrine secretions of the gonads and adrenal cortex.

Urine Fluid excreted by the kidneys. The quantity excreted in 24 hours varies with the amount of fluid consumed but averages between 1000 and 1500 ml. It is slightly acid in reaction and has a specific gravity of 1.005 to 1.030. The amount of solids varies with the diet, although urine collection normally contains from 40 to 75 gm solids/24 hours. Urine formation is the result of three processes that occur in the nephron: *filtration* through the glomerular capillaries; *reabsorption* of fluid and solutes in the proximal tubule, the loop of Henle, and the distal tubule; and *secretion* into the lumen of the distal tubule. See also Normal constituents of urine, Appendix R.

Urobilin Also called stercobilin; a brownish pigment derived from the oxidation of urobilinogen, a derivative of the bile pigment bilirubin. This is found in the feces and sometimes in the urine after exposure to air. It is primarily responsible for the brown color of the feces.

Urobilinogen Also called stercobilinogen; a

colorless reduction product of bilirubin by the intestinal bacteria. When urine is allowed to stand, it is oxidized in the air to *urobilin*.

Urocanic acid Acid formed from the deamination of histidine; found in dog urine.

Urochrome The chief yellow pigment of the urine, which is believed to be a compound of urobilin and a peptide of unknown structure. Other urinary pigments are *uroerythrin* and *uroporphyrin*.

Urocortisone One of the major urinary adrenal cortical steroids together with urocortisol and cortisone.

Urocyanosis Blue discoloration of the urine resulting from the presence of *indican*, which is oxidized to indigo blue.

Uroerythrin Red pigment found in urine that is responsible for its reddish yellow color. It is believed to be derived from melanin.

Urogastrone A substance found in the urine similar to enterogastrone. It also inhibits gastric secretion and motility.

Urolith A stone or calculus in the urine. The formation of urinary calculi is called *urolithiasis* and the removal of a calculus from the urinary tract is *urolithotomy*. See *Urinary calculi*.

Urology Branch of medicine that deals with the study and treatment of diseases and defects in the urinary and genital organs in the male and the urinary organs in the female. A specialist in urology is called a *urologist*.

Uronic acid The sugar acid that results if the primary alcohol group farthest removed from the aldehyde (i.e., at the opposite end of the chain) is oxidized to the carboxyl group. An example is glucuronic acid.

Uroporphyrin A porphyrin found in small amounts in the urine. It is excreted in abnormally large amounts in lead poisoning, congenital porphyria, and porphyrinuria.

USDA Abbreviation for *United States Department of Agriculture*.

USP Abbreviation for *United States Pharmacopeia*.

Uterus The womb; a pear-shaped hollow muscular organ in the female that receives and nourishes the fertilized ovum during its fetal development. It is about 3 inches long, 2 inches wide, and 1 inch thick and includes the *fundus* (the upper and broad portion) the *body*, which gradually narrows down to the *cervix* and extends down to the *vagina*.

V

Vaccination Inoculation with a vaccine for protection or immunity against a given disease. A *vaccine* is a suspension of killed or weakened microorganisms that produces immunization against a specific disease on introduction into the body. Examples of vaccines are those against smallpox, poliomyelitis, cholera, and rabies.

Vacuole Small space or cavity in a cell.

Vagina 1. A sheath. 2. Canal that runs from the external female organ to surround the neck of the womb. Its wall consists of muscle, fibrous tissue, and mucous membrane.

Vagus The tenth and largest cranial nerve originating from the brain and carrying impulses to many organs in the head, neck, chest, and abdomen. Resection of the vagus nerve is called *vagotomy*.

Valence 1. In chemistry, the combining power of an element; the capacity of an atom to combine with other atoms. 2. In immunology, the number of reactive sites on the surface of molecules of a homologous antigen and antibody.

Valine Alpha-aminoisovaleric acid; an *essential* amino acid necessary for growth and maintenance of tissues. Deficiency in rats causes hyperesthesia and muscular incoordination.

Vanadium Trace element found in the human body. Its biologic function has not yet been established. Vanadium salts reduce tissue sterol content, although the relationship between vanadium, body cholesterol, and heart disease is not clear. It is also believed that vanadium is needed for the calcification of bones and teeth during prenatal life. In rats and guinea pigs, vanadium promotes mineralization of bones and teeth and reduces dental caries. For further details, see Summary of minerals, Appendix H.

van den Bergh reaction Test for the detection of bile pigments in blood serum. In the presence of Ehrlich diazo reagent, bilirubin gives a typical red color, the color intensity being proportional to the pigment concentration. There are two types of reactions: direct and indirect. An *indirect* van den Bergh reaction is suggestive of hemolytic or prehepatic jaundice, whereas a *direct* reaction is suggestive of obstructive and posthepatic jaundice.

van't Hoff's law At constant temperature the osmotic pressure of a dilute solution is equal to the pressure that it would exert if present as gas and occupying the same volume as that of the solution.

Vapor Gaseous form of a substance that is either liquid or solid at ordinary temperatures. *Vaporization* is the conversion of a solid or liquid into a vapor.

Vapor pressure Pressure of a liquid, solid, or solution that is exerted by a vapor when a state of equilibrium has been reached between the liquid, solid, or solution and its vapor.

Varicose Descriptive word for blood vessels that are swollen, dilated, knotted, and tor-

233

tuous, as *varicose veins*. The surgical removal of a varicose vein is called *varicotomy*.

Vascular Relating to or referring to blood or lymphatic vessels and ducts. Most often refers to blood vessels. The vascular bed is the total blood supply (i.e., arteries, capillaries, and veins) of an organ or region.

Vasoconstriction Constriction of the blood vessels, leading to a reduction in the caliber of the vessels, particularly the arterioles. A *vasoconstrictor* is any nerve, drug, or agent that causes constriction of the blood vessels.

Vasodepression Lowering of the blood pressure caused by relaxation of the blood vessels. Any drug, nerve, or agent that relaxes the blood vessels is called a *vasodepressor*.

Vasodilation Dilation or increase in the caliber of a blood vessel, especially the arterioles, leading to an increased blood supply. This effect is brought about by a *vasodilator agent*.

Vasomotor Regulating the movements of the walls of the blood vessels, i.e., their contraction (vasoconstriction) and expansion (vasodilation).

Vasopressin A posterior pituitary hormone that exerts both pressor and antidiuretic action. Its *pressor* action is a result of peripheral vasoconstriction in the systemic arterioles and capillaries. There is constriction of the coronary and pulmonary vessels and dilation of cerebral and renal vessels. The *antidiuretic effect* is exerted in the collecting tubules of the kidney, accelerating the rate of water reabsorption and causing an increase in urine volume with high concentrations of sodium, chloride, phosphate, and total nitrogen. A lack of this hormone results in diabetes insipidus. This is characterized by excessive renal loss of water and excessive thirst. Release of vasopressin is stimulated by a variety of neurogenic stimuli such as pain, trauma, and emotional stress.

Vasotonic 1. Relating to the normal tension or tone of the blood vessels. 2. A vasostimulant.

Vasotonin A vasoconstrictor substance present in the blood. See *Vasoconstriction*.

VC Symbol for acuity of color vision; abbreviation for *vital capacity*.

VDM A vasodepression material; identified as ferritin, which is released in the liver, spleen, and skeletal muscles under anaerobic conditions. It causes relaxation of the vascular beds and lowering of the blood pressure. See also *VEM*.

Vector A carrier; an arthropod that carries an infective agent from one infected person to another.

Vegan (**vegetarian**) Person subsisting entirely or in large part on plants. A *pure vegetarian* is one who eats only foods of plant origin without specific restrictions as to kind. A *fruitarian* is one who restricts the variety of plant foods he eats to fruits and nuts, with or without the addition of grains and legumes. In addition to grains, legumes, vegetables, and fruits, some vegetarians also consume milk (lacto-vegetarian), or eggs (ovo-vegetarian), or both (lacto-ovo–vegetarian).

Vegetable protein mixture Blend of processed vegetable protein foods with or without skim milk powder and with added vitamins and minerals. It is a cheap source of protein-rich food in developing countries where animal protein foods are expensive or unavailable. See Protein food mixtures, Appendix P-2.

Vein Blood vessel that carries blood from the tissues to or toward the heart.

VEM Vasoexcitor material formed in the kidneys under anaerobic conditions. It is a protein with pressor activity and enhances the constriction of the precapillary sphincters. The effect of **VEM** is counteracted by a vasodepressor material (VDM). It is postulated that a VEM/VDM imbalance may be related to the development of shock and hypertension.

Venesection Blood letting; opening of a vein to remove blood.

Venoclysis Injection of a nutrient, medicine, or other substance into a vein.

Venomotor Influencing the movements of the walls of the vein, as contraction and dilation.

Ventricle A pouch or small cavity, as the left and right ventricles of the heart or one of the several cavities of the brain.

Verdoflavin Name given to a substance isolated from grass; later shown to be riboflavin.

Verdoglobin Also called *choleglobin*. See *Choleglobin*.

Verdohemoglobin Intermediate compound formed in the breakdown of hemoglobin by the opening of one porphyrin ring. It is a biliverdin-iron-protein complex that has a green color.

Vernier Device attached to a graduated scale or measuring apparatus for measuring to finer or smaller subdivisions of the scale, e.g., into tenths or fractions.

Vertebra Any one of the 33 bones forming the spinal or vertebral column.

Vesicle A blister; small bladder or sac containing liquid.

Vessel Tube, duct, or canal for conveying fluids in the body, as the blood vessels.

Vestibule Space or cavity at the entrance of a canal, as the vestibule of the ear.

Villi Small, fingerlike projections on the surface of a mucous membrane, as in the walls of the small intestine, where absorption takes place.

Viosterol Vitamin D_2, an artificial product of plants, resulting from the irradiation of ergosterol. See *Ergocalciferol*.

Virilism Masculinity; the development of male characteristics in the female.

Virology Study of viruses and the diseases they produce. A specialist in this field is a *virologist*.

Virulent Exceedingly noxious, deleterious, or pathogenic.

Virus Disease-producing agent smaller than the ordinary germ; consists of a nucleic acid, RNA or DNA, enclosed in a protein layer. It is a living pathogen that can multiply only in the presence of living, healthy host cells. Some viruses are visible under the ordinary microscope; others, the ultraviruses, are visible only under the ultramicroscope. Some can pass through porcelain filters, whereas the nonfilterable viruses cannot pass through.

Viscera Organs enclosed within the four great cavities: the cranium, thorax, abdomen, and pelvis. Pertains most commonly to the digestive organs within the abdominal cavity.

Viscid Viscous; of a thick, mucous, or gelatinous nature, e.g., egg white.

Viscosity Resistance of a liquid to flow. The viscosity of a liquid is measured by an instrument called a *viscosimeter*.

Vision Sense of sight; considered the most important of all senses. Man relies on vision for protection, equilibrium, coordination, creation, and pleasure. In vision, light from objects in the environment stimulates the receptor cells in the retina to send nervous impulses to the brain, where the mental image is formed. Vision is multifaceted, involving physics, anatomy, physiology, biochemistry, and psychology.

Visual process The photoreceptors of the eye transmit the photostimulation to two receptors (rods and cones) located in the retina. The rods are involved in vision in dim light (scotopic vision), and the cones function in vision in bright light (photopic vision). The light sensitivity of these receptors is a result of two photosensitive pigments: *rhodopsin* (in the rods) and *iodopsin* (in the cones), which are protein complexes of *vitamin A*. On exposure to light, rhodopsin is bleached through a series of intermediate compounds, giving as end products *opsin* (a protein) and *retinaldehyde* (vitamin A aldehyde, retinal, or retinene). Since retinaldehyde has an all-*trans* configuration, it cannot recombine with opsin to regenerate rhodopsin, which is of the 11-*cis* structure. Retinaldehyde is therefore reduced to *retinol* (vitamin A$_1$ alcohol) by the enzyme retinaldehyde reductase with nicotinamide adenine dinucleotide as the coenzyme. This is brought into the circulation, taken up by the liver, and converted to *neo-b* vitamin A$_1$, which has the 11-*cis* configuration. The retina then selectively reabsorbs 11-*cis* retinol, which is oxidized to 11-*cis* retinaldehyde. The latter recombines with opsin to regenerate rhodopsin.

Visual purple Also called rhodopsin; a conjugated protein containing vitamin A. It is a pigment in the retina of the eye that is bleached to visual yellow by light. See *Rhodopsin.*

Visual threshold Minimal light intensity required to evoke a visual sensation.

Visual yellow Colorless substance formed in the retina when visual purple (rhodopsin) is exposed to light. It is a mixture of retinaldehyde (formerly called retinene) and a protein, opsin.

Vital capacity (VC) Volume of air that can be breathed out by the deepest possible expiration following the deepest possible inspiration.

Vital statistics Figures on births, deaths, longevity, disease rates, and other data that indicate the state of health of a population. See also *Crude birth rate, Crude death rate, Maternal mortality rate,* and *Morbidity.*

Vitamer 1. Substance structurally related to a vitamin and capable of producing the same biologic activity. 2. One of the early names given to vitamins.

Vitamin General term originally given to a group of organic substances that are present in food in minute quantities and that perform specific functions for normal nutrition. At present it is rather difficult to formulate a completely satisfactory statement of what the term really means. It has been suggested that an organic compound should have all of the following characteristics in order to be considered a vitamin: (a) a compound in natural foods but distinct from carbohydrate, fat, or protein, (b) present in normal food in extremely small concentrations, (c) essential for normal health and growth, (d) causing a specific deficiency disease when not adequately supplied by the diet, and (e) not synthesized in sufficient amounts by the host and therefore obtained exclusively from the diet. This last characteristic is the one used to distinguish a vitamin from a hormone. However, it is possible that the same compound is a vitamin in one species and a hormone in another. For example, ascorbic acid is a vitamin for man, other primates, and guinea pigs and a hormone for other animals, since they are able to synthesize it. On the other hand, para-aminobenzoic acid (PABA) and meso-inositol are vitamins for certain microorganisms but not for man. The following are old terms suggested for vitamin: accessory food factor, advitant, biocatalyst, catalin, ergin, ergon, exogenous hormone, nutrilite, vitamer, vitamine, and vitazyme.

Vitamin A A highly complex alcohol that is soluble in fat and organic solvents. It exists in two forms: *retinol* (vitamin A$_1$), which predominates in mammals and saltwater fish, and *dehydroretinol* (vitamin A$_2$), which predominates in freshwater fish. The vitamin is colorless and occurs preformed only in foods of animal origin. It is present in yellow and green leafy plants as provitamin A, of which there are several forms, but the most important in human nutrition are alpha- and beta-carotene and cryptoxanthin. These are converted to the active vitamin in the intestinal wall and liver. Vitamin A is necessary for normal growth and development, maintenance of the normal structure of tissues, and other physiologic functions, including vision and reproduction. Recent evidence indicates that the vitamin may be needed for mucopolysaccharide biosynthesis. Deficiency symptoms vary with the animal species. In man the most common signs are poor growth, lowered resistance to infection, night blindness, and rough, scaly skin. Severe deficiency leads to keratomalacia and xerophthalmia. Vitamin A is not normally excreted and can accumulate in the body. Excessive intake (hypervitaminosis A) causes headache, dry skin, loss of hair, and softening of bones. The vitamin was formerly called axerophthol and antixerophthalmic vitamin. For further details, see Summary of vitamins, Appendix I-1.

Vitamin B complex Group of water-soluble vitamins generally found together in nature and somewhat related in function, although unrelated chemically. These include vitamin B$_1$ (thiamin), vitamin B$_2$ (riboflavin), vitamin B$_6$ group (pyridoxine, pyridoxal, and pyridoxamine), vitamin B$_{12}$ group (the cobalamins), nicotinic acid (niacin), pteroylglutamic acid (PGA or folic acid), pantothenic acid, and biotin. These vitamins have the following characteristic features: (a) they function as coenzymes and are essential for metabolism in living cells (except vitamin B$_{12}$, which is not required by plants); (b) there is very little storage, and the small amount stored is related to the ability to saturate an apoenzyme; (c) most of them occur in bound form in nature and must first be liberated from the bound form before they can be absorbed; (d) absorption is an active process, requiring energy; (e) there is competition between host and parasite, since intestinal microorganisms also need the B vitamins; and (f) early manifestations of a deficiency state are the same. (In advanced deficiency states the impairment of a vitamin's specific function[s] produces differential manifestations.)

Vitamin B$_1$ Also called thiamin; originally designated as water-soluble vitamin B or the antiberiberi or antineuritic factor found in rice polishings. It was given the subscript number 1 when the B vitamin was discovered to be not a single factor but a complex composed of several factors. The vitamin was identified and synthesized by R. R. Williams et al., who coined the word "thiamine" to indicate its structure —containing both sulfur and an amino

group. Other names given to this vitamin are aneurine and vitamin F. See *Thiamin*.

Vitamin B$_2$ Also called riboflavin; name given to the heat-stable fraction of vitamin B to differentiate it from the heat-labile fraction, designated vitamin B$_1$. Originally mistaken as the P-P (pellagra-preventive) factor because of its close relationship to nicotinic acid. It was recognized to be a yellowish green fluorescent pigment belonging to a group of compounds known as flavin and given the names Warburg's "yellow enzyme," vitamin G, and lactoflavin; ovoflavin; hepatoflavin; or verdoflavin; since it was isolated from milk, egg, liver, and grass. The compound was later called *riboflavine* because it contains a ribose conjugated to a protein plus a pigment, flavin. The final "e" was recently dropped from the spelling because the vitamin is not really an amine. See *Riboflavin*.

Vitamin B$_3$ Also called filtrate factor and chick pellagra factor; an undetermined factor necessary for the growth of pigeons; possibly the same as pantothenic acid. Found to occur in yeast, liver, and grain.

Vitamin B$_4$ Undetermined factor claimed to prevent muscular weakness and paralysis in rats and chicks; described as a mixture of arginine and glycine but could be a mixture of riboflavin and pyridoxine. It is said to occur in wheat germ, yeast, and liver.

Vitamin B$_5$ Heat-stable factor necessary for the growth of pigeons. As yet undetermined; could be nicotinic acid.

Vitamin B$_6$ Also called pyridoxine; a member of the B complex vitamins capable of preventing dermatitis in young rats and man. Formerly known as the eluate factor, rat acrodynia factor, adermin, and vitamin Y. The vitamin is now recognized to be composed of three chemically related compounds designated as *pyridoxine* (the alcoholic form), *pyridoxal* (the aldehyde form), and *pyridoxamine* (the amine form). See *Pyridoxine*.

Vitamin B$_7$ Also called rice polish factor and vitamin I; a factor in rice polishings necessary for growth and feathering; prevents digestive disturbances in pigeons.

Vitamin B₈ Adenylic acid, a participant in phosphate transfer in many types of organisms; no longer classified as a vitamin.

Vitamin B₉ Number unused because nine B vitamins were recognized when vitamins B_{10} and B_{11} were announced.

Vitamin B₁₀ and B₁₁ Factors that promote feathering and growth in chicks; probably a mixture of folic acid and vitamin B_{12}.

Vitamin B₁₂ Also called cobalamin; the antipernicious anemia factor found to be identical with the extrinsic factor of Castle, erythrocyte maturation factor, and animal protein factor. It has a characteristic red color and contains cobalt as an essential mineral constituent. The vitamin has various physiologic functions such as stimulation of red blood cell formation, synthesis of nucleic acids and nucleoproteins, and metabolism of nervous tissue as well as iron, sulfur-containing amino acids, carbohydrate, fat, and protein. It is present only in animal foods. The richest sources are kidney, liver, eggs, and milk. Failure to absorb the vitamin because of absence of an intrinsic factor in the gastric juice results in a condition called *pernicious anemia*. For further details, see Summary of vitamins, Appendix I-1. See also *Cobalamin*.

Vitamin B₁₃ Unidentified factor that promotes growth in rats and chickens. Recovered in distiller's dried solubles.

Vitamin B₁₄ Crystalline compound isolated from wine originally thought to be a metabolite of xanthopterin; claimed to check the growth of cancer cells.

Vitamin B₁₅ Factor that facilitates uptake of oxygen in anoxic rabbits; pangamic acid.

Vitamin Bₑ Chicken antianemic factor identified as pteroylheptaglutamic acid, a folic acid derivative.

Vitamin Bₚ An antiperosis factor for chickens replaceable by manganese and choline.

Vitamin Bₜ Factor identical to carnitine and required for the growth and survival of the mealworm *Tenebrio molitor*.

Vitamin Bᵥᵥ Name applied to biotin.

Vitamin Bₓ Name alternately applied to pantothenic acid and para-aminobenzoic acid.

Vitamin C Water-soluble vitamin that exists in many forms, of which the two most active are L-*ascorbic acid* and L-*dehydroascorbic acid*. It is synthesized from glucose or galactose by most animals except man, monkey, guinea pig, Indian fruit-eating bat, red-vented bulbul bird, and apparently elephants. It is the most unstable vitamin, readily oxidized on exposure to air and light and destroyed by high temperatures, alkali, and copper. Vitamin C functions in a wide variety of roles. It is involved in the formation and maintenance of the intercellular cementing substance; is necessary for the metabolism of tyrosine and phenylalanine; facilitates the absorption of iron; stimulates the conversion of folic acid to its metabolically active form, folinic acid; may be involved in the synthesis of steroid hormones; increases body resistance to infection; and acts as a good antioxidant. Deficiency of the vitamin results in *scurvy*, anemia, delayed or incomplete wound healing, and reduced resistance to infection. Richest sources are *acerola* and *camu-camu;* other good sources include citrus fruit, cabbage, green pepper, and tomato. Old names given to the vitamin include antiscorbutic vitamin and cevitamic acid. For further details, see Summary of vitamins, Appendix I-1.

Vitamin D Fat-soluble vitamin formed by irradiation of sterols. Ergocalciferol (vitamin D_2) is obtained by irradiating the provitamin ergosterol found in plants, and cholecalciferol (vitamin D_3) is produced by irradiation of the provitamin 7-dehydrocholesterol found underneath the skin. The vitamin is metabolized in the liver into 25-hydroxycholecalciferol (25-HCC) and then in the kidney to 1,25-dihydroxycholecalciferol. This metabolite returns to the intestinal mucosal cells, where it initiates the production of a calcium-binding protein. Because of this action, it has been suggested that vitamin D acts like a hormone rather than like a cofactor for an enzyme. The 1,25-dihydroxycholecalciferol also promotes bone resorption. It is also believed that the vitamin regulates the level of alkaline phosphatase in the serum, although the exact relationship between vitamin D and alkaline phosphatase is not clearly understood. Deficiency in the vitamin leads to *rickets* in children and *osteomalacia* in adults. In contrast to the almost universal distribution of provitamins D, the vitamin itself is limited in nature. It is found abundantly in fish liver oils and in fair amounts in the flesh of sardines and salmon. Excessive intake of the vitamin (hypervitaminosis D) causes anorexia, nausea, calcification of soft tissues, and renal damage. Obsolete names for the vitamin include antirachitic vitamin and rachitamin. For further details, see Summary of vitamins, Appendix I-1.

Vitamin E Originally known as the antisterility vitamin. It is a fat-soluble vitamin required by many species for normal reproduction. A derivative of chromanol, it is composed of several substances designated collectively as *tocopherols*. The significance of vitamin E in human nutrition is not clearly understood. It is a good antioxidant that preserves easily oxidizable vitamins and unsaturated fatty acids in foods or in the body. It also prevents hemolysis of red blood cells and seems to be concerned with the structural integrity of a number of unrelated tissues such as the muscles, liver, reproductive organs, and nervous and vascular systems. Dietary deficiency in humans is unlikely to occur. Tocopherols are present in practically every component of the diet, particularly in vegetable oils, cereals, and egg yolk. Results of deficiency in animals are varied: sterility (male rats); resorption gestation (female rats); muscular dystrophy (cattle, lambs, chickens, rabbits, guinea pigs, and rats); and liver necrosis, exudative diathesis, and encephalomalacia (chickens). In humans, therapeutic doses of the vitamin have been used in menstrual disorders, muscular dystrophy, cardiovascular diseases, and prevention of abortion. For further details, see Summary of vitamins, Appendix I-1.

Vitamin F Obsolete term for vitamin B_1; former designation for essential fatty acids.

Vitamin G Obsolete name for vitamin B_2 or riboflavin.

Vitamin H Obsolete name for biotin.

Vitamin I Same as vitamin B_7.

Vitamin J Antipneumonia principle found to be necessary for guinea pigs.

Vitamin K Group of fat-soluble 2-methyl-1,4-naphthoquinone derivatives necessary for the prevention of hemorrhagic conditions. The naturally occurring vitamins K are vitamin K_1 (or *phylloquinone*), found in plants, and vitamin K_2 (or *farnoquinone*), formed by bacterial synthesis in the intestine. Vitamins K_3 to K_7 are synthetic preparations, of which the most active is vitamin K_3 (or *menadione*). The vitamin participates indirectly in the blood clotting mechanism by influencing the concentration of prothrombin, proconvertin, and thromboplastin in the plasma. It has also been suggested that the vitamin probably functions in photosynthetic phosphorylation and in the respiratory enzyme system by participating in the coupled electron transport. Deficiency of the vitamin results in a delayed blood clotting time and hemorrhagic tendency. Because of its wide distribution in plants and intestinal synthesis by bacteria, deficiency resulting from dietary lack in human adults is rare. It may, however, occur in the presence of conditioning factors such as sulfonamide therapy, inadequate intestinal absorption, and hepatic injury. Infants are susceptible to vitamin K lack because of small prenatal vitamin K storage and inadequate intestinal flora for its synthesis. For further details, see Summary of vitamins, Appendix I-1.

Vitamin L Uncharacterized factor necessary for lactation. Reported to be related to anthranilic acid and adenosine.

Vitamin M Obsolete name for folic acid. A factor found to be necessary for the prevention of anemia and loss of weight in monkeys.

Vitamin N Obsolete term for factors from brain or stomach reported to inhibit cancer growth.

Vitamin P Group of factors that decrease capillary fragility. No longer considered a vitamin.

Vitamin R Factor that promotes bacterial growth; found necessary for proper development of chickens; possibly one of the folic acid group.

Vitamin S Name applied to a chicken growth factor related to the bacterial growth factor strepogenin; probably biotin.

Vitamin T Termite factor reported to improve protein assimilation in rats and produce gigantism in insects.

Vitamin U Factor in cabbage juice presumably effective for treatment of peptic ulcer; also promotes bacterial growth. It is probably folic acid.

Vitamin W Unidentified factor that promotes bacterial growth; probably biotin.

Vitamin X Promotes bacterial growth, probably biotin.

Vitamin Y Factor identical with pyridoxine.

Vitamine Original spelling of *vitamin* as proposed by Funk in 1911 to designate that the *accessory food factor* necessary for life is a vital amine. The final letter "e" was dropped when the chemical nature of several of these factors showed that not all of them are amines.

Vitamin-like substances Substances that, on the basis of current information, fail to meet all the criteria necessary to be classified as vitamins but still have some properties of vitamins. In some cases they are present in larger amounts than vita-

mins; in others the body can synthesize sufficient amounts to meet body needs if precursors are present; and for others it has been impossible to determine any essential biologic role. Examples of these substances are inositol, choline, lipoic acid, and ubiquinone.

Vitamin nomenclature As suggested by Osborne and Mendel and McCollum and Davis, vitamins were originally classified according to their solubility, e.g., fat-soluble vitamin A and water-soluble vitamin B. Successive letters were assigned to new vitamins as they were characterized and isolated. Later it became evident that vitamin B was not a single vitamin but a group of vitamins, and subscripts were added for identification. The nomenclature became confusing when new factors thought to be new vitamins were so named only to be found to be duplicates of other vitamins already named. The present trend is to call the vitamins by their chemical names. To date we recognize 13 vitamins essential to human nutrition: four fat-soluble vitamins (vitamins A, D, E, and K) and nine water-soluble vitamins (ascorbic acid, thiamin, riboflavin, nicotinic acid, pyridoxine, cobalamin, pantothenic acid, pteroylglutamic acid, and biotin). *Fat-soluble vitamins* have the following general properties: (a) soluble in fat and fat solvents; (b) not absolutely necessary in the diet every day; (c) have precursors or provitamins; (d) intake in excess of daily need is not excreted but stored in the body; and (e) deficiencies are slow to develop. *Water-soluble vitamins* have the following general properties: (a) soluble in water; (b) must be supplied every day in the diet; (c) generally do not have precursors; (d) intake in excess of daily need is excreted in the urine with minimal storage in the body; and (e) deficiency symptoms often develop rapidly.

Vitazyme 1. A vitamin-containing enzyme. 2. Old term for vitamin.

Vitellin Phosphoprotein found in egg yolk.

Vitreous humor Transparent gel-like fluid that fills the posterior chamber of the eye. The gel component consists of hyaluronic acid within a protein framework called vitrein.

Vivonex-100 Elemental diet low in residue; consisting of synthetic amino acids, safflower oil, simple sugars, vitamins, and minerals. It can be used for drinking or tube feeding. Also available as Vivonex 100-HN, which has twice the nitrogen content of the standard formula. (Eaton.) See Proprietary foods: composition, features, and uses, Appendix P-1.

von Gierke's disease Inborn error of carbohydrate metabolism characterized by excessive deposition of glycogen in the tissues, especially the liver and kidneys. It results from a deficiency of *glucose-6-phosphatase,* a branching enzyme.

Vulnerability Susceptibility to injury or contagion. In nutrition, the phrase *vulnerable group* refers to infants, children, pregnant or lactating women, and elderly people, a group particularly prone to develop nutritional disorders.

W

Wallace-Diamond test Used for the detection of *urobilinogen* in the urine. The quantity of urobilinogen in the urine is estimated by noting the rapidity and intensity of color development.

Warburg's apparatus Small vessel attached to a manometer in which reactions that involve gas exchange can be followed. The vessel is immersed in a constant-temperature bath and shaken to equilibrate the gas in solution. It is useful in studying respiration of microorganisms and living tissues (slices, minces, or homogenates).

Warburg's respiratory enzyme Cytochrome oxidase, also called cytochrome "a_3." See *Cytochrome oxidase* and *Cytochromes*.

Warburg's yellow enzyme See *Yellow enzyme*.

Warfarin From *W*isconsin *A*lumni *R*esearch *F*oundation; an anti-vitamin K compound used as a rat poison and therapeutically as an anticoagulant.

Water One of the major nutrients needed by the body. It comprises about 60% to 70% of total body weight and performs varied functions. Water is second only to oxygen in maintaining life. The body can live for several days, even months, without food but dies within 5 to 10 days without water. Loss of body water to an extent of 20% results in death. All chemical reactions in the body take place in the presence of water. It acts as a solvent for products of digestion, as a lubricant of moving body parts, and as a regulator of body temperature. Blood is 90% water and urine is 97% water. It is also important for the proper elimination of waste products.

Bound w Portion of water in food and body tissues that is attached to the colloids and is therefore more difficult to release than *free water*.

Demineralized w Also called purified water; water freed from mineral salts.

Distilled w Water that has been purified by distillation.

Endogenous w Also called metabolic water; water derived from the metabolism of food in the body.

Exogenous w Water in the body coming from dietary sources either as liquid or as a food component.

Free w That portion of the water in the body or food that is not closely bound by attachment to the colloids.

Hard w Water that contains soluble salts of calcium or magnesium; does not readily form lather with soap.

Heavy w D_2O; also called deuterium oxide, a compound analogous to water but containing deuterium. It differs from ordinary water in having a higher freezing point (3.8° C) and boiling point (101.4° C).

Metabolic w Also called water of combustion; water in the body that is provided by the combustion of foodstuffs (i.e., carbohydrate, protein, and fat). Oxidation of 1 gm of carbohydrate, protein, and fat yields approximately 0.60, 0.41, and 1.07 gm water, respectively.

Mineral w Water containing mineral salts in solution in sufficient quantity to give it special properties and taste.

Potable w Water that is suitable for drinking purposes.

Purified w Water obtained by distillation or deionization; used for pharmaceutical or other purposes requiring a mineral-free water.

Serum w Mixture of blood serum and distilled water with sugar and indicator added. It is used to prepare bacteriologic culture media.

Soft w Water that contains little or no mineral matter.

Water balance Balance between water input and output. Water intake comes from fluids and beverages (free water), as part of the food molecule (bound water), or as a product of the oxidation of foods in the body (metabolic water). The channels of water output are through the kidney (urine), the skin (sweat and insensible perspiration), the lungs (expired air), and the gastrointestinal tract (saliva and feces). Water intake must equal output, the difference resulting in edema or dehydration, depending on whether intake is greater or less than the output. Control of water intake is by the thirst center in the hypothalamus. Water output is controlled by the hormone vasopressin, which is secreted by the pituitary gland. Release of this hormone decreases water excretion by the kidney by increasing the rate of water reabsorption from the tubules. The urine is an important medium for the elimination of excess water. Abnormal losses of water, however, may occur in diarrhea, excessive vomiting, and severe burns. See also *Balance study.*

Water compartment, body Water inside the body exists in two main compartments: within the cells (intracellular water) or outside of the cells (extracellular water). Water outside the cells is found within the blood vessels (intravascular water) or between the vascular spaces and the cells (interstitial water). Smaller amounts are in cerebrospinal fluid, synovial fluid, aqueous and vitreous humors, and lymph.

Water determination, body The two general methods of measuring body water are direct and indirect. The direct method is obviously feasible only in human autopsy studies. The indirect methods of estimating the volume of each of the various water compartments are essentially the same. A material, previously found to be distributed almost exclusively within the compartment to be measured, is given intravenously in known amounts. After a sufficient time for mixing, a sample of plasma is obtained and the concentration of the administered material is measured. *Total body water* can be measured by the use of a substance such as heavy water or antipyrine that passes freely through capillary walls, cell membranes, and the blood-brain barrier. Determination of this material in any available fluid, e.g., plasma or urine, indicates the amount of total body water. Determination of total *extracellular fluid* requires a substance such as inulin, thiocyanate, or thiosulfate that can cross capillary walls and distribute itself uniformly in the plasma and interstitial fluid without entering the cell. *Estimation* of *plasma volume* requires the administration of dyes or iodine 131, which will be retained only within the vascular spaces. The volume of the *interstitial water,* together with the specialized extracellular fluids, is calculated as the difference between the volume of total extracellular fluid and plasma volume.

Water intoxication Condition that results from excessive intake of fluids without an equivalent amount of salt, as in glucose administration to persons with inadequate renal function. The accumulated water enters all the fluid compartments, including the cells and tissues, which become waterlogged. Serious symptoms develop, including vomiting, convulsions, coma, and even death.

Water requirement Two vital needs of the

243

body demand a continual expenditure of water. They are removal of body heat by vaporization of water through the skin and lungs and excretion of urea and other products of metabolism in the urine. There is an obligatory daily loss of approximately 1500 ml of water. Of this amount, about 600 ml is lost through the skin as insensible perspiration, 400 ml in expired air, and 500 ml in urine. Any excess of water intake over this obligatory water loss appears as an increase in urine volume, and any deficit under the obligatory water loss is taken at the expense of total body water, resulting in dehydration. The need for water is increased in hot climates or with excessive exercise because of the loss of water through sweat and in burns, fever, and other pathologic conditions that increase the need for water over and above the normal requirement. An allowance of 1 ml water/calorie is generally considered sufficient.

Waxes Simple lipids; esters of fatty acids with certain alcohols. Some waxes are sperm oil, beeswax, carnauba oil, and lanolin. See Classification of lipids, Appendix C-3.

WBC Abbreviation for *white blood cell.* See *Leukocyte.*

Wean To stop breast feeding when the infant is capable of taking substantial nourishment from sources other than breast milk. Weaning earlier than this period is indicated when there is insufficiency of breast milk or when the mother is in poor health or becomes pregnant again.

Weanling diarrhea Diarrhea associated with weaning of malnourished infants. It is commonly seen in underdeveloped countries where a low standard of sanitation exists and the incidence of food-borne infections is high. Malnutrition lowers body resistance to disease, thus making these infants more susceptible to such infections.

Weende food analysis See *Proximate analysis.*

Weight Force with which a body is attracted to the earth. In reference to body weight the word "weight," if used unqualified, means the *actual* body weight as measured on a weighing scale. *Standard weight* is the average weight for each sex for different statures at various ages. *Ideal or desirable weight* (taken as the standard weight at age 25) is the weight associated with the most favorable mortality. Standard weight tables imply that average weights are "normal." Although the increase in body weight with age is a statistical fact, it is not considered biologically desirable. Desirable weight tables therefore have only one set of values for adult men and women; weights are given as ranges and according to body build as small, medium, or large to make allowances for individual variations.

Weight Watchers Commercial organization that is concerned with the problem of weight reduction. The program involves a weight reducing plan to reach a weight goal, a leveling plan to provide an incentive when the person is 10 pounds away from that goal, and a maintenance plan to help one stay at the weight goal.

Wernicke's encephalopathy Disease caused by an acute biochemical lesion in the brain because of thiamin deficiency. The syndrome was originally described by Wernicke among alcoholics and can be considered as the human counterpart of the encephalopathy produced in animals by acute deprivation of thiamin. It is characterized by paralysis or weakness of eye movements, ataxia, and mental disturbances.

Wet nurse A lactating woman who breast-feeds an infant deprived of his own mother's milk.

Wetting agent Agent that lowers interfacial tension, thus causing liquid to spread more readily on a solid surface.

Wetzel grid Technique for measuring and evaluating child growth. It consists of nine physique channels that range from the very fat to the very thin. The height-weight data of a child is plotted throughout his growth period. The rate of growth is thought to be a more accurate measure of nutritional status than one weight measurement. The grid can be used to detect children who are failing to develop normally.

Whey "Milk serum," the liquid that remains after the curd and cream are removed from coagulated milk. It contains most of the lactose of the original milk but has little protein and almost no fat.

White blood cell (WBC) See *Leukocyte*.

White House Conference on Food, Nutrition and Health As a result of the concern for hunger and malnutrition in the United States, a conference was held in December 1969 in Washington. Its objectives were to advise the President and to create a national nutrition policy. The areas discussed at the conference included methods for continual evaluation of (a) the nutritional status of the American people; (b) nutritional needs of special vulnerable groups such as children, pregnant and lactating women, adolescents, and the aged; (c) foods to meet the nutritional needs of the people; (d) nutrition education; and (e) the role of voluntary groups in improving the nutritional state of the American people.

White matter White nervous tissue composed mostly of myelinated nerve fibers; the conducting portion of the brain and spinal cord.

WHO Abbreviation for *World Health Organization*.

Wills factor Hematopoietic principle present in autolyzed yeast and in crude liver extract that is effective in the treatment of certain patients with macrocytic anemia that do not respond to administration of vitamin B_{12}. It has been found to be identical to *folic acid*.

Wilson's disease Rare inherited disorder of copper metabolism characterized by a decrease in plasma *ceruloplasmin* concentration and an increase in copper concentration in the liver and brain, leading to neurologic changes and liver damage. See *Diet, copper-restricted*.

Witch's milk Lay term for milk secreted in the breasts of a newly born infant; milk secretion is stimulated by the lactating hormone circulating in the mother.

World Health Organization (WHO) International organization that aims to eliminate all kinds of diseases. In the field of nutrition, WHO has been involved in developing and testing new protein-rich foods; combating protein-calorie malnutrition, nutritional anemias, vitamin A deficiency, endemic goiter, and rickets; assessing nutritional status; determining nutritional requirements; and developing coordinated applied nutrition programs and training personnel for them. WHO was created in 1948 and is composed of about 90 member countries with headquarters in Geneva, Switzerland.

WSB Wheat-soy blend; a mixture of 74% wheat flour and 24% soy flour with a protein concentrate, vitamins, and minerals. It is used in developing countries as a dietary supplement.

W-T low residue food An *elemental diet* low in residue; contains chemically defined amino acids, safflower oil, dextrin, vitamins, and minerals. (Warren-Teed.) See Proprietary foods: composition, features, and uses, Appendix P-1.

❧ X Y Z ❧

Xanthine An intermediate product in the catabolism of adenine and guanine. It is formed by the oxidation of hypoxanthine or by the hydrolytic deamination of guanine. Oxidation of xanthine by *xanthine oxidase* yields uric acid, the major end product of purine metabolism in man and higher apes.

Xanthine oxidase Flavoprotein enzyme found in liver and milk. It contains iron, molybdenum, and flavin mono- or dinucleotide as a prosthetic group. It catalyzes the oxidation of hypoxanthine to xanthine and of the latter to uric acid. It also catalyzes the oxidation of various aldehydes.

Xanthinuria Hereditary disorder in man resulting from a lack of *xanthine oxidase* and characterized by the excretion of xanthine in the urine.

Xanthoma Yellowish or orange growth on the skin occurring as flat or slightly raised patches due to deposits of lipids.

Xanthomatosis Condition characterized by yellow lipoid deposits in the skin, tendon sheaths, and internal organs. The condition is associated with lipemia and hypercholesterolemia.

Xanthophyll Yellow plant pigment occurring with carotene in green leaves and other vegetables. It has no vitamin A activity.

Xanthoproteic test Test for the presence of tyrosine and tryptophan. A yellowish derivative formed with concentrated nitric acid turns orange on the addition of ammonia.

Xanthopterin Yellow pigment present in the liver and urine that has folic acid activity in several animal species. It has antianemic activity in large doses and may be regarded as a possible precursor of folic acid.

Xanthosis Yellowish discoloration of the skin due to the deposition of carotenoid pigment; often results from excessive intake of yellow fruits and vegetables such as carrots and squash, or it may follow quinacrine (Atabrine) administration in the treatment of malaria. The skin discoloration is reversible.

Xanthurenic acid Compound formed in the metabolism of tryptophan to niacin. It is excreted in large amounts in the urine in pyridoxine deficiency. Thus the *xanthurenic acid index* in the urine after a standard dose of tryptophan is used to determine the degree of pyridoxine deficiency. A high index in pregnancy can be reduced by pyridoxine administration.

Xanthylic acid Metabolite formed in the synthesis of guanylic acid from inosinic acid.

Xeroderma Sometimes called "fish skin" or "alligator skin"; the skin becomes dry and rough and comes off in fine or branny scales. Sometimes a layer of "lacquer" appears on the surface that, on drying, breaks up into individual "islands" or patches of varying sizes. There is often some desquamation from the borders of each island, while the intervening gaps become fissured. Xeroderma is often associated with vitamin A deficiency, although exposure to dirt and alternate heat and moisture often contribute to its causation.

Xerophthalmia Dry and lusterless condition of the eyeball characterized by atrophy of the paraocular glands, hyperkeratosis of the conjunctiva, and finally involvement of the cornea. The cornea becomes dry but later becomes inflamed and edematous. This is followed by cloudiness and infection, leading to ulceration, softening, and blindness. Xerophthalmia is associated with severe vitamin A deficiency; it may also follow chronic conjunctivitis and other diseases of the tear-producing gland.

Xerosis Abnormal dryness of the skin, mucous membranes, or conjunctiva.

Xylan A hemicellulose of the pentosan type occurring in woody tissues, corncobs, peanut shells, and straw. Yields xylose on hydrolysis.

Xylose Wood sugar; a pentose obtained from the hydrolysis of *xylan*. It is very poorly digested and used medicinally in diabetic foods.

Yeast Microscopic, unicellular, fungal plant extensively used by man for fermentation processes and for bread making. In medicine, it is used as a supplementary source of the B vitamins and protein. There are several varieties and strains; the food yeast *Torula utilis* is an excellent source of protein and can be grown on a commercial scale to produce a satisfactory source of food protein.

Yeast adenylic acid Adenosine-3-phosphate.

Yeast eluate factor Obsolete name for vitamin B_6.

Yeast extract Preparation of the water-soluble fraction of autolyzed yeast; valuable as a rich source of the B vitamins.

Yeast filtrate factor Obsolete name for pantothenic acid.

Yellow enzyme Flavin-containing enzyme isolated by Warburg et al. from yeast. It is involved in biologic oxidations and has been found to contain riboflavin as a prosthetic group.

Yogurt Curdled, fermented milk, resulting in the formation of lactic acid from lactose. Lactic acid in milk is believed to encourage a favorable intestinal flora, lessen fermentation, and act as an antiseptic.

Zeaxanthin One of the carotenoid pigments in maize and egg yolk; used as a coloring agent and exhibits no vitamin A activity.

Zein Protein from maize; soluble in alcohol but insoluble in water and dilute alkali. It is an incomplete protein deficient in lysine and low in tryptophan. As the sole source of protein, zein can neither support growth nor maintain life.

Zinc Essential trace mineral found in minute amounts in hair, skin, nails, bones, liver, kidneys, muscles, pancreas, spleen, and testes. It is essential for growth and is a constituent of several enzymes that are involved in digestion and metabolism. Zinc is needed for the action of insulin. Zinc is widely distributed in plant and animal tissues. Retarded growth, delayed sexual maturity, and delayed wound healing have been found in Iranians and Egyptians deficient in zinc. Zinc-deficient animals show poor growth, loss of hair, and marked skin abnormalities.

Zoology Study of animals.

Zoopherin Name of a factor necessary for the growth of rats. Zoopherin means "to carry on animal species." The factor has been demonstrated to be vitamin B_{12}.

Zwischenferment Glucose-6-phosphate dehydrogenase, an enzyme involved in the pentose phosphate pathway. It catalyzes the reaction converting glucose-6-phosphate to 6-phosphogluconolactone.

Zwitterion A dipolar ion or doubly charged ion containing a positive and a negative charge and hence electrically neutral. Amino acids may form zwitterions in solution by migration of a hydrogen ion from the carboxyl group to the basic nitrogen atom of the amino group.

Zygote The fertilized ovum before cleavage.

Zymase 1. An enzyme. 2. A mixture of enzymes in yeast that results in alcoholic fermentation.

Zymogen A proenzyme or the inactive form of an enzyme. The conversion of a zymogen to its active form is affected by various agents such as hydrogen ions, specific enzymes, or proteolytic enzymes. In many instances the active enzyme, once formed, can act as an activator of its own zymogen.

Zymogenic Causing fermentation.

Zymosis Fermentation.

Zymosterol An intermediate product in the biosynthesis of cholesterol. It arises from lanosterol.

❦ Bibliography ❦

BOOKS

Albanese, A.: Newer methods of nutritional biochemistry, New York, 1963, Academic Press, Inc., vol. 1.

Albanese, A.: Newer methods of nutritional biochemistry, New York, 1965, Academic Press, Inc., vol. 2.

Arnow, L. E.: Introduction to physiological and pathological chemistry, ed. 8, St. Louis, 1972, The C. V. Mosby Co.

Aykroyd, W. R.: Conquest of deficiency diseases. Achievements and prospects, WHO Basic Study No. 24, Geneva, Switzerland, 1970, World Health Organization.

Aykroyd, W. R., and Doughty, J.: Legumes in human nutrition, Rome, 1964, Food & Agriculture Organization.

Bajusz, E., et al.: Physiology and pathology of adaptation mechanisms: neural-neuroendocrine-humoral, New York, 1969, Pergamon Press, Inc.

Beaton, G., and McHenry, E., editors: Nutrition: a comprehensive treatise. Macronutrients and nutrient elements, New York, 1964, Academic Press, Inc., vol. 1.

Beaton, G., and McHenry, E., editors: Nutrition: a comprehensive treatise. Vitamins, nutrient requirements and food selection, New York, 1964, Academic Press, Inc., vol. 2.

Beaton, G., and McHenry, E., editors: Nutrition: a comprehensive treatise. Nutritional status, assessment and application, New York, 1966, Academic Press, Inc., vol. 3.

Beck, I. T., and Sinclair, D. G.: The exocrine pancreas, Baltimore, 1969, The Williams & Wilkins Co.

Beck, W. S.: Human design: molecular, cellular, and systematic physiology, New York, 1971, Harcourt Brace Jovanovich, Inc.

Becker, G. C.: Introductory concepts of biology, New York, 1972, Macmillan, Inc.

Bell, G. H., Davidson, J., and Emslie-Smith, D.: Textbook of physiology and biochemistry, ed. 8, Baltimore, 1972, The Williams & Wilkins Co.

Best, C., and Taylor, E.: The physiological basis of medical practice, ed. 8, Baltimore, 1966, The Williams & Wilkins Co.

Bourne, G., editor: World review of nutrition and dietetics, New York, 1971, S. Karger AG, vol. 14.

Bourne, G., editor: World review of nutrition and dietetics, New York, 1972, S. Karger AG, vol. 15.

Bowen, E. P.: Biology of human behavior, New York, 1968, Appleton-Century-Crofts.

Burgess, A., and Dean, R. F. A.: Malnutrition and food habits, London, 1962, Tavistock Publications, Ltd.

Cantarow, A., and Schepartz, B.: Biochemistry, ed. 4, Philadelphia, 1967, W. B. Saunders Co.

Chaney, M., and Ross, M.: Nutrition, ed. 8, Boston, 1971, Houghton Mifflin Co.

Church, C. F., and Church, H. N.: Food values of portions commonly used, ed. 11, Philadelphia, 1970, J. B. Lippincott Co.

Comar, C. L., and Bronner, F.: Mineral metabolism, New York, 1962, Academic Press, Inc.

Committee on Food Protection: Food chemicals codex committee on specifications, ed. 2, Washington, D. C., 1972, National Academy of Sciences, National Research Council.

Committee on Maternal Nutrition: Maternal nutrition and the course of pregnancy, Washington, D. C., 1970, National Academy of Sciences, National Research Council.

Conn, E. E., and Stumpf, P. K.: Outlines of biochemistry, ed. 3, New York, 1972, John Wiley & Sons, Inc.

Davidson, L., and Passmore, R.: Human nutrition and dietetics, ed. 5, Baltimore, 1973, The Williams & Wilkins Co.

The dietary management of hyperlipoproteinemia: a handbook for physicians, Bethesda, Md., 1971, National Heart & Lung Institute.

Eppright, E., Pattison, M., and Barbour, H.: Teaching nutrition, ed. 2, Ames, 1970, Iowa State University Press.

Fabry, P.: Feeding pattern and nutritional adaptations, London, 1969, Butterworth & Co. (Publishers), Ltd.

Fleck, H.: Introduction to nutrition, ed. 2, New York, 1971, Macmillan, Inc.

Fomon, S.: Infant nutrition, Philadelphia, 1967, W. B. Saunders Co.

Food and Nutrition Board: Recommended dietary allowances, 1973 revision, ed. 8, Washington, D. C., 1973, National Academy of Sciences, National Research Council.

Food fortification—protein calorie malnutrition, Report 8 of Joint FAO/WHO Expert Committee on Nutrition, WHO Tech. Rep. Ser. No. 477 and FAO Nutr. Meet. Rep. Ser. No. 49, Geneva, Switzerland, 1971, World Health Organization.

Gifft, H. H., Washbon, M. B., and Harrison, G. G.: Nutrition, behavior and change, Englewood Cliffs, N. J., 1972, Prentice-Hall, Inc.

Goldblith, S., and Joslyn, M.: Milestones in nutrition, Westport, Conn., 1964, Avi Publishing Co., vol. 2.

Goldsmith, G.: Nutritional diagnosis, Springfield, Ill., 1959, Charles C Thomas, Publisher.

Gontzea, I., and Sutzescu, P.: Natural antinutritive substances in foodstuffs and forages, New York, 1968, S. Karger AG.

Gould, R.: World protein reserves, Washington, 1966, American Chemical Society.

Guidelines for food fortification in Latin America and the Caribbean, Report of the PAHO Technical Group meeting, Washington, D. C., 1972, Pan American Health Organization.

Guthrie, H. A.: Introductory nutrition, ed. 2, St. Louis, 1971, The C. V. Mosby Co.

Guyton, A. C.: Basic human physiology: normal function and mechanisms of disease, Philadelphia, 1971, W. B. Saunders Co.

Halpern, S. L., guest editor: Current concepts in clinical nutrition, Philadelphia, 1970, W. B. Saunders Co.

Hansten, P. D.: Drug interactions: clinical significance of drug-drug interactions and drug effects on clinical laboratory results, Philadelphia, 1971, Lea & Febiger.

Harper, H.: Review of physiological chemistry, ed. 13, Los Altos, Calif., 1971, Lange Medical Publications.

Health maintenance organizations. The concept and structure, Washington, D. C., 1971, U. S. Department of Health, Education, & Welfare.

Hoch, F. L.: Energy transformations in mammals: regulatory mechanisms, Philadelphia, 1971, W. B. Saunders Co.

Hopps, H. C., and Cannon, H. L., editors: Geochemical environment in relation to health and disease, Ann. N. Y. Acad. Sci. 199:entire issue, 1972.

Human development and public health, Report of a WHO Group of Experts, WHO Tech. Rep. Ser. No. 485, Geneva, Switzerland, 1972, World Health Organization.

Interdepartmental Committee on Nutrition for National Defense: Manual for nutrition surveys, Washington, D. C., 1963, U. S. Government Printing Office.

Jellife, D.: The assessment of the nutritional status of the community, WHO Monogr. Ser. No. 53, Geneva, Switzerland, 1966, World Health Organization.

Jennings, I. W.: Vitamins in endocrine metabolism, London, 1970, William Heinemann, Ltd.

Jollife, N., editor: Clinical nutrition, ed. 2, New York, 1962, Harper & Row, Publishers.

Kaldor, G.: Physiological chemistry of proteins and nucleic acids in mammals, Philadelphia, 1969, W. B. Saunders Co.

Keys, A., et al.: The biology of human starvation, Minneapolis, 1950, University of Minnesota Press, vols. 1 and 2.

King, T. E., and Klingenberg, M., editors: Electron and coupled energy transfer in biological systems, New York, 1971, Marcel Dekker, Inc.

Krause, M. V., and Hunscher, M. A.: Food, nutrition and diet therapy, ed. 5, Philadelphia, 1972, W. B. Saunders Co.

Kruse, H. D.: Nutrition: its meaning, scope and significance, Springfield, Ill., 1969, Charles C Thomas, Publisher.

Latham, M. C., McGandy, R. P., McCann, M. B., and Stove, F. S.: Scope manual on nutrition, Kalamazoo, Mich., 1970, The Upjohn Co.

Liener, I. E., editor: Toxic constituents of plant foodstuffs, New York, 1969, Academic Press, Inc.

Lowenberg, M. E., et al.: Food and man, New York, 1968, John Wiley & Sons, Inc.

Mahler, H. R., and Cordes, E. H.: Biological chemistry, ed. 2, New York, 1971, Harper & Row, Publishers.

Manocha, S. L.: Malnutrition and retarded human development, Springfield, Ill., 1972, Charles C Thomas, Publisher.

Martin, E. A.: Nutrition in action, ed. 3, New York, 1971, Holt, Rinehart & Winston, Inc.

Martini, L., and James, V. H. T., editors: Current topics in experimental endocrinology, New York, 1971, Academic Press, Inc., vol. 1.

Masoro, E. J., and Siegel, P. D.: Acid-base regulation: its physiology and pathophysiology, Philadelphia, 1971, W. B. Saunders Co.

Mateles, R. I., and Tannenbaum, S. R., editors: Single-cell protein, Cambridge, Mass., 1968, The M.I.T. Press.

Maynard, L., and Loosli, J.: Animal nutrition, ed. 5, New York, 1962, McGraw-Hill Book Co.

Mertz, W., and Cornatzer, W. E., editors: Newer trace elements in nutrition, New York, 1971, Marcel Dekker, Inc.

Metabolic adaptation and nutrition, Proceedings of the special session held during the ninth meeting of the PAHO Advisory Committee on Medical Research, Washington, D. C., 1971, Pan American Health Organization.

Mitchell, H. H.: Comparative nutrition of man and domestic animals, New York, 1962, Academic Press, Inc., vol. 1.

Mitchell, H. H.: Comparative nutrition of man and domestic animals, New York, 1964, Academic Press, Inc., vol. 2.

Mitchell, H. S., Rynbergen, H., Anderson, L., and Dibble, M.: Cooper's nutrition in health and disease, ed. 15, Philadelphia, 1968, J. B. Lippincott Co.

Nizel, A.: The science of nutrition and its application in clinical dentistry, ed. 2, Philadelphia, 1966, W. B. Saunders Co.

Norris, T.: Dietary surveys: their techniques and interpretation, Washington, D. C., 1949, Food & Agriculture Organization.

Nutritional anemias, Report of a WHO Group of Experts, WHO Tech. Rep. Ser. No. 503, Geneva, Switzerland, 1972, World Health Organization.

Official methods of analysis, ed. 10, Washington, D. C., 1965, Association of Official Agricultural Chemists.

Pelczar, M., and Reid, R.: Microbiology, ed. 2, New York, 1965, McGraw-Hill Book Co.

Pike, R., and Brown, M.: Nutrition, an integrated approach, New York, 1967, John Wiley & Sons, Inc.

Pritchard, J. A.: Maternal nutrition and the course of pregnancy, Washington, D. C., 1970, National Academy of Sciences.

Rafelson, M. E., Binkley, S. B., and Hayashi, J. A.: Basic biochemistry, ed. 3, New York, 1971, Macmillan, Inc.

Reh, E.: Manual on household food consumption surveys, Rome, 1962, Food & Agriculture Organization.

Requirements of ascorbic acid, vitamin D, vitamin B_{12}, folate and iron, Report of Joint FAO/WHO Expert Group, WHO Tech. Rep. Ser. No. 452, Geneva, Switzerland, 1970, World Health Organization.

Richard, N., editor: Biology of nutrition; the evolution and nature of living systems; the organization and nutritional methods, ed. 1, Elmsford, N. Y., 1972, Pergamon Press, Inc.

Robinson, C. H.: Fundamentals of normal nutrition, ed. 2, New York, 1973, Macmillan, Inc.

Robinson, C. H.: Normal and therapeutic nutrition, ed. 14, New York, 1972, Macmillan, Inc.

Robson, J. R.: Malnutrition: its causation and control, New York, 1972, Gordon & Breach, Science Publishers, Inc., vols. 1 and 2.

Rowe, A. H.: Food allergy: its manifestations and controls, and the elimination diets—a compendium, Springfield, Ill., 1972, Charles C Thomas, Publisher.

Sapeika, N.: Food pharmacology, Springfield, Ill., 1969, Charles C Thomas, Publisher.

Schottelius, B. A., and Schottelius, D. D.: Textbook of physiology, ed. 17, St. Louis, 1973, The C. V. Mosby Co.

Scrimshaw, N. S., and Gordon, J. E., editors: Malnutrition, learning and behavior, Cambridge, Mass., 1968, The M.I.T. Press.

Scrimshaw, N. S., Taylor, C. E., and Gordon, J. E.: Interactions of nutrition and infection, WHO Monogr. Ser. No. 57, Geneva, Switzerland, 1968, World Health Organization.

Sebrell, W. H., and Harris, R. S., editors: The vitamins: chemistry, physiology, pathology, methods, ed. 2, New York, 1971, Academic Press, Inc., vol. 5.

Seminar on malnutrition in early life and subsequent mental development, PAHO Scientific Publ. No. 251, Washington, D. C., 1972, Pan American Health Organization.

Stedman's medical dictionary, ed. 22, Baltimore, 1972, The Williams & Wilkins Co.

Todhunter, E. N.: A guide to nutrition terminology for indexing and retrieval, Washington, D. C., 1970, U. S. Government Printing Office.

Turner, D.: Handbook of diet therapy, ed. 5, Chicago, 1970, University of Chicago Press.

Underwood, E. J.: Trace elements in human and animal nutrition, New York, 1962, Academic Press, Inc.

Watt, B. K., and Merrill, A. L.: Composition of foods—raw, processed and prepared, Handbook No. 8, Washington, D. C., 1968, U. S. Department of Agriculture.

White, A., Handler, P., and Smith, E. L.: Principles of biochemistry, ed. 5, New York, 1973, McGraw-Hill Book Co.

Williams, S. R.: Nutrition and diet therapy, ed. 2, St. Louis, 1973, The C. V. Mosby Co.

Wilson, H. T.: Intestinal absorption, Philadelphia, 1962, W. B. Saunders Co.

Winick, M., editor: Nutrition and development, New York, 1972, John Wiley & Sons, Inc.

JOURNALS

American Family Physician
American Journal of Clinical Nutrition
American Journal of Digestive Diseases
American Journal of Medicine
Archives of Internal Medicine
British Journal of Nutrition
Circulation
Diabetes
FDA Consumer
Federation Proceedings
Gastroenterology
Geriatrics
Hospitals
Journal of the American Dietetic Association
Journal of the American Medical Association
Journal of Home Economics

Journal of Nutrition
Journal of Nutrition Education
Journal of Pediatrics
Lancet
Metabolism
New England Journal of Medicine
Nutrition Abstracts and Reviews
Nutrition and Metabolism
Nutrition Reviews
Nutrition Today
Pediatric Clinics of North America
Postgraduate Medicine
Proceedings of the Nutrition Society
Science
Vitamins and Hormones
WHO Chronicle

❧ Appendices ❧

Recommended daily dietary allowances*[1]
(Designed for maintenance of good nutrition of practically all healthy people in

	Age (yr)	Weight		Height		Energy (kcal)[2]	Protein (gm)	Fat-soluble vitamins			
								Vitamin A activity		Vita-min D (IU)	Vita-min E activity[5] (IU)
		kg	lb	cm	in.			RE[3]	IU		
Infants	0-½	6	14	60	24	kg × 117	kg × 2.2	420[4]	1400	400	4
	½-1	9	20	71	28	kg × 108	kg × 2.0	400	2000	400	5
Children	1-3	13	28	86	34	1300	23	400	2000	400	7
	4-6	20	44	110	44	1800	30	500	2500	400	9
	7-10	30	66	135	54	2400	36	700	3300	400	10
Males	11-14	44	97	158	63	2800	44	1000	5000	400	12
	15-18	61	134	172	69	3000	54	1000	5000	400	15
	19-22	67	147	172	69	3000	54	1000	5000	400	15
	23-50	70	154	172	69	2700	56	1000	5000		15
	51+	70	154	172	69	2400	56	1000	5000		15
Females	11-14	44	97	155	62	2400	44	800	4000	400	10
	15-18	54	119	162	65	2100	48	800	4000	400	11
	19-22	58	128	162	65	2100	46	800	4000	400	12
	23-50	58	128	162	65	2000	46	800	4000		12
	51+	58	128	162	65	1800	46	800	4000		12
Pregnancy						+300	+30	1000	5000	400	15
Lactation						+500	+20	1200	6000	400	15

*From Recommended dietary allowances (revised 1973), Food and Nutrition Board, National Academy of Sciences/
[1]The allowances are intended to provide for individual variations among most normal persons as they live in the United
other nutrients for which human requirements have been less well defined.
[2]Kilojoules (KJ) = 4.2 × kcal.
[3]Retinol equivalents.
[4]Assumed to be all as retinol in milk during first 6 months of life. All subsequent intakes are assumed to be one-half as
as retinol and one-fourth as beta-carotene.
[5]Total vitamin E activity, estimated to be 80% as alpha-tocopherol and 20% other tocopherols.
[6]Folacin allowances refer to dietary sources as determined by *Lactobacillus casei* assay. Pure forms of folacin may be
[7]Although allowances are expressed as niacin, it is recognized that on the average 1 mg of niacin is derived from each 60
[8]This increased requirement cannot be met by ordinary diets; therefore the use of supplemental iron is recommended.

Water-soluble vitamins							Minerals					
Ascorbic acid (mg)	Folacin[6] (μg)	Niacin[7] (mg)	Riboflavin (mg)	Thiamin (mg)	Vitamin B6 (mg)	Vitamin B12 (μg)	Calcium (mg)	Phosphorus (mg)	Iodine (μg)	Iron (mg)	Magnesium (mg)	Zinc (mg)
35	50	5	0.4	0.3	0.3	0.3	360	240	35	10	60	3
35	50	8	0.6	0.5	0.4	0.3	540	400	45	15	70	5
40	100	9	0.8	0.7	0.6	1.0	800	800	60	15	150	10
40	200	12	1.1	0.9	0.9	1.5	800	800	80	10	200	10
40	300	16	1.2	1.2	1.2	2.0	800	800	110	10	250	10
45	400	18	1.5	1.4	1.6	3.0	1200	1200	130	18	350	15
45	400	20	1.8	1.5	1.8	3.0	1200	1200	150	18	400	15
45	400	20	1.8	1.5	2.0	3.0	800	800	140	10	350	15
45	400	18	1.6	1.4	2.0	3.0	800	800	130	10	350	15
45	400	16	1.5	1.2	2.0	3.0	800	800	110	10	350	15
45	400	16	1.3	1.2	1.6	3.0	1200	1200	115	18	300	15
45	400	14	1.4	1.1	2.0	3.0	1200	1200	115	18	300	15
45	400	14	1.4	1.1	2.0	3.0	800	800	100	18	300	15
45	400	13	1.2	1.0	2.0	3.0	800	800	100	18	300	15
45	400	12	1.1	1.0	2.0	3.0	800	800	80	10	300	15
60	800	+2	+0.3	+0.3	2.5	4.0	1200	1200	125	18+8	450	20
60	600	+4	+0.5	+0.3	2.5	4.0	1200	1200	150	18	450	25

National Research Council.
States under usual environmental stresses. Diets should be based on a variety of common foods in order to provide

retinol and one-half as beta-carotene when calculated from international units. As retinol equivalents, three-fourths are

effective in doses less than one fourth of the RDA.
mg of dietary tryptophan.

Comparative dietary standards for adults in selected countries and FAO

Country	Sex	Age (yr)	Wt (kg)	Activity	Calories	Protein (gm)	Calcium (gm)	Iron (mg)	Vitamin A (IU)	Thiamin (mg)	Riboflavin (mg)	Niacin equivalent	Ascorbic acid (mg)
FAO[a]	M	25	65	FN[b]	3200	46[c]	0.4-0.5[d]		750[e]	1.3[f]	1.8[f]	21.1[f]	
	F	25	55	FN[b]	2300	39[c]	0.4-0.5[d]		750[e]	0.9[f]	1.3[f]	15.2[f]	
Australia[a]	M	18-35	70	FN[b]	2800	70[e]	0.4-0.8	10	750[d]	1.1[e]	1.4[e]	18[e]	30
	F	18-35	58	FN[b]	2000	58[e]	0.4-0.8	12	750[d]	0.8[e]	1.0[e]	13[e]	30
Canada[a]	M	Adult	72	FN[b]	2850	48[c]	0.5	6	3700[d]	0.9[e]	1.4[e]	9[e]	30
	F	Adult	57	FN[b]	2400	39[c]	0.5	10	3700[d]	0.7	1.2	7	30
Central America and Panama[a]	M	25	55	MA	2700	65[b]	0.45	10	4333[c]	1.1	1.6	17.8	60
	F	25	50	MA	2000	60[b]	0.45	10	4333[c]	0.8	1.2	13.2	50
Colombia[a]	M	20-29	65	FN[b]	2850	68	0.5[c]	10[d]	5000[e]	1.1[f]	1.7[f]	18.8[f]	50
	F	20-29	55	FN[b]	1900	60	0.5[c]	15[d]	5000[e]	0.8[f]	1.1[f]	12.5[f]	50
Japan[a]	M	26-29	56[b]	MA	3000	70[c]	0.6	10	2000[d]	1.5	1.5	15	65
	F	26-29	49[b]	MA	2400	60[c]	0.6	10	2000[d]	1.2	1.2	12	60
Netherlands[a]	M	20-29	70	LA	3000	70[b]	1.0	10	5500[c]	1.2	1.8	12	50
	F	20-29	60	LA	2400	60[b]	1.0	12	5500[c]	1.0	1.5	10	50
Norway[a]	M	25	70	NS	3400	70	0.8	12	2500[b]	1.7	1.8	17	30
	F	25	60	NS	2500	60	0.8	12	2500[b]	1.3	1.5	13	30
Philippines[a]	M	25	56	MA	2500	63[b]	0.5	8	5000[c]	1.3	1.3[d]	16	75
	F	25	49	MA	1900	55[b]	0.5	18	5000[c]	1.0	1.0[d]	13	70
South Africa[a]	M	NS	73	MA	3000	65	0.7	9	4000[b]	1.0	1.6	15	40
	F	NS	60	MA	2300	55	0.6	12	4000[b]	0.8	1.4	12	40
United Kingdom[a]	M	18-35[b]	65[c]	MA	3000	75[d]	0.5	10	750[e]	1.2[f]	1.7	18	30
	F	18-55[b]	55[c]	MA	2200	55[d]	0.5	12	750[e]	0.9[f]	1.3	15	30
United States[a]	M	23-50	70	FN[b]	2700	56	0.8	10	5000	1.4	1.6	18[c]	45
	F	23-50	58	FN[b]	2000	46	0.8	18	4000	1.0	1.2	13[c]	45

FN = footnote; MA = moderate activity; LA = light activity; NS = not specified.

EXPLANATIONS

The purpose for establishing a national dietary standard is not the same in all countries. Some variation in nutrient allowances from country to country should therefore be expected. The "reference" individual varies in different countries, and even in instances where presumed similar objectives exist among countries as to the purpose and usefulness of proposed dietary standards, the table shows that there is no uniform agreement as to the nutrient allowance that may be considered desirable.

FAO (Food and Agriculture Organization)

[a]Calorie requirements, FAO, FAO Nutr. Stud. No. 15, 1957; Protein requirements, FAO/WHO, FAO Nutr. Meet. Rep. Ser. No. 37, WHO Tech. Rep. Ser. No. 301, 1965; Calcium requirements, FAO/WHO, FAO Nutr. Meet. Rep. Ser. No. 30, WHO Tech. Rep. Ser. No. 230, 1962; Requirements of vitamin A, thiamine, riboflavin and niacin, FAO/WHO, FAO Nutr. Meet. Rep. Ser. No. 41, WHO Tech. Ser. No. 362, 1967. Mean annual temperature, 10° C.

[b]The activity for the reference man is described as "on each working day he is employed 8 hours in an occupation which is not sedentary, but does not involve more than occasional periods of hard physical labor. When not at work, he is sedentary for about 4 hours daily and may walk for up to 1½ hours. He spends about 1½ hours on active recreations and household work." The activity of the reference woman is described as "she may be engaged either in general

household duties or in light industry. Her daily activities include walking for about 1 hour and 1 hour of active recreation, such as gardening, playing with children, or non-strenuous sport." (Calorie requirements, FAO, FAO Nutr. Stud. No. 15, 1957.)

[c]The protein value is defined as a safe practical allowance designed to cover the needs of all but a small percent of the population. It is based on 0.71 gm/kg, representing a level 20% above the requirements for reference protein.

[d]The value of 0.4 gm is the recommended minimum amount for a safe practical allowance. A range is given to emphasize that knowledge does not permit any greater accuracy as to a safe allowance.

[e]One microgram of beta-carotene is equivalent to 0.167 μg of retinol.

[f]The allowances for vitamins are based on the following: thiamin, 0.4 mg/1000 kcal; riboflavin, 0.55 mg/1000 kcal; and niacin equivalent, 6.6 mg/1000 kcal.

Australia

[a]Dietary allowances for Australians (1970 revision), Med. J. Aust. 1:1289, 1971. The allowances are designed to be used as a basis for planning menus for individuals and groups.

[b]Activity is based on an average of the weekly schedule. On each working day, activity consists of 8 hours of physical work; 4 hours of sedentary activity; 2 hours of walking slowly on the level; and at least 2 hours out-of-doors. On each nonworking day, exercise and sport are not extremely strenuous.

[c]A practical protein allowance is calculated on the basis of 10% to 12% of the kilocalories being derived from protein.

[d]Value is for "retinol activity" in micrograms. This includes all compounds having vitamin A activity. To calculate the retinol activity, it is necessary to add the amount of retinol to a fraction (one sixth) of the beta-carotene equivalent.

[e]The calculations for vitamins are based on the following allowances: thiamin, 0.4 mg/1000 kcal; riboflavin, 0.5 mg/1000 kcal; and niacin equivalent, 6.6 mg/1000 kcal.

Canada

[a]Recommended daily intakes of calories and nutrients for Canadians, Can. J. Public Health 61:198, 1970.

[b]Activity is equivalent to doing most household chores, office work, and most mechanical trades and crafts.

[c]In terms of the average protein Canadian food supply (reference protein multiplied by 1.43). Reference protein is defined as an ideal protein completely utilizable in anabolic processes and equivalent in quality to the protein in human milk and egg; then 30% is added to allow for individual variability.

[d]The average Canadian diet supplies vitamin A in about equal amounts as international units of carotene and of the preformed vitamin. The recommendations are based on those proportions. Corresponding amounts of only preformed vitamin A would be about two thirds of the amount shown.

[e]The recommended amounts of thiamin, riboflavin, and niacin are, respectively, 0.3, 0.5, and 3 mg/1000 kcal.

Central America and Panama

[a]Publicaciones cientificas del Instituto de Nutricion de Centro America y Panama, Recopilacion No. 5, pp. 75-76, 1966. The figures for nutrients are designed to meet the needs of nearly all individuals. Average annual temperature, 20° C.

[b]The figure assumes 30% protein of high biologic value.

[c]Listed in the table as 1.3 mg of vitamin A alcohol and assuming that one fifth of the total is preformed vitamin A and four fifths is beta-carotene. International units shown were derived by converting as follows: 1 IU = 0.0003 mg (0.3 μg) of vitamin A.

Colombia

[a]Archivos latinoamericanos de nutricion, 17:255, 1967. Values listed are those tabulated at 20° C.

[b]Activities for reference man are described as farming and day laborer; activities for reference woman include housework, factory work, office work, and minding children.

[c]Based on Calcium requirements, FAO/WHO, FAO Nutr. Meet. Rep. Ser. No. 30, WHO Tech. Rep. Ser. No. 230, 1962.

[d]Based on National Research Council recommendations with allowances for differences in weights.

[e]Based on National Research Council recommendations.

[f]The allowances for vitamins are based on the following: thiamin, 0.4 mg/1000 kcal; riboflavin, 0.6 mg/1000 kcal; and niacin equivalent, 6.6 mg/1000 kcal.

Japan

[a]Nutrition in Japan, Ministry of Health and Welfare, 1965. Data adopted by the Council on Nutrition in 1960. The allowances are believed to be sufficient to establish and maintain a good nutritional state in typical individuals.

[b]Based on 1961 weight averages.

[c]Higher intakes are specified for heavy and very hard work.

[d]Requirement for both sexes specified as 2000 IU of preformed vitamin A or 6000 IU of carotene.

Netherlands

[a]Recommended quantities of nutrients, Committee on Nutritional Standards of the Netherlands Nutrition Council. The figures for calories are average requirements. The figures for nutrients are set to cover individuals having high requirements.

[b]Assumes one third is from animal sources. Protein is increased for heavy and very heavy work.

[c]Assumes 1500 IU as preformed vitamin A and 4000 IU as beta-carotene.

Norway

[a]Evaluation of nutrition requirements, State Nutrition Council, 1958. Figures are somewhat higher than average requirements.

[b]Vitamin A as present in animal foods.

Philippines

[a]Recommended daily allowances for specific nutrients, Food and Nutrition Research Center Publication No. 75 (1970 revision).

[b]Estimated at 1.1 gm/kg body weight based on a net protein utilization value of 63%.

[c]Assumes two-thirds contributed by carotene.

[d]Riboflavin allowance of 0.5 mg/1000 kcal, which is the same allowance for thiamin.

South Africa

[a]Recommended minimum daily dietary standards, National Research Council, S. Afr. Med. J. 30:108, 1956.

[b]Assumes two-thirds contributed by carotene.

United Kingdom

[a]Recommended daily intakes of energy and nutrients for the United Kingdom, Rep. Public Health Med. Subj. No. 120, 1970.

[b]The figures refer to age 25 years for the age range 18 to 35 years for men, and age 35 years for the age range 18 to 55 years for women.

[c]The body weights do not represent average values. They are those of the FAO reference man and woman (1957).

[d]Recommended intakes calculated as providing 10% of energy needs.

[e]Figure is given in retinol equivalents. One retinol equivalent = 1 μg retinol or 6 μg beta-carotene.

[f]Recommended intake of thiamin is 0.4 mg/1000 kcal.

United States

[a]Recommended dietary allowances, National Academy of Sciences, Washington, D. C., 1973. The allowances are designed for the maintenance of good nutrition of practically all healthy people in the U. S. A.

[b]Allowances are intended for persons normally active in a temperate climate.

[c]Niacin equivalents include sources of the vitamin itself plus 1 mg equivalent for each 60 mg of dietary tryptophan.

■ APPENDIX B-1

Four basic food groups (U. S. Department of Agriculture)

Milk group

Children: 3 or more glasses (8 ounces) of milk
Teenagers: 4 or more glasses of milk
Adults: 2 or more glasses of milk

Cheese, ice cream, and other foods made with milk can be used in place of milk.

Meat group

Two or more servings: the following are equivalent to one serving:

   Meat, poultry, or fish, 2-3 ounces
   Two eggs
   Cooked dried peas or beans, 1 cup
   Peanut butter, 4 tablespoons

Vegetable-fruit group

Four or more servings: one serving equals $\frac{1}{2}$ cup (raw or cooked); include the following:

   Citrus fruits or tomatoes for vitamin C
   Dark green and deep yellow vegetables for vitamin A
   Other fruits and vegetables, including potatoes

Bread and cereal group

Four or more servings: the following are equivalent to one serving:

   Enriched bread (1 slice) or roll
   Ready-to-eat cereal, 1 ounce
   Cooked cereal, $\frac{1}{2}$-$\frac{3}{4}$ cup

■ APPENDIX B-2

Food grouping systems in different countries*†

	Number of groups	Milk	Cheese	Fish	Meat	Eggs	Pulses	Seeds	Nuts	Fats, oils	Bread
Australia	5	A	B	B	B	B	B		B	C	D
Brazil	—										
Bulgaria	7	A	A	B	B	B	C		C	D	E
Canada	5	A	B	B	B	B	B				C
Central America	3	A	A	A	A	A	B			B	B
Chile	4	A	A	B	B	B	C			C	C
Czechoslovakia	5	A	A	B	B	B	B			C	D
Denmark	6	A	A	B	B	B	C			D	C
Ecuador	4	A	A	B	B	B	C	C	C	C	C
Egypt	3	A	A	A	A	A	A		A		B
Finland	6	A	A	B	B	B	C			D	E
France	6	A	A	B	B	B				C	D
Ghana	6	A	A	A	A	A	B	B	B	C	D
Great Britain	—										
Greece	—										
Iceland	—										
India	5	A	A	A	A	A	A		A	B	C
Indonesia	4										
Italy	3	A	A	A	A	A	C			B	B
Italy	5	A	A	B	B	B				C	C
Italy	7	A	A	B	B	B	C			D	E
Japan	6	A		A, B	B	B	B		C	C	D
Korea	5	A		A, B	B	B	B	C	C	C	D
Lebanon	8	A	A	B	B	B		C	C	D	E
Malaysia	3										
Mexico	7										
Netherlands	5	A	B	B	B	B	B			C	D
New Zealand	4	A	B	B	B	B					C
Norway	—										
Peru	3	A	A	A	A	A	B			B	B
Philippines	6	A		A	A	A	A		A	B	C
Poland	6	A	A	B	B	B	C			D	C
Poland	12	A	A	B	B	C	D			E, F	G
Puerto Rico	5	A		B	B					C	
Senegal	3	A		A	A	A	A	A	A	B	B
South Africa	4	A	A	B	B	B	B		B	C	C
South Africa	5	A	A	B	B	B	B		B	C	D
Soviet Union	6	A	A	B	B	B				C	D
Spain	7	A	A	B	B	B	C	C	C	D	E
Sweden	7	A	A	B	B	B				C	D
Taiwan	5	A		A	A	A	A			B	
Thailand	5	A	A	A	A	A	A			B	C
Turkey	4	A	A	B	B	B	B				C
United States	4	A	A	B	B	B	B		B		C
Venezuela	4	A	A	B	B	B	C			C	C
West Germany	7	A	A	B	B	B				C	D

*From Ahlström, A.: J. Nutr. Ed. 5:15, 1973.

†The table includes only those foods that could unanimously be grouped on the basis of the information given. Foods belonging in several groups for some reason, it is given all the respective letters.

Cereals	Rice	Sugar, sweets	Tubers, roots	Potato	Vege- tables	Fruits, berries	Notes
D			E	E	E	E	
					F	G	
C				D	D	E	
B	B	B	B	B	C	C	Costa Rica, Guatemala, Honduras, Nicaragua, Panama, El Salvador
C	C	C		D	D	D	
D	D		E	E	E	E	
C			E	E	E, F	F	
C	C		D	D	D	D	
B					C	C	Also basic four grouping system in use
E			F	F	C	C	
D					E, F	E, F	Fresh and cooked vegetables and fruits
D	D		E	E	F	F	
							Swedish and Danish groupings in use
C	C	B			D, E	E	Grouping system unknown
B	B	B	C	C	C	C	Ministry of the Interior
C	C	C	D	D	D	E	Also basic four grouping system in use
E	E		F		F, G	G	Ministry of Agriculture
D	D		E	D	E, F	F	Popular nutrition education
D	D		E	D	E	E	
E	F	G		F	H	H	Grouping system unknown
							Grouping system unknown, new being planned
D	D			E	E	E	
C	C			D	D	D	
B		B		B	C	C	
C	C		C, E		D-F	E, F	Also FAO grouping in use
C		E	F	F	F	F	Popular nutrition education
G		H	I-K	L	I-K	I-K	Guide for diet planning
	C	C			D	D, E	
B	B		B		C	C	FAO grouping
C	C				D	D	High-income groups
D	D				E	E	Low-income groups
D	D	D		D	E	F	
E	E	E	F	C	F	G	
D	D		E	E	F	G	
C			C		D	E	
C	C	C	C		D	E	
C	C	C			D	D	Fat and sugar as an additional group
C	C		D	D	D	D	
C	C	C	C, D	C	D	D	
D		D		E	F	G	New grouping being planned

to the same group are marked by the same letter; thus the letters do not indicate order of groups. If a food component appears

Classification of carbohydrates

Carbohydrate	Occurrence	Characteristics
Monosaccharides (simple sugars)		
Hexoses		
Glucose	Honey, fruits, corn syrup, sweet grapes, and sweet corn; hydrolysis of starch and of cane sugar	Physiologically the most important sugar; the "sugar" carried by the blood and the principal one used by tissues
Fructose	Honey, ripe fruits, and some vegetables; hydrolysis of sucrose and inulin	Can be changed to glucose in the liver and intestine; an intermediate metabolite in glycogen breakdown
Galactose	Not found free in nature; digestive end product of lactose hydrolysis	Can be changed to glucose in the liver; synthesized in body to make lactose; constituent of glycolipids
Mannose	Legumes; hydrolysis of plant mannosans and gums	Constituent of polysaccharide of albumins, globulins, and mucoids
Pentoses		
Arabinose	Derived from gum arabic and plum and cherry gums; not found free in nature	Has no known physiologic function in man; used in metabolism studies of bacteria
Ribose	Derived from nucleic acid of meats and seafoods	Structural element of nucleic acids, ATP, and coenzymes, e.g., NAD and FAD
Ribulose	Formed in metabolic processes	Intermediate in direct oxidative pathway of glucose breakdown
Xylose	Wood gums, corncobs, and peanut shells; not found free in nature	Very poorly digested and has no known physiologic function; used medicinally as a diabetic food
Oligosaccharides (2 to 10 sugar units)		
Disaccharides		
Sucrose	Cane and beet sugar, maple syrup, molasses, and sorghum	Hydrolyzed to glucose and fructose; a nonreducing sugar
Maltose	Malted products and germinating cereals; formed from diastatic hydrolysis of starch; an intermediate product of starch digestion	Hydrolyzed to two molecules of glucose; a reducing sugar; does not occur free in tissue
Lactose	Milk and milk products; formed in body from glucose	Hydrolyzed to glucose and galactose; may occur in urine during pregnancy; a reducing sugar
Trisaccharides		
Raffinose	Cottonseed meal, molasses, and sugar beets and stems	Only partially digestible but can be hydrolyzed by enzymes of intestinal bacteria to glucose, fructose, and galactose
Melizitose	Honey, poplars, and conifers	Composed of one fructose unit and two glucose units

Classification of carbohydrates—cont'd

Carbohydrate	Occurrence	Characteristics
Polysaccharides (more than 10 sugar units) Digestible		
Glycogen	Meat products and seafoods	Polysaccharide of the animal body, often called animal starch; storage form of carbohydrate in body, mainly in liver and muscles
Starch	Cereal grains, unripe fruits, vegetables, legumes, and tubers	Most important food source of carbohydrate; storage form of carbohydrate in plants; composed chiefly of two constituents—amylose and amylopectin; completely hydrolyzable to glucose
Dextrin	Toasted bread; intermediate product of starch digestion	Formed in course of hydrolytic breakdown of starch
Partially digestible Inulin	Tubers and roots of dahlias, artichokes, dandelions, onions, and garlic	Hydrolyzable to fructose; used in physiologic investigation for determination of rate of glomerular filtration
Mannosan	Legumes and plant gums	Hydrolyzable to mannose but digestion incomplete; further splitting by bacteria may occur in large bowel
Indigestible Cellulose	Skins of fruits, outer coverings of seeds, and stalks and leaves of vegetables	Not subject to attack of digestive enzyme in man, hence an important source of "bulk" in diet; may be partially split to glucose by bacterial action in large bowel
Hemicellulose	Pectins, woody fibers, and leaves	Less polymerized than cellulose; may be digested to some extent by microbial enzymes, yielding xylose

■ APPENDIX C-2

Classification of proteins*

Protein	Occurrence	Characteristics
Simple proteins		
Albumins	Blood (serum albumin); milk (lactalbumin); egg white (ovalbumin); lentils (legumelin); kidney beans (phaseolin); wheat (leucosin)	Globular protein; soluble in water and dilute salt solutions; precipitated by saturated solution and coagulated by heat; found in both plant and animal tissues
Globulins	Blood (serum globulin); muscle (myosin); potato (tuberin); Brazil nuts (excelsin); hemp (edestin); lentils (legumin)	Globular protein; sparingly soluble in water; soluble in dilute neutral solutions; precipitated by dilute ammonium sulfate and coagulated by heat; distributed in both plant and animal tissues
Glutelins	Wheat (glutenin); rice (oryzenin)	Insoluble in water and dilute salt solutions; soluble in dilute acids; found in grains and cereals
Prolamines	Wheat and rye (gliadin); corn (zein); rye (secaline); barley (hordein)	Insoluble in water and absolute alcohol; soluble in 70% alcohol; high in amide nitrogen and proline; occur in grain seeds
Protamines	Sturgeon (sturine); mackerel (scombrine); salmon (salmine); herring (clupeine)	Soluble in water; not coagulated by heat; strongly basic; high in arginine; associated with DNA and occur in sperm cells
Histones	Thymus gland, pancreas; nucleoproteins (nucleohistone)	Soluble in water, salt solutions, and dilute acids; insoluble in ammonium hydroxide; yields large amounts of lysine and arginine; combined with nucleic acids within cells
Scleroproteins or albuminoids	Connective tissue and hard tissues	Fibrous protein; insoluble in all solvents and resistant to digestion
Collagen	Connective tissues, bones, cartilage, and gelatin	Resistant to digestive enzymes but altered to digestible gelatin by boiling water, acid, or alkali; high in hydroxyproline
Elastin	Ligaments, tendons, and arteries	Similar to collagen but cannot be converted to gelatin
Keratin	Hair, nails, hooves, feathers, and horn	Partially resistant to digestive enzymes; contains large amounts of sulfur, as cystine
Conjugated proteins		
Nucleoproteins	Cytoplasm of cells (ribonucleoprotein); nucleus of chromosomes (deoxyribonucleoprotein); viruses and bacteriophages	Contains nucleic acids, nitrogen, and phosphorus; present in chromosomes and in all living forms as a combination of protein with either DNA or RNA

*Based on solubility and other physical properties.

Classification of proteins—cont'd

Protein	Occurrence	Characteristics
Mucoproteins or Glycoproteins	Saliva (mucin); egg white (ovomucoid)	Proteins combined with amino sugars, sugar acids, and sulfates
	Bone (osseomucoid); tendons (tendomucoid); cartilage (chondromucoid)	Containing more than 4% hexosamine, mucoproteins; if less than 4%, glycoproteins
Phosphoproteins	Milk (casein); egg yolk (ovovitellin)	Phosphoric acid joined in ester linkage to protein
Chromoproteins	Hemoglobin; myoglobin; flavoproteins; respiratory pigments; cytochromes	Protein compounds with nonprotein pigment such as heme; colored proteins
Lipoproteins	Serum lipoprotein; brain, nerve tissues, milk, and eggs	Water-soluble proteins conjugated with lipids; found dispersed widely in all cells and all living forms
Metalloproteins	Ferritin; carbonic anhydrase; ceruloplasmin	Proteins combined with metallic atoms that are not parts of a nonprotein prosthetic group
Derived proteins		
Proteans	Edestan (from edestin) and myosan (from myosin)	Results from short action of acids or enzymes; insoluble in water
Proteoses	Intermediate products of protein digestion	Soluble in water, uncoagulated by heat, and precipitated by saturated ammonium sulfate; result from partial digestion of protein by pepsin or trypsin
Peptones	Intermediate products of protein digestion	Same properties as proteoses except that they cannot be salted out; of smaller molecular weight than proteoses
Peptides	Intermediate products of protein digestion	Two or more amino acids joined by a peptide linkage; hydrolyzed to individual amino acids

Classification of lipids

Lipid	Occurrence	Characteristics
Simple lipids		
Triglycerides, neutral fats	Adipose tissue, butterfat, lard, suet, fish oils, olive oil, corn oil, etc.	Esters of three molecules of fatty acids and one molecule of glycerol; the fatty acids may all be different
Waxes	Beeswax, head oil of sperm whale, cerumen, carnauba oil, and lanolin	Composed of esters of fatty acids with alcohol other than glycerol; of industrial and medicinal importance
Compound lipids		
Phospholipids (phosphatides)	Chiefly in animal tissues	Substituted fats consisting of phosphatidic acid; composed of glycerol, fatty acid, and phosphoric acid bound in ester linkage to a nitrogenous base
Lecithin	Brain, egg yolk, and organ meats	Phosphatidyl choline; phosphatide linked to choline; a lipotropic agent; important in fat metabolism and transport; used as emulsifying agent in food industry
Cephalin	Occurs predominantly in nervous tissue	Phosphatidyl ethanolamine; phosphatide linked to serine or ethanolamine; plays a role in blood clotting
Plasmalogen	Brain, heart, and muscle	Phosphatidal ethanolamine or choline; phosphatide containing an aliphatic aldehyde
Lipositol	Brain, heart, kidneys, and plant tissues together with phytic acid	Phosphatidyl inositol; phosphatide linked to inositol; rapid synthesis and degradation in brain; evidence for role in cell transport processes
Sphingomyelin	Nervous tissue, brain, and red blood cells	Sphingosine-containing phosphatide; yields fatty acid, choline, sphingosine, phosphoric acid, and no glycerol; source of phosphoric acid in body
Glycolipids		
Cerebroside	Myelin sheaths of nerves, brain, and other tissues	Yields on hydrolysis fatty acids, sphingosine, galactose (or glucose), but not fatty acid; includes kerasin and phrenosin
Ganglioside	Brain, nerve tissue, and other selected tissues, notably spleen	Contains a ceramide linked to hexose (glucose or galactose), neuraminic acid, sphingosine, and fatty acids
Sulfolipid	White matter of brain, liver, and testicle; also plant chloroplast	Sulfur-containing glycolipid; sulfate present in ester linkage to galactose

Classification of lipids—cont'd

Lipid	Occurrence	Characteristics
Proteolipids	Brain and nerve tissues	Complexes of protein and lipids having solubility properties of lipids
Terpenoids and steroids		
Terpenes	Essential oils, resin acids, rubber, plant pigments such as carotenes and lycopenes, vitamin A, and camphor	Large group of compounds made up of repeating isoprene units; vitamin A of nutritional interest; fat-soluble vitamins E and K also related chemically to terpenes
Sterols		
Cholesterol, ergosterol, and 7-dehydrocholesterol	Cholesterol found in egg yolk, dairy products, and animal tissues; ergosterol found in plant tissues, yeast, and fungi; 7-dehydrocholesterol found in animal tissues and underneath skin	Derivatives of a ring structure known as cyclopentanoperhydrophenanthrene; cholesterol, constituent of bile acids and precursor of vitamin D; ergosterol and 7-dehydrocholesterol, converted to vitamin D_2 and D_3, respectively, on irradiation
Sex hormones		
Androgens and estrogens	Ovaries and testes	(See Summary of endocrine glands, Appendix K.)
Adrenal cortical steroids	Adrenal cortex, blood	(See Summary of endocrine glands, Appendix K.)
Derived lipids		
Fatty acids	Occur in plant and animal foods; also exist in complex forms with other substances	Obtained from hydrolysis of fats; in natural fats usually contain an even number of carbon atoms and are straight chain derivatives; may be saturated or unsaturated

Utilization of carbohydrates

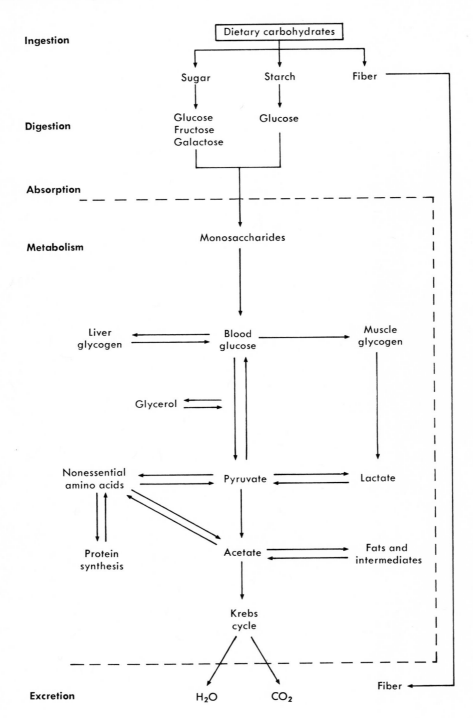

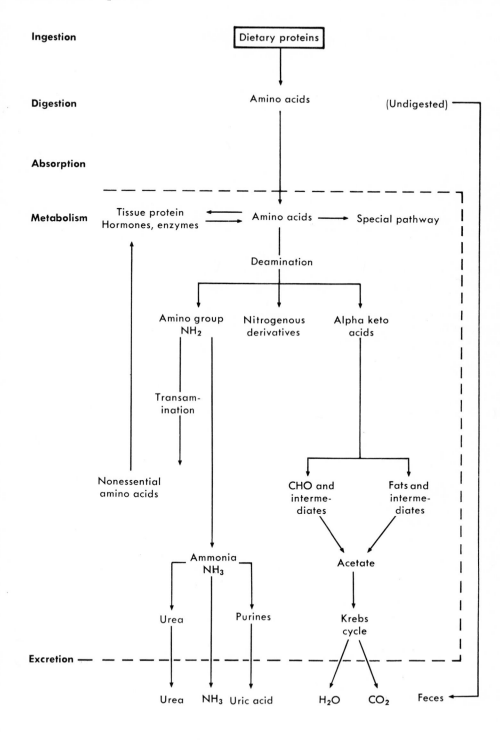

Utilization of fats

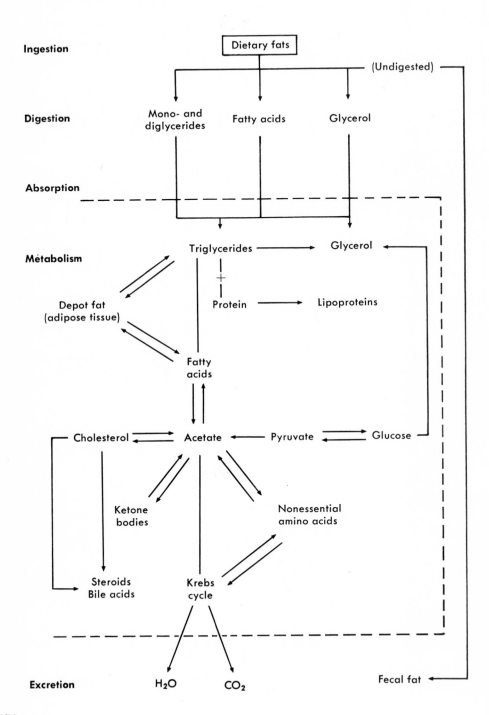

■ **APPENDIX D-4**

Utilization of food energy

Gross energy of food	(less energy in feces) →	Digestible energy	(less energy in urine) →	Available or metabolizable energy
CHO, 4.1 kcal/gm		CHO, 4.0 kcal/gm		CHO, 4.0 kcal/gm
Pro, 5.65 kcal/gm		Pro, 5.2 kcal/gm		Pro, 4.0 kcal/gm
Fat, 9.4 kcal/gm		Fat, 9.0 kcal/gm		Fat, 9.0 kcal/gm

■ **APPENDIX E**

Interrelationship of carbohydrate, protein, and fat

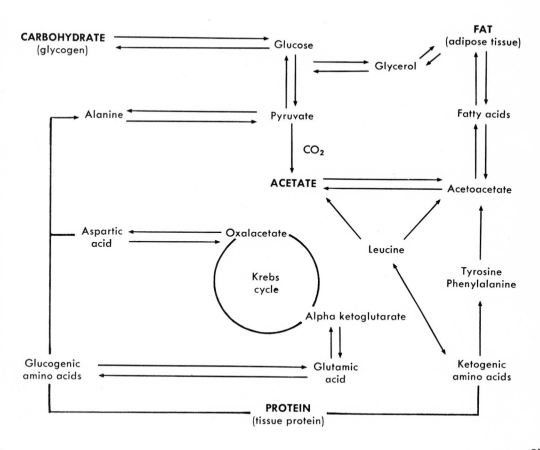

Embden-Meyerhof pathway

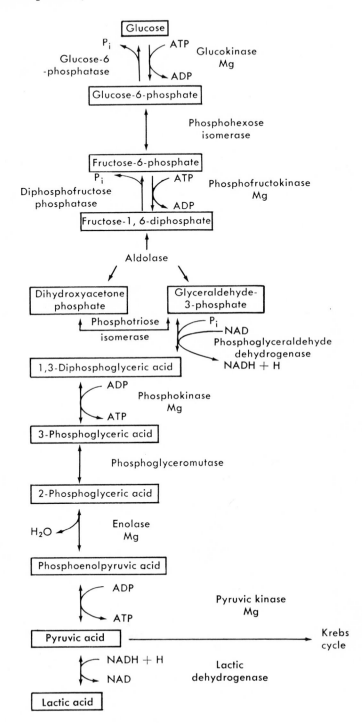

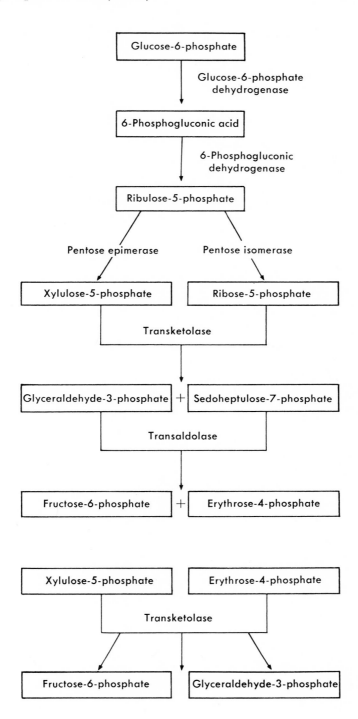

Krebs cycle (tricarboxylic acid cycle)

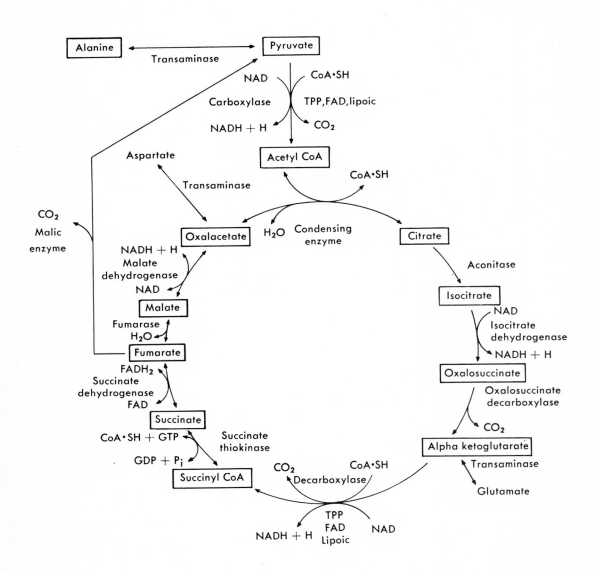

■ APPENDIX F-4

Electron transport system and coupled oxidative phosphorylation

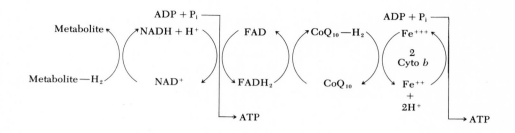

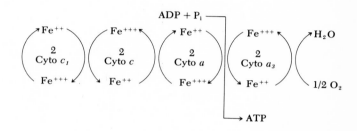

■ APPENDIX G

Inborn errors of metabolism

Disorder	Enzyme defect and characteristic features
Disorders in protein metabolism	
Albinism	Lack of tyrosinase; inability to form pigment melanin; lack of pigmentation of hair, skin, and eyes
Alkaptonuria	Lack of homogentisic acid oxidase; incomplete oxidation of tyrosine and phenylalanine; urinary excretion of homogentisic acid; darkening of urine
Arginosuccinic aciduria	Lack of arginosuccinase; elevated arginosuccinic acid in blood, urine, and cerebrospinal fluid; ammonia intoxication; mental retardation
Citrullinemia	Lack of arginosuccinic acid synthetase; elevated citrulline in blood, urine, and cerebrospinal fluid; mental retardation; ammonia intoxication
Cystathioninuria	Probably a defect of the enzyme cystathioninase; elevated cystathionine in tissues, blood, and spinal fluid; mental retardation; pituitary disease
Cystinuria	Defect in renal tubular reabsorption; high urinary excretion of cystine, lysine, arginine, and ornithine; cystine renal stones
Fanconi's syndrome	Defective renal tubular reabsorption of amino acids, glucose, phosphate, and bicarbonate; results in rickets or osteomalacia, renal glycosuria, aminoaciduria, phosphaturia, and often acidosis
Glycinuria	Probably failure of conversion of glycine to glyoxalate; elevated glycine in blood and urine; acidosis; seizures; mental retardation
Hartnup disease	Lack of tryptophan pyrrolase; gross aminoaciduria, particularly valine, leucine, isoleucine, threonine, serine, citrulline, tryptophan, and phenylalanine; ataxia; pellagra-like skin rash; mental retardation
Histidinemia	Lack of histidase; elevated histidine in blood and urine; mental retardation; speech and hearing defects
Homocystinuria	Lack of cystathionine synthetase in liver and brain; excretion of homocystine in urine; elevated blood methionine and homocysteine; dislocated lenses, glaucoma, and cataracts; shuffling gait; osteoporosis; curvature of spine
Hydroxyprolinemia	Lack of hydroxyproline oxidase; elevated levels of hydroxyproline in blood and urine; severe mental retardation; hematuria
Hyperammonemia	Lack of ornithine transcarbamylase in liver; ammonia intoxication and cerebral and cortical atrophy
Hyperprolinemia	Probably due to lack of proline dehydrogenase; elevated levels of proline in blood and urine; increased urinary levels of hydroxyproline and glycine; fever, vomiting, diarrhea, drowsiness, frequent convulsions, and hearing loss
Lysine intolerance	Inability to hydrolyze lysine; interference with urea cycle; slightly elevated blood and urine levels of lysine and arginine
Maple syrup urine disease (branched chain ketoaciduria)	Deficiency in oxidative decarboxylation of leucine, isoleucine, and valine; high levels of valine, leucine, and isoleucine in blood and urine; maple syrup urine odor; mental retardation; spasticity; seizures; convulsions
Ornithinemia	Elevated ornithine in blood; ammonia intoxication; mental retardation
Phenylketonuria	Lack of phenylalanine hydroxylase; elevated phenylalanine in blood and urine; mental retardation; fair complexion; convulsions; eczema
Tyrosinosis	Lack of para-hydroxyphenylpyruvic acid oxidase; gross aminoaciduria, particularly tyrosine, proline, serine, and threonine; renal tubular damage; liver cirrhosis

Inborn errors of metabolism—cont'd

Disorder	Enzyme defect and characteristic features
Disorders in carbohydrate metabolism	
Carbohydrate intolerance	Lack of intestinal saccharidases such as maltase, isomaltase, invertase, lactase, and trehalase; diarrhea most outstanding symptom; disappears when sugar not tolerated is eliminated from diet
Galactosemia	Lack of galactose-1-phosphate uridyl transferase; elevated galactose in blood and urine; jaundice; edema; enlarged liver; mental retardation; cataract formation
Gargoylism (Hurler's syndrome)	Excessive excretion of chondroitin sulfate B; abnormal mucopolysaccharide formation and degradation; stiff joints; mental retardation
Glycogen storage disease	
Type I (von Gierke's disease)	Lack of glucose-6-phosphatase; glycogen accumulation in liver and other organs; hypoglycemia; convulsions; coma
Type II (generalized glycogenosis)	Lack of alpha glucosidase; massive glycogen infiltration in tissue, particularly heart; cardiac distress; heart failure
Type III (limit dextrinosis)	Lack of amylo-1,6-glucosidase; accumulation of glycogen (with abnormal structure and short outer chains) in liver and muscle
Type IV (diffuse glycogenosis)	Lack of amylo-$(1,4\rightarrow1,6)$-transglucosidase; glycogen with less branches but longer chain length; accumulation in organs, stimulating tissues to "foreign body" reaction
Type V (McArdle's disease)	Lack of myophosphorylase; muscle glycogen accumulation leading to weakness
Type VI (Hers' disease)	Lack of hepatophosphorylase; glycogen accumulation in liver; ascites; cirrhosis
Hyperoxaluria	Inability to metabolize glyoxylic acid, resulting in increased urinary excretion of oxalate, calcium oxalate nephrolithiasis, nephrocalcinosis, and renal failure
Leucine-induced hypoglycemia	Unknown cause; hypoglycemia on ingestion of leucine
Pentosuria	Most likely a defect in the oxidation of glucuronic acid, resulting in excretion of L-xylulose in urine; no disturbance in any other metabolic reaction and no other symptoms
Disorders in lipid metabolism	
Fabry's disease (glycolipid liposis)	Exact cause unknown; accumulation of glycolipids in tissues; skin lesions, corneal opacities, fever, burning pain in extremities, peripheral edema, and renal dysfunction in hemizygous males; corneal opacities in heterozygous females
Familial high-density lipoprotein deficiency (Tangier disease)	Probably due to defective synthesis of high-density lipoprotein; storage of large amounts of cholesterol esters in foam cells, enlargement of tonsils, and orange color in pharyngeal and rectal mucosa
Familial hyperlipoproteinemia	
Type I	Hyperchylomicronemia with normal or elevated cholesterol levels; eruptive xanthomas, hepatosplenomegaly, abdominal pain, and lipemia retinalis
Type II	Elevated beta-lipoproteins and cholesterol; xanthelasma, tendon and tuberous xanthomas, juvenile corneal arcus, and accelerated atherosclerosis

Continued.

Inborn errors of metabolism—cont'd

Disorder	*Enzyme defect and characteristic features*
Type III	Elevated prebeta-lipoproteins, plasma cholesterol, and triglycerides; xanthoma planum tuberoeruptive and tendon xanthomas, and accelerated atherosclerosis of coronary and peripheral vessels
Type IV	Elevated levels of prebeta-lipoproteins and triglycerides and normal or slightly elevated cholesterol levels; accelerated coronary vessel disease, abnormal glucose tolerance, and hyperuricemia
Type V	Elevated hyperchylomicronemia, prebeta-lipoproteinemia, cholesterol, and triglycerides; eruptive xanthomas, hepatosplenomegaly, abdominal pain, hyperglycemia, hyperuricemia, and lipemia retinalis
Gaucher's disease (cerebroside lipidosis)	Defect in cerebroside metabolism; accumulation of cerebroside in liver, spleen, and bone marrow; hepatosplenomegaly and bone lesions
Niemann-Pick disease (sphingomyelin lipidosis)	Defect in sphingomyelin metabolism; exact cause not known; accumulation of phosphatides, chiefly sphingomyelin and lecithin, in liver, spleen, and various organs of central nervous system; mental and physical retardation, hepatosplenomegaly, and cherry red spot on retina
Tay-Sachs disease (ganglioside lipidosis)	Probably due to a block in catabolism of gangliosides; retardation of growth, hyperacusis, dementia, motor loss, and blindness with a cherry red spot on the retina

■ APPENDIX H
Summary of minerals

CALCIUM

Occurrence Comprises 1.5% to 2% of adult body weight. About 99% in bones and teeth, the rest in soft tissues.

Function Builds bones and teeth. Needed for muscle contraction, normal heart rhythm, nerve irritability, water and acid-base balance, and blood clotting. Activates pancreatic lipase. Cofactor of enzymes that release energy from carbohydrate, fat, and protein. Promotes iron and vitamin B_{12} absorption. Regulates cell permeability. Reduces uptake of radioactive strontium 90. Prevents rickets.

Utilization Absorbed in intestines with the following factors favorable for its absorption: vitamin D, acid medium, lactose, ascorbic acid, a 2:1 to 1:1 phosphorus:calcium ratio, and emotional stability. Factors that interfere with absorption include excess fat, laxatives, phytates and oxalates, lack of exercise, and any condition that increases gastrointestinal motility. Stored mainly in the trabeculae. Metabolism regulated by vitamin D, parathormone, and phosphatase. Excreted chiefly in the feces.

Deficiency Retarded growth, osteoporosis, osteomalacia, tetany, and rickets.

Toxicity Hypercalcuria, hypercalcemia, renal calculi, deposition of calcium in soft tissues. Depressing effect on utilization of fat, phosphorus, iodine, iron, magnesium, and zinc.

Allowance See Recommended Daily Dietary Allowances, Appendix A-1.

Sources Milk and milk products, except butter and cream. Sardines, salmon, oyster, crab, soybeans, and green leafy vegetables that do not have much phytate and oxalate.

CHLORINE

Occurrence Comprises about 0.15% of adult body weight. Widely distributed in the body, but is in highest concentration in the cerebrospinal fluid and gastrointestinal secretions, especially gastric juice. Commonly combined with sodium in extracellular fluid and with potassium in intracellular fluid in the form of chloride.

Function Needed for maintaining acid-base balance and osmotic pressure. As part of HCl, it maintains normal acidity in stomach for optimal action of gastric enzymes. Chloride ions readily pass in and out of red blood cells

Summary of minerals—cont'd

(chloride shift), which is important in buffer action and maintenance of blood pH.

Utilization Readily absorbed in gastrointestinal tract. Excreted chiefly in the urine; the amount excreted parallels intake. Whenever sodium loss is excessive, as in diarrhea, vomiting, sweating, etc., chloride is concurrently lost.

Deficiency Occurs only after prolonged vomiting, profuse sweating, diarrhea, or excessive loss of extracellular fluids.

Sources Table salt, meats, seafoods, milk, and eggs.

COBALT

Occurrence Comprises 4% of vitamin B_{12}.

Function As part of vitamin B_{12}, it is needed for blood formation, normal appetite, and prevention of pernicious anemia. Acts as cofactor of enzyme systems in energy metabolism. See also Summary of vitamins (vitamin B_{12}), Appendix I-1.

Utilization Readily absorbed in gastrointestinal tract. Excreted mainly in urine with little body storage.

Deficiency Not known.

Toxicity In animals: polycythemia, hyperplasia, and goitrogenic effect.

Sources Meats, especially liver, kidney, and lean muscle meat; milk; shellfish, e.g., clams and oysters; and saltwater fish.

COPPER

Occurrence The body has about 100 mg of copper concentrated in the liver, spleen, kidney, and heart. Traces are found in all other cells.

Function Needed for the metabolism of iron. Promotes maturation of red blood cells and prevents anemia. Affects iron and ascorbic acid absorption. Maintains integrity of myelin sheath that surrounds nerve fibers. Cofactor of certain enzymes (catalase and cytochrome oxidase) involved in cellular respiration. Involved in melanin formation. Has unexplained role in bone formation.

Utilization Absorbed in the intestines. Transported in the form of ceruloplasmin in the blood plasma and quickly distributed to the liver, bone marrow, kidney, cerebrospinal fluid, and other tissues. Within the red blood cell, occurs as protein complex (erythrocuprein) and in another form not yet identified. Stored in the liver, spleen, kidney, and bone marrow.

Excreted mainly in the feces as a result of bile secretion and direct loss from the intestinal walls and from food as unabsorbed copper. Only 4% of total copper metabolized is excreted in the urine. Zinc increases excretion; a high molybdenum–high sulfate intake decreases absorption or increases excretion.

Deficiency Not noted in humans, unless due to iron deficiency or induced by excessive loss of copper and disturbances of protein metabolism. Hypocupremia is seen in Wilson's disease, a hereditary disorder involving the central nervous system. Anemia, usually of the hypochromic microcytic type.

Toxicity Appears to be toxic at levels ten times that found in a normal diet. Dietary copper is about 2.5 mg in the daily diet.

Allowance About 0.08 mg/kg body weight.

Sources Organ meats, shellfish, nuts, cocoa, whole grain cereals, and legumes (over 8 ppm). Green leafy vegetables, eggs, lean meats, poultry, and fish (2 to 8 ppm).

CHROMIUM

Occurrence About 20 ppb in blood and higher in glandular organs. Not accidentally introduced as contaminant but present in very small traces; higher at birth than in later life. Biologically active form: trivalent chromate.

Function Appears to be part of digestive enzymes. Interrelated with insulin. Catalyzes reactions involving energy release, particularly in the first steps of glucose metabolism by facilitating transfer of glucose from plasma to cell. Stimulates the synthesis of fatty acids and cholesterol in liver. Rats and mice: promotes growth and prolongs life.

Utilization Readily absorbed in the gastrointestinal tract. Once absorbed into the blood, it enters tissues rapidly and is easily released back to the blood, especially after glucose ingestion. About 50% of chromium ingested appears in the urine.

Deficiency Deficiency state hard to attain even in experimental nutrition. The diet of lowest known concentration still has 50 ppb of chromium. Rats and mice: impaired growth, increased mortality rate, and elevated blood glucose with excretion in urine.

Toxicity As hexavalent chromate, it is easily concentrated in tissues of animals and exerts toxic effects. As trivalent chromate, it is toxic only when injected intravenously at a level 10,000 times the dose required to improve glucose tolerance of chromium-deficient rats.

Allowance Has not been studied as yet, since it is the latest microelement added to the list of essential minerals.

Sources Fats have the highest concentration (about 500 ppb in corn oil). Meats, cereals, fruits, and vegetables are good sources. Drinking water may furnish as much as 10 μg/L.

FLUORINE

Occurrence Constituent of bones and teeth.

Function Prevents dental caries; mode of action is probably by displacing some calcium phosphate crystals of hydroxyapatite during tooth formation. The fluoroapatite seems less soluble in acid and appears more resistant to cariogenic factors. Another explanation is the inhibitory effect of fluorine on certain enzymes that hasten caries formation and on the growth of oral bacteria that act on carbohydrates.

Utilization Readily absorbed in gastrointestinal tract as fluoride; 90% appears in the blood and 50% of this is excreted in urine. The rest is deposited in bones and teeth; traces in body fluids but none in soft tissues. A dose of 50 mg/day improves calcium balance and prevents osteoporosis.

Deficiency Susceptibility to dental decay.

Toxicity Mottling of enamel or dental fluorosis; acute gastroenteritis with diarrhea, vomiting, and abdominal pain. Marked fall in blood pressure; convulsions. As much as 6000 ppm in bones is not yet toxic. Growth is depressed at 50 ppm; fatal poisoning may occur at an intake of 2500 times the recommended level.

Allowance Fluoridation of drinking water at 1 to 1.5 ppm (dental fluorosis occurs from 2 to 8 ppm).

Sources Found naturally in some water supplies or by adding it to water low in fluorine. Fluorine content of cereals, meats, milk, eggs, fruits, and vegetables vary according to water supply. In addition to water content, a normal diet may contribute 1.5 mg fluorine/day from solid foods.

IODINE

Occurrence About 0.00004% of body weight or a total of about 20 mg in human adult. About 80% of total iodine is in the thyroid gland (see also *Thyroid hormones*). The rest is in blood, hair, skin, and other tissues.

Function Constituent of thyroxine and other hormones (See *Thyroxine*.); prevents simple goiter.

Utilization Inorganic iodide is absorbed mainly in the intestines; can be absorbed by epithelial cells of skin. Goitrogenic substances interfere with absorption. Immediately after absorption, it enters the "iodide pool" in the blood; 30% is "trapped" by the thyroid gland, reducing the iodide to iodine to be incorporated in thyroid hormones. The rest of the iodide stays in the plasma or is relayed to the kidneys where some may be excreted. The excretion in the urine helps in preventing accumulation of iodine in tissues and thus protects the body from toxicity.

Deficiency Simple goiter, cretinism, myxedema.

Allowance See Recommended Daily Dietary Allowances, Appendix A-1.

Sources Food and water supply iodine in the diet at varying amounts that parallel iodine content in the soil. Seafoods are the richest source; fruits, vegetables, milk, and eggs in nongoiter areas. The most practical way is to iodize table salt in the form of potassium iodide at 1 part/10,000 parts salt.

IRON

Occurrence About 0.004% of body weight or a total of 3 to 5 gm, of which 60% is in hemoglobin, 10% to 20% in myoglobin, and the rest in storage depots.

Function Constituent of hemoglobin and myoglobin; carrier of O_2 and CO_2. Involved in blood formation and prevention of anemia. Cofactor in enzymes (e.g., cytochrome, catalase, and peroxidase) for cellular oxidation.

Utilization Regulated absorption of iron from the upper part of the small intestine, since there is no mechanism for the excretion of iron. Iron occurs in food primarily as the ferric ion, but it is reduced to the ferrous form, which is more efficiently utilized than the ferric ion. Factors that interfere with absorption include oxalates, phytates, excess phosphorus, and high bulk content of diet. Diarrhea, steatorrhea, and low altitudes decrease amount of iron absorbed. Transported by blood as transferrin, iron-protein complex; removed from blood either by cells for use by respiratory enzymes or as cell constituent; bone marrow for red blood cell synthesis; or iron storage depots. About 1 gm iron is normally stored by the body at any one time (30% in the liver, 30% in bone marrow, and the rest in muscles and other glandular organs) in the form of hemosiderin and ferritin. Although iron released from the breakdown of hemoglobin is utilizable, losses occur from desquamated epithelial cells of the gastrointestinal tract (above 0.5 mg/day is lost this way through the feces). Other routes of iron loss are urine, nails, hair, sloughed-off skin linings, and sweat. In adult men, total iron losses that need replacement amount to 1 mg/ day. In adult women, menstrual losses should be considered (about 5 to 32 mg/month).

Deficiency Anemia, especially of the hypochromic microcytic type; easy fatigability; dysphagia; sore mouth and tongue; liver damage; and retarded growth and loss of weight.

Toxicity Hemosiderosis; hemochromatosis.

Allowance See Recommended Daily Dietary Allowances, Appendix A-1.

Sources Liver and other glandular organs; lean meats, seafoods, dried fish and dried fruits, whole-grain or enriched cereals, egg yolk, green leafy vegetables without phytates and oxalates, and legumes.

MAGNESIUM

Occurrence Total amount in the adult body is 21 to 28 gm; about 60% of this is in bones and teeth and the rest in soft tissues and body fluids.

Function Builds bones and teeth. Activates enzymes involved in the release of energy from carbohydrate, protein, and fat. Needed for the production of adenosine triphosphate. Maintains muscle contractility, nerve irritability, and acid-base balance. Influences secretion of thyroxine and helps maintain normal basal metabolic rate.

Utilization Phytates and oxalates decrease absorption in the intestines. High intakes of vitamin D and alcohol increase magnesium requirement.

Deficiency Tetany, as seen in some alcoholics and postoperative patients, after prolonged diarrhea and vomiting, and in infants with kwashiorkor. Affects renal, cardiovascular, nervous, and muscle systems.

Allowance See Recommended Daily Dietary Allowances, Appendix A-1.

Sources Widely spread in food; richest sources are nuts, cocoa, soybeans, and whole grains. Good sources are clams, other legumes, and green leafy vegetables with little phytates or oxalates.

MANGANESE

Occurrence Comprises about 0.0002% of body weight; concentrated in liver, pancreas, kidney, skin, muscles, and bones.

Function A catalyst to a number of enzymes for glucose and fatty acid metabolism. Part of arginase; needed for urea and thyroxine production. Adequate manganese increases thiamin utilization.

Utilization Limited especially in the presence of excess calcium and phosphorus.

Deficiency No report of dietary lack in man. In chickens, lack of manganese results in perosis.

Toxicity Workers exposed to manganese dust manifest asthenia, apathy, anorexia, headache, muscle cramps, speech disturbance, reduced hemoglobin regeneration, and decreased iron absorption.

Allowance About 0.3 mg/kg body weight.

Sources Nuts, legumes, whole-grain cereals, tea, dried fruits, and green leafy vegetables.

MOLYBDENUM

Occurrence Found in all cells, especially in liver, pancreas, kidneys, and bones.

Function Constituent of the enzymes xanthine oxidase and aldehyde oxidase; involved in purine metabolism and mobilization of iron from storage depots.

Deficiency Not observed in man or animals.

Toxicity Excess molybdenum causes severe diarrhea, anemia, retarded growth, loss of weight, weakness, stiffness, and loss of hair color in animals.

Sources Requirements not known; modybdenum is widely distributed in foods, particularly liver, kidney, legumes, cereals, and green leafy vegetables.

PHOSPHORUS

Occurrence Comprises about 1% of body weight or about 650 gm in an adult; of this, 85% is in bones and teeth and the rest in soft tissues, especially striated muscles.

Function Builds bones and teeth; part of the nucleus and cytoplasm of every cell. Practically all biologic reactions need phosphorus for use in adenosine triphosphate and enzyme systems for energy metabolism. Maintains acid-base balance; aids in fat solubility and absorption of many nutrients in the intestines that require phosphorylation.

Utilization Regulated by vitamin D, parathormone, and phosphatase.

Deficiency Same as in calcium deficiency.

Allowance See Recommended Daily Dietary Allowances, Appendix A-1. During growth, phosphorus intake must equal calcium needs.

Sources Present in a wide variety of foods, hence dietary lack is unlikely. All foods rich in protein and calcium are good sources of phosphorus. These are milk, cheese, meats, legumes, nuts, whole-grain cereals, eggs, and leafy greens without phytates and oxalates.

POTASSIUM

Occurrence About 250 gm in an adult body; concentrated inside cells (intracellular fluids).

Function Regulates acid-base and water balance. Maintains muscle and nerve irritability. Regulates normal heart rhythm. Acts as catalyst in many biologic reactions, especially those involving the release of energy, glycogen, and protein synthesis.

Utilization Excreted chiefly in the urine and perspiration.

Deficiency Muscle weakness, especially cardiac and respiratory muscles; glycogen depletion; poor intestinal tonus; nausea and lack of appetite.

Allowance Amount present in normal diet is more than sufficient for minimal potassium needs (about 2 to 4 gm/day for adults).

Sources Widely distributed in many foods (meats, legumes, nuts, cereals, fruits, and vegetables).

SELENIUM

Occurrence Concentrated in liver and other glandular organs, blood, and muscles.

Function An integral part of factor 3, a selenium-containing compound related to the function of vitamin E as catalyst in oxidation-reduction reactions (electron transport). Selenium is effective in treating muscular dystrophy in animals.

Deficiency Not observed in man. In calves, white muscle disease; in lambs, stiff lamb's disease; in chickens, exudative diathesis; in rats and mice, necrotic liver.

Toxicity Occurs when selenium in the diet is over 3 ppm. In man, gastric and hepatic disorders occur; in grazing animals, alkali disease and blind stagger. Toxic effect may be due to the ability of selenium to replace sulfur in the body; high protein intake will reduce selenium toxicity.

Sources Variable, depending on level in soil where plants are grown. Cereals have greater ability to take up selenium than other vegetables.

SODIUM

Occurrence About 50% of total body sodium is in extracellular fluids; 40% is in the skeleton; and the rest is inside the cells. In a 70 kg man the total amount of sodium is 105 gm (or 0.15% of total body weight).

Function Regulates osmotic pressure, water and acid-base balance, nerve irritability, muscle contraction, and absorption of glucose. Sodium is the major cation in extracellular fluids.

Utilization Readily absorbed in gastrointestinal tract; amount in body is regulated by the kidneys and the adrenal cortical hormones. Stored temporarily in the bones. Estrogens promote retention. Excreted in the feces, urine, sweat, and digestive contents, as in vomiting.

Deficiency Nausea, vomiting, muscle cramps, disturbed acid-base balance, and diarrhea.

Toxicity High intake not yet proved to be harmful to a healthy person, since the body can excrete excess sodium readily in urine. In experimental animal studies, a prolonged high salt diet correlated with hypertension. Large sodium intakes may aggravate a tendency toward high blood pressure.

Sources Salt, baking powder, baking soda, and all processed foods containing these as ingredients. Meats, fish, poultry, milk, eggs, certain vegetables, and food additives. (For details, see *Diet, sodium-restricted.*)

SULFUR

Occurrence Comprises about 0.25% of body weight (175 gm in a 70 kg man). Present in every cell, especially hair, nails, cartilage, insulin, glutathione, melanin, and the amino acids cystine, cysteine, and methionine.

Function In addition to its structural function as an integral part of cells and substances listed above, sulfur is part of vitamin B_1, pantothenic acid, biotin, and lipoic acid. It forms a high energy compound and also combines with toxic substances.

Utilization Ingested mainly as protein, excreted chiefly as sulfates in the urine.

Deficiency and sources No dietary deficiency if protein intake is adequate. Constitutes about 1% of protein. All foods rich in protein provide sulfur.

ZINC

Occurrence Widely distributed in the body; an adult has about 2 gm of zinc. Concentrated in hair, skin, nails, testes, and especially in the retina of the eye. In the blood, red blood cells have more zinc than the serum. Also found in the liver, muscles, and bones.

Function Component of carbonic anhydrase and several digestive enzymes; part of insulin; involved in muscle movement and synthesis of red blood cells.

Utilization High calcium intake interferes with absorption; excreted mainly in the feces and some in the urine.

Deficiency In humans, dwarfism and hypogonadism.

Toxicity Zinc poisoning results in increased losses of iron and copper.

Allowance See Recommended Daily Dietary Allowances, Appendix A-1.

Sources Seafood, shellfish, liver, cereal germ, egg yolk, etc. Widely distributed; usual daily intake is 12 mg.

■ APPENDIX I-1
Summary of vitamins

VITAMIN A

Nomenclature Retinol (vitamin A_1); dehydroretinol (vitamin A_2); retinaldehyde (vitamin A_1 aldehyde); retinoic acid (vitamin A_1 acid). Obsolete names: axerophthol; antixerophthalmic vitamin; anti-infective vitamin; biosterol; ophthalmin.

Assay Biologic; chemical; spectrophotometric.

Unit One IU = 0.3 μg vitamin A_1 alcohol; 0.344 μg vitamin A_1 acetate; 0.6 μg beta-carotene.

Characteristics Soluble in organic solvents; insoluble in water. Unstable in air but can be stabilized by addition of antioxidants. Stable to high temperature in the absence of oxygen. Stable to acid, alkali, and ordinary cooking methods. Occurs only in lipids of animals. Provitamins A in plants exist in several isomeric forms. Most important are alpha- and beta-carotene and cryptoxanthin, of which beta-carotene is the most potent. No losses in cooking and ordinary storage.

Physiology Absorbed from the intestines and transported via the lymph. Bile is necessary for absorption. Conversion of provitamins A occurs chiefly in the intestinal wall; some conversion occurs in the liver and kidneys. Stored chiefly in the liver as an ester, primarily vitamin A acetate. Transported as retinol (alcohol form) and active as retinaldehyde.

Functions Bone and skeletal growth. Maintenance of normal epithelial tissue structure. Rhodopsin regeneration for vision. Related to biosynthesis of steroids. Normal functioning of nervous and reproductive systems.

Deficiency Man: poor growth; faulty bone and tooth development; lowered resistance to infection; keratinization of epithelial tissues, mucous membranes, and skin; night blindness; Bitot's spots; xerophthalmia and keratomalacia in severe cases. Rat: xerophthalmia. Chicken: ataxia. Cattle: nerve degeneration. Pig: paralysis of hind legs.

Toxicity Violent headache; nausea; peeling and thickening of skin; swelling and pain of long bones; coarse sparse hair; hepatomegaly; splenomegaly.

Requirement Related to body weight (20 IU vitamin A or 40 IU carotene/kg body weight). See Recommended Daily Dietary Allowances, Appendix A-1, for allowance. It is based on the premise that approximately two thirds of the vitamin A value of the average diet is contributed by carotene and that carotene has half or less than half the value of vitamin A.

Sources Animal sources (as preformed vitamin A): fish liver oils; liver; egg yolk; milk; butter; cheese. Plant sources (as provitamins A): dark green leafy vegetables and yellow fruits and vegetables such as squash and carrots.

Summary of vitamins—cont'd

VITAMIN D

Nomenclature Ergocalciferol (vitamin D_2, calciferol, viosterol, irradiated ergosterol); cholecalciferol (vitamin D_3, irradiated 7-dehydrocholesterol). Obsolete names: antirachitic factor; rachitamin; sunshine vitamin.

Assay Biologic; chromatographic; calcium line test.

Unit One IU or USP $= 0.025$ μg vitamin D_3.

Characteristics Soluble in fat; insoluble in water. Stable to heat, acid, alkali, and oxidation. Of 15 forms, six are considered major; most important are vitamins D_2 and D_3. Ergosterol is the most abundant plant precursor; converted to ergocalciferol on irradiation. Man can synthesize provitamin D_3 in the body; it is activated on exposure of skin to ultraviolet light.

Physiology Absorbed via the lacteals; both fat and bile salts necessary for absorption. Stored to a limited extent in the liver; also some storage in bones and soft tissues, particularly spleen, lungs, and brain. Placental transfer to fetus is not great but enough to supply the fetus. Metabolized in the liver to 25-hydroxycholecalciferol and in the kidney to 1,25-dihydroxycholecalciferol. The latter metabolite initiates the production of a protein that binds calcium in the intestines.

Functions Promotes normal bone and teeth formation. Regulates the absorption, transport, and deposition of calcium and phosphorus in the body. Relationship between vitamin D and alkaline phosphatase is not clear, except that phosphatase level in the blood increases in rickets.

Deficiency Infants: tetanic convulsions due to low blood calcium levels. Children: rickets (soft and fragile bones; pigeon breast and rachitic rosary; bone deformities in chest, spine, and pelvis; enlarged joint; bowlegs and knock knees; pot belly due to weak abdominal muscles; delayed dentition and closure of fontanelles). Adults: osteomalacia (softening of bones; skeletal deformities; fractures; pain of rheumatic type in bones).

Toxicity Nausea, diarrhea, weight loss, and polyuria in mild cases. Demineralization of bones, calcification of soft tissues, renal damage, and uremia in severe cases.

Requirement Not known for adults—probably very little and met by ordinary diet and casual exposure to sunlight. Allowance of 300 to 400 IU daily is sufficient for growing infants; also probably adequate during pregnancy and lactation.

Sources Animal sources: fish liver oils; vitamin D–fortified milk; activated sterols. Small amounts in liver, egg yolk, butter, sardines, and salmon. Plant sources: none comparable to animal sources. Incidental source: exposure to sunlight.

VITAMIN E

Nomenclature Tocopherols (alpha-, beta-, gamma-, and delta-). Obsolete names: antisterility vitamin; factor X.

Assay Chromatographic; chemical; prevention of fetal resorption in rats.

Unit One IU $= 1$ mg dl-alpha-tocopherol.

Characteristics Fat soluble. Stable to high temperature and acid. Readily oxidized in the presence of lead, iron salts, and rancid fat. Decomposes in ultraviolet light. Derivative of chromanol and structurally related to vitamin K and ubiquinone. Eight naturally occurring tocopherols have been isolated; four are biologically active, of which alpha-tocopherol is the most potent.

Physiology Absorbed via the lymphatics. Bile is needed for optimal absorption. Not stored in the body to a great extent. Found mainly in fatty tissues and liver. No evidence of intestinal synthesis; vitamin E synthesis is a function of plants. Has sparing effect on vitamin A and essential fatty acids.

Functions Its function in humans is not clearly understood. It seems to prevent hemolysis of red blood cells and reduce oxidation of vitamin A, carotene, and polyunsaturated fatty acids. Recent investigations, however, suggest that tocopherol may be more than just an antioxidant. It appears important in ensuring stability and integrity of biologic membranes. Among the observations seen in animals deficient in vitamin E are the following: (1) loss of integrity of membranes, (2) hemolysis of red blood cells, (3) decreased lipogenesis, (4) decline in respiration, (5) altered DNA/RNA ratio, and (6) disruption in electron transport system.

Deficiency Man: increased tendency to hemolysis; anemia. Rat: infertility in males; resorption gestation in females; liver necrosis; muscular dystrophy. Chicken: exudative diathesis; encephalomalacia; muscular dystrophy. Mouse:

multiple necrotic degeneration of heart, liver, and muscles. Cattle: muscular dystrophy. Swine: liver necrosis. Turkey: hock disorder; embryonic abnormalities; exudative diathesis; encephalomalacia. In animals, vitamin E deficiency manifestations may be prevented by dietary selenite, cystine, antioxidants, and redox dyes.

Toxicity No reported case.

Requirement For infants, 0.5 mg/kg has been suggested as the minimum requirement. Adult requirement may vary from 10 to 20 mg/day; the higher level is suggested when intake of vegetable oils high in polyunsaturated fatty acids is substantial.

Sources Animal sources: except for egg yolk, liver, and milk, animal foods are poor sources. Plant sources: vegetable oils (wheat germ, corn, cottonseed, soybean); unmilled cereals; green leafy vegetables; and nuts and legumes.

VITAMIN K

Nomenclature Phylloquinone (vitamin K_1); farnoquinone (vitamin K_2); menadione (vitamin K_3). Obsolete names: Koagulations vitamin; antihemorrhagic factor.

Assay Clotting time; prevention of hemorrhage in chickens.

Unit Menadione is reference standard. One unit vitamin $K = 1$ μg menadione.

Characteristics Soluble in fat. Stable to heat, oxygen, and moisture. Unstable to alkali and oxidizing agents. No appreciable loss in ordinary cooking. Compounds with vitamin K activity are all related to 2-methyl-1,4-naphthoquinone.

Physiology Optimal absorption requires the presence of bile. Level in blood is low and storage is small. There is some placental transport to fetus but not stored prenatally. Synthesized by a large number of bacteria in the digestive tract. Intestinal synthesis prevented by sulfonamides and antibiotics. Not synthesized by infants due to absence of intestinal flora.

Functions Functions chiefly in maintaining blood plasma prothrombin level. Possible role in respiratory enzyme system, photosynthesis, and oxidative phosphorylation. Used therapeutically in treating neonatal bleeding, impaired intestinal obstruction, and postoperative conditions.

Deficiency Hemorrhagic disease in newborn because of lack of bacterial synthesis. Delayed blood clotting time seen in adults. However, direct dietary deficiency of the vitamin in human adults has never been seen. Conditioned vitamin K deficiency may be caused by a number of factors such as (1) faulty intestinal synthesis, (2) hepatic injury, (3) sulfonamide and antibiotic therapy, (4) poor intestinal absorption, and (5) obstruction in bile duct.

Antivitamins Dicumarol; sulfaquinoxaline; warfarin.

Toxicity Vomiting; albuminuria; hemolytic anemia; kernicterus. Menadione and other synthetic preparations are more toxic than the naturally occurring vitamins K_1 and K_2.

Requirement Not known because of variability in intestinal synthesis and inconsistent distribution in foods.

Sources Animal sources: none comparable to plant sources. Plant sources: vitamin K_1 is found in vegetables, notably green leaves. Other sources: vitamin K_2 is produced by intestinal bacteria, and vitamins K_3 to K_7 are synthetic forms.

ASCORBIC ACID

Nomenclature Vitamin C. Obsolete names: antiscorbutic vitamin; cevitamic acid.

Assay Chemical.

Unit Milligram.

Characteristics Very soluble in water. Most unstable of all vitamins; readily destroyed by heat, alkali, and light. Oxidized on exposure to air. Quite stable in dry form but destroyed during storage and processing. Of several forms; the most active biologically are L-ascorbic acid and L-dehydroascorbic acid.

Physiology Almost completely absorbed. Very limited storage and deficiency results readily. Highly concentrated in glandular organs; found in greatest concentration in adrenals, eye lens, and liver. Excess intake readily eliminated after tissue saturation. Synthesized by all plants and animals except man, guinea pig, monkey, Indian fruit bat, red-vented bulbul bird, and probably elephant.

Functions Necessary in the formation of intercellular cementing substance. Important in the metabolism of tyrosine and phenylalanine. Facilitates the absorption of iron and reduction of ferric to ferrous iron. Stimulates the conversion of folic acid to its metabolically active form, folinic acid. May be involved in the synthesis of collagen and steroid hormones. A good antioxidant.

Deficiency Scurvy (swollen and bleeding gums; petechial or cutaneous hemorrhages; pain and tenderness on thighs and joints; poor wound healing; reduced resistance to infection; improper bone formation; anemia; stunted growth).

Antivitamin D-Glucose ascorbic acid.

Toxicity None. Excess has no effect.

Allowance See Recommended Daily Dietary Allowances, Appendix A-1. Opinions differ widely regarding intakes that may be regarded as satisfactory or approximately optimal. Minimal levels of intake are approximately one third to one sixth of the recommended allowances. These low intakes, however, are not satisfactory when the body is subjected to stress.

Sources Animal sources: appreciable amounts in adrenals and spleen; not comparable to plant sources. Plant sources: citrus fruits (e.g., orange), acerola; strawberry; cabbage family; tomatoes; green pepper; guava; ripe papaya, etc. Content in plants varies with part of plant, maturity, variety, and climatic conditions.

THIAMIN

Nomenclature Thiamine; vitamin B_1. Obsolete names: aneurine, antiberiberi vitamin; antineuritic factor; vitamin F; oryzamin; "morale vitamin."

Assay Thiochrome method; microbiologic.

Unit Milligram or microgram.

Characteristics Very soluble in water. Stable in dry form and slightly acid medium. Readily destroyed in neutral or alkaline medium. Destroyed by sulfite treatment. Great cooking losses if cooking liquid is discarded and high temperature and prolonged heating are employed.

Physiology Absorbed primarily from the duodenum and carried to the liver via the portal system. Absorption is an active process, requiring energy. Very limited storage in the body; only enough to last a few days. Largest concentration found in liver, heart, kidneys, brain, and muscles. Fat, protein, sulfonamides, and antibiotics have "thiamin sparing action" and reduce the need for this vitamin. Closely related to lipoic acid. Evidence of intestinal synthesis in man but apparently not available to the body. The kidney has no known threshold; large doses eliminated in the urine.

Functions Component of coenzyme (thiamin pyrophosphate) that functions in oxidative decarboxylation of keto acids and in the transfer of "active glycoaldehyde" in the hexose monophosphate shunt. Helps maintain normal appetite. Regulates muscle tone of the gastrointestinal tract. Necessary for normal functioning of nerves.

Deficiency Man: beriberi, affecting chiefly the nervous and cardiovascular systems. Symptoms include anorexia, easy fatigue, lassitude, numbness of the legs, constipation or indigestion in early stages. Later manifestations include mental confusion, loss of ankle and knee jerk reflexes, painful calf muscles, peripheral neuritis, dyspnea and palpitation on exertion, and edema (wet beriberi); generalized polyneuropathy and muscular paralysis (dry beriberi); and cyanosis, tachycardia, and cardiac failure (infantile beriberi). Animals: growth retardation; muscle spasm; convulsive seizures; and death within 3 to 6 weeks. Opisthotonus occurs in chickens, and Chastek paralysis or bracken fern poisoning is seen in foxes and cattle due to thiaminase intake.

Antivitamins Pyrithiamine; oxythiamine; thiaminase.

Toxicity None. No adverse effect of excessive intake, although 100 mg injection in man causes an allergic reaction.

Requirement Evidence that minimal requirement approximates 0.2 mg/1000 calories. (See Recommended Daily Dietary Allowances, Appendix A-1). Thiamin needs increase in fever, hyperthyroidism, cardiac conditions, polyneuropathies, alcoholism, and constipation.

Sources Animal sources: lean pork; liver and other organ meats; egg yolk. Plant sources: whole-grain cereals; enriched rice; peanuts; legumes; mungo; peas; collard greens. Dried yeast is richest source.

RIBOFLAVIN

Nomenclature Riboflavin; vitamin B_2. Obsolete names: ovoflavin, lactoflavin; hepatoflavin; verdoflavin; vitamin G.

Assay Fluorometric; microbiologic.

Unit Milligram or microgram.

Characteristics A yellowish pigment with a greenish fluorescence. Slightly soluble in water. Readily destroyed in the presence of light. Unstable in alkaline medium. Relatively resistant to dry heat, acid, and oxidizing agents. Very little loss in ordinary cooking methods because of stability in heat and limited solubility in water. Occurs in bound form in plant and animal tissues and not made available unless binding is liberated by cooking.

Physiology Absorbed through the intestinal walls; phosphorylation needed for absorption. Transported either attached to protein or linked with a phosphate molecule (as FAD or FMN). Little storage in the body; amount stored depends on saturation of protein. Excreted in urine and feces; excretion is increased when protein is catabolized. Occurs in coenzyme form; free riboflavin found only in milk, retina of eye, and urine. Intestinal synthesis not available unless coprophagy is practiced. Coefficient of food digestibility and intestinal disorders affect its availability and absorption.

Functions Important in carbohydrate, fat, and protein metabolism as essential component of flavin mononucleotide and flavin adenine dinucleotide, which serve as carriers in the electron transport system, leading to the formation of high energy ATP. Involved in the conversion of tryptophan to nicotinic acid. Necessary for normal growth and development. Plays a role in normal skin tone, normal vision, and light adaptation.

Deficiency Man: ariboflavinosis. Symptoms are cheilosis, magenta-colored tongue, angular stomatitis, nasolabial dermatitis, corneal vascularization, dimness of vision, photophobia, growth retardation, and congenital malformation (if deficiency occurs during period of conception). Rat: alopecia; scaly brown dermatitis. Chicken: curled toe paralysis; poor hatchability. Dog: dermatitis; weak hind legs; fatty liver. Swine: cataract; abnormal gait; nerve degeneration. Cat: fatty liver; cataract; skin changes. Monkey: loss of weight; scaly dermatitis; decrease in white blood cells.

Antivitamins Quinacrine; isoriboflavin; araboflavin; galactoflavin.

Toxicity Not produced by oral doses. Riboflavin is not very soluble and is excreted in the feces. Toxicity occurs if given in massive doses by injection.

Requirement Minimum requirement appears to be closely related to energy expenditure (0.3 mg/1000 calories). Allowance may be computed as twice the requirement (0.6 mg/1000 calories). See Recommended Daily Dietary Allowances, Appendix A-1.

Sources Animal sources: milk; egg; liver and other organ meats; lean meat. Plant sources: whole grain cereals; dried beans; leafy green vegetables.

NICOTINIC ACID

Nomenclature Niacin; niacinamide; nicotinamide. Obsolete names: Pellagra-preventive factor; PP factor; antiblacktongue factor.

Assay Microbiologic; chemical.

Unit Milligram.

Characteristics Nicotinic acid (or niacin) is present in plant tissues. It is soluble in hot water and ethanol, stable to heat, acid, and alkali. Niacinamide (or nicotinamide) is present in animal tissues. It is very soluble in water and acetone and converted to nicotinic acid by acid or base. Probably the most stable of all vitamins, being resistant to heat, light, air, acid, and alkali. Not destroyed by ordinary cooking methods, although small amounts are lost in discarded cooking liquid.

Physiology Hydrolyzed in the gut into the free acid and the amide. Present in the blood as both acid and amide. Present in the tissues in coenzyme form. Excreted largely as methylated products. Stored to a limited extent, depending on tissue saturation. Synthesized by mammalian cells from tryptophan (60 mg tryptophan equivalent to 1 mg nicotinic acid).

Functions Acts as hydrogen and electron acceptor as constituent of coenzyme I (nicotinamide adenine dinucleotide [NAD]) and coenzyme II (nicotinamide adenine dinucleotide phosphate [NADP]). Functions in carbohydrate metabolism (aerobic and anaerobic oxidation of glucose), lipid metabolism (glycerol synthesis and breakdown, fatty acid synthesis and oxidation), and protein metabolism (synthesis and degradation of amino acids, oxidation of carbon chains). Also functions in rhodopsin synthesis and in CO_2 fixation (photosynthesis). Used therapeutically to lower blood cholesterol levels.

Deficiency Man: pellagra. Symptoms are bilateral dermatitis sensitive to solar radiation; glossitis with fiery red tongue; angular stomatitis; and mental changes (anxiety, confusion, delirium, and dementia). Rat: porphyrin-caked whiskers; alopecia; rough hair coat.

Dog: black tongue; oral lesions; bloody diarrhea; inflamed gums. Chicken: perosis; poor growth and feathering. Swine: stomatitis; anemia; diarrhea. Rabbit: leukopenia; terminal diarrhea.

Antivitamins 6-Aminonicotinamide; 3-acetylpyridine; isonicotinic acid hydrazide (INH).

Toxicity Large intakes of nicotinic acid increase gastrointestinal motility and secretion of acid, causing epigastric pain and reactivation of peptic ulcer. Niacinamide is more toxic, causing flushing and tingling sensations and, in excessive amounts, paralysis of the respiratory center (5 to 7 mg/kg body weight in rats).

Requirement Based on body weight and caloric intake. Averages 4.4 mg/1000 calories (including that formed from tryptophan). A 50% factor of safety is added for dietary allowance.

Sources Animal sources: organ meats, especially pork liver; poultry; fish; lean meat. Plant sources: rice polishings; enriched rice, bread, and cereals; peanuts; dried beans; green vegetables.

PANTOTHENIC ACID

Nomenclature Name from Greek word meaning "from everywhere." Obsolete names: chick antidermatitis factor; filtrate factor.

Assay Microbiologic. No suitable chemical method.

Unit Milligram or microgram.

Characteristics Extremely soluble in water. Unstable at high temperatures. Easily hydrolyzed in hot acid or base. Commercially available as white crystalline calcium or sodium salt. Widely distributed in plants and animals in bound form; the free acid has never been isolated. Fairly stable during ordinary storage and processing.

Physiology Readily absorbed from small intestines and excreted chiefly via the urine. There may be some destruction in the gut. Host and intestinal organisms compete for the use of the vitamin. Occurs in the tissues and blood in bound form; liberated by proteolytic enzymes. Stored to some extent in liver and kidneys. There is close correlation between pantothenic acid level and adrenal cortex function. Utilization depends on the presence of folic acid and biotin. Evidence of intestinal synthesis by bacteria.

Functions A constituent of coenzyme A, which plays an important role in acetylation and acylation reactions; oxidation of keto acids and fatty acids; synthesis of triglycerides, steroids, phospholipids, and fatty acids; formation of acetylcholine; and synthesis of porphyrin for hemoglobin formation. As acetyl CoA, the vitamin plays a key role in the metabolism of carbohydrate, protein, and fat. Also necessary for the maintenance of normal skin and development of the central nervous system. Large amounts of pantothenic acid help man withstand stress, perhaps due to its effect on the adrenal gland.

Deficiency Man: not observed with natural diet since the vitamin is widely distributed in foods. Experimental deficiency states in humans fed an antagonist (omega-methylpantothenic acid) produce a syndrome characterized by sleep disturbances; easy fatigue, abdominal cramps; vomiting; paresthesia in extremities (burning feet syndrome) and muscle cramps. Rat: achromotrichia; porphyrin-caked whiskers; scaly dermatitis; alopecia. Chicken: poor feathering and hatchability; severe dermatitis around the eyes; foot lesions; myelin degeneration. Dog: convulsions; necrotic adrenals; gastrointestinal tract disorders; fatty liver; nervous symptoms. Swine: goose-stepping; excessive lacrimation. Calf and duck: death ensues rapidly.

Antivitamins Omega-methylpantothenic acid; pantoyl taurine; phenyl pantothenate.

Requirement Not exactly known. About 5 to 15 mg/day; this amount is apparently satisfied by the daily diet. Needs presumably increase during stress, injury, antibiotic therapy, and severe illness.

Sources Universally present in all living cells. Animal sources: liver is highest source. Plant sources: yeast is highest source.

VITAMIN B₆ GROUP

Nomenclature Pyridoxine is the class name given to include three compounds with vitamin B_6 activity: pyridoxine (alcohol form), pyridoxal (aldehyde form), and pyridoxamine (amine form). Obsolete names: adermin; eluate factor.

Assay Microbiologic; fluorometric.

Unit Milligram or microgram.

Characteristics Extremely soluble in water. Stable in acid and alkaline solution. Rapidly destroyed by light in neutral and alkaline solution. Fairly stable to heat. Pyridoxal and pyridoxamine occur in animal tissues; pyridoxine occurs in plants. Some losses in food processing, especially in milk.

Physiology Readily and completely absorbed from the gut. Level in the blood is extremely low and storage is very limited. Found in the blood as pyridoxal phosphate, the coenzyme form. The biologic activities of the three forms in mammals are equal; all can be converted to the coenzyme form. Evidence of intestinal synthesis, although apparently not much utilized by man.

Functions Pyridoxal phosphate is a coenzyme in a number of reactions involving degradation, interconversion, and integration of amino acids (e.g., decarboxylation, transamination, racemization, desulfuration, dehydration, etc.). Involved in the metabolism of a number of amino acids, such as serine, cysteine, and tryptophan. Necessary for conversion of tryptophan to nicotinic acid, urea production, and metabolism of essential fatty acids. Used therapeutically to control nausea and vomiting of pregnancy and to alleviate the peripheral neuritis of INH medication.

Deficiency Man: adult human deficiency has not been produced by dietary means. An increase in xanthurenic acid excretion in the urine is observed, although no other abnormalities appear. Administration of an antagonist, deoxypyridoxine, produces the following symptoms: nausea and vomiting; oxaluria; glossitis; stomatitis; conjunctivitis; seborrheic dermatitis; and depression. Infants: vitamin B_6 deficiency has been induced with milk formula deficient in the vitamin, causing hyperirritability, poor growth, anemia, and convulsions. Monkey: anemia; skin lesions. Rat: acrodynia; epileptic fits. Dog: skin lesions; epileptic fits; anemia. Swine: anemia. All symptoms are accentuated by high protein intake.

Antivitamins Deoxypyridoxine; toxopyrimidine; isoniazid; methoxypyridoxine.

Toxicity Not toxic if given orally unless tremendous levels are given. Quite toxic if injected; 3 gm/kg body weight in rats can cause death.

Requirement Minimal daily requirement is about 0.65 to 0.75 mg. Requirement increases with protein intake. See Recommended Daily

Dietary Allowances, Appendix A-1, for allowance.

Sources Animal sources: muscle meats; liver; kidneys and other organ meats; small amount in milk. Plant sources: whole-grain cereals; soybeans and peanuts; green vegetables.

VITAMIN B_{12} GROUP

Nomenclature Cobalamins; cyanocobalamin (cobamide cyanide). Obsolete names: antipernicious anemia factor; animal protein factor; zoopherin; extrinsic factor; erythrocyte maturation factor.

Assay Microbiologic; biologic.

Unit Milligram or microgram.

Characteristics Dark red crystalline solid containing cobalt. Slightly soluble in water, soluble in ethanol, and insoluble in organic solvents. Relatively stable in solution, especially at pH 4.0 to 7.0. Destroyed by oxidizing and reducing agents and exposure to sunlight. Occurs bound to protein in foods of animal origin; there is very little in vegetables. Of several forms such as cyano-, hydroxo- and nitrito-, of which the cyanide form is the most active.

Physiology Absorbed from the ileum; needs the intrinsic factor for absorption. Unusual storage in the liver; amount stored may last 3 to 4 years in the absence of additional supply. Circulates in the blood bound to alpha globulins; found in the mitochondria combined with ammonia and amino-containing groups. The fetus concentrates the vitamin. There are at least five different coenzyme forms; the most frequently encountered is adenylcobamide.

Functions Promotes growth. Exact role in metabolism is not clearly understood, although required in several enzyme systems. Normal development and maturation of red blood cells. Normal function of nervous tissue, bone marrow, and gastrointestinal tract. Synthesis of nucleic acids, possibly in the conversion of ribose to deoxyribose and formation of methyl group of thymine. Single carbon metabolism (methyl group synthesis) and in metabolism of carbohydrate, protein, and fat.

Deficiency Man: pernicious anemia. Generally due to lack of intrinsic factor. Dietary deficiency occasionally seen in strict vegetarians. Conditioned deficiency seen in gastrectomy and parasitism. Symptoms are sore tongue; paresthesia; anorexia; abdominal discomfort; coldness of extremities; general weakness; neurologic changes. Chicken: poor growth; poor hatchability; no anemia. Rat: brain damage; uremia; no anemia. Swine: incoordinated gait; poor growth. Ruminant: wasting disease; poor growth; anemia.

Antivitamins None known.

Toxicity None. As much as 100 million times requirement produce no effect. Only minute amounts can be bound to protein; the free form is excreted.

Requirement About 3 μg/day (assuming 30% absorption). Intake of 15 μg/day will replenish body stores if depleted. Average diets appear to meet these requirements.

Sources Widely distributed in minute amounts in foods of animal origin. Excellent sources are meat, milk, liver, eggs, and fish. Plants are practically devoid of the vitamin.

PTEROYLGLUTAMIC ACID

Nomenclature PGA; folic acid; folinic acid; folacin; citrovorum factor; leucovorin. Obsolete names: Will's factor; vitamin M; factor U; factor SLR; factor R; vitamin B_{11}; vitamin B_c; Norite eluate factor; *L. casei* factor; rhizopterin.

Assay Microbiologic; colorimetric.

Unit Milligram or microgram.

Characteristics Orange-yellow crystal slightly soluble in water. Sensitive to light and heat in acid solution; stable between pH 4.0 and 12. Present in foods as conjugates of glutamic acid. Appreciable losses during storage and cooking.

Physiology Readily absorbed from both upper and lower gastrointestinal tract. Bound to protein and often conjugated. Stored primarily in the liver. Folic acid is converted to folinic acid in the presence of ascorbic acid. The physiologically active form is tetrahydrofolic acid. Excess excreted in the urine and feces. Synthesized by intestinal bacteria in most mammals; apparently not in man.

Functions Single carbon metabolism (interconversion of serine and glycine; synthesis of purines and pyrimidines; synthesis of methyl group of methionine, choline, and thymine; degradation of histidine). Together with vitamin B_{12} and ascorbic acid, necessary for regeneration of red blood cells. Used therapeutically in tropical sprue, nutritional macrocytic anemia of infancy, and macrocytic anemia of pregnancy.

Deficiency Man: not produced by dietary lack, but occurs secondary to disease (as sprue), folic acid antagonist, or following prolonged therapy with Dilantin and phenobarbital. Symptoms include glossitis and other oral lesions; gastrointestinal disturbances; megaloblastic anemia; granulocytopenia. Chicken: poor growth and feathering; perosis; low hemoglobin; macrocytic anemia. Turkey: cervical paralysis. Monkey: marked weight loss; leucopenia; macrocytic anemia; gingivitis.

Antivitamins Aminopterin; amethopterin; tetrahydroaminopterin; pteroylaspartic acid.

Toxicity Quite toxic in large doses. May plug the kidney. Animals die of uremia. Sale without prescription of vitamin preparations recommending doses of more than 0.1 mg/day is prohibited.

Requirement Not known; probably 0.1 to 0.2 mg/day.

Sources Widely distributed in nature. Animal sources: organ meats, especially liver and kidneys; lean beef. Plant sources: green vegetables; dried beans; nuts and cereals.

BIOTIN

Nomenclature Obsolete names: Vitamin H; bios II; coenzyme R; anti-egg white injury factor.

Assay Microbiologic; biologic.

Unit Microgram.

Characteristics White crystalline solid. Soluble in water and alcohol. Stable to heat and light. Inactivated by strong acid, alkali, and oxidizing agent. Present in animal products as water-insoluble protein complexes; present in plants in water-soluble form.

Physiology Not readily absorbed. Absorption prevented by avidin, a protein in raw egg white that is inactivated by heat. Bound to protein and liberated largely during digestion. Evidence of intestinal synthesis, although its contribution to tissue needs is probably small.

Functions Primary function is CO_2 fixation, which is an important cellular synthetic mechanism. Indirectly plays a role in synthesis of purines, citrulline, and aspartic acid, metabolism of fatty acids, and carboxylation and decarboxylation reactions.

Deficiency Man: true dietary deficiency is unlikely to occur even with a poor diet. Deficiency in man can be induced by large intakes of raw egg white, producing a syndrome characterized by dry, scaly dermatitis, nausea, lassitude, depression, and muscular or nervous disorders. Rat: spectacle eye; greasy, scaly dermatitis; spastic gait; paralysis of hind legs. Chicken: perosis; dermatitis around mouth, eyes, and feet. Swine: alopecia; dermatitis; spastic gait; cracks in feet.

Antivitamins Biotin sulfone. While not really an antivitamin, avidin binds biotin, making it unavailable for use.

Toxicity No evidence of toxic effects.

Requirement Not exactly known; probably between 150 and 300 μg/day. Apparently no dietary requirement; intestinal synthesis is presumed to be adequate.

Sources Wide distribution in nature. Animal sources: liver; eggs; fish; muscle meat; milk. Plant sources: whole-grain cereals; legumes and nuts; most fruits and vegetables.

■ APPENDIX I-2

Vitamins as coenzymes

Vitamin	Coenzyme form	Functions
Thiamin	Thiamin pyrophosphate or diphosphothiamin	Oxidative decarboxylation of alpha keto acids; transketolase reaction of hexose monophosphate shunt
Riboflavin	Flavin mononucleotide; flavin adenine dinucleotide	Hydrogen acceptor or carrier in electron transport system; also involved in specific dehydrogenation of adjacent carbon atoms
Nicotinic acid	Nicotinamide adenine dinucleotide; nicotinamide adenine dinucleotide phosphate	Hydrogen acceptor of dehydrogenases; designated as NADH and NADPH in the reduced state
Pantothenic acid	Coenzyme A	Acetyl or other acyl group transfer; fatty acid oxidation and synthesis; synthesis of cholesterol and phospholipid
Pyridoxine (vitamin B_6)	Pyridoxal phosphate	Nonoxidative degradation of amino acids; transamination, deamination, decarboxylation, etc.; metabolism of unsaturated fatty acids
Cobalamin (vitamin B_{12})	Cobamide	Interconversion of single carbon units by oxidoreduction; nucleic acid synthesis; methyl group transfer
Pteroylglutamic acid	Tetrahydrofolic acid	Carrier for single carbon groups; purine and pyrimidine synthesis
Biotin	Biotin	CO_2 transfer; not identified with any specific enzyme but probably a prosthetic group in combination with specific proteins

■ APPENDIX J-1

Summary of digestive enzymes

Source and secretion	Enzyme	Substrate	Products
Mouth			
Saliva	Salivary amylase (ptyalin)	Cooked starch	Dextrins and maltose
Stomach			
Gastric juice	Pepsin	Protein	Proteoses and peptones
	Rennin	Casein of milk	Calcuim caseinate
	Gastric lipase	Emulsified fat	Fatty acids and glycerol
Pancreas			
Pancreatic juice	Trypsin	Protein	Proteoses, peptones, and polypeptides
	Chymotrypsin	Protein	Proteoses, peptones, and polypeptides
	Pancreatic amylase (amylopsin)	Starch and dextrins	Dextrins and maltose
	Pancreatic lipase (steapsin)	Fat	Simple glycerides, fatty acids, and glycerol
Small intestines			
Intestinal juice (succus entericus)	Enterokinase	Trypsinogen	Trypsin
	Peptidases (amino-peptidase, carboxy-peptidase, and dipeptidase)	Peptones, polypeptides, and dipeptides	Amino acids
	Nucleases	Nucleic acids and derivatives	Phosphoric acid, pentose, purine, and pyrimidine bases
	Sucrase	Sucrose	Glucose and fructose
	Maltase	Maltose	Glucose
	Lactase	Lactose	Glucose and galactose
	Intestinal lipase	Fat	Fatty acids and glycerol

■ APPENDIX J-2
Summary of enzymes*

Name and class	Action
Hydrolases	Hydrolysis; i.e., introduction of the elements of water to a specific bond of the substrate
Carbohydrases	
Amylase	Splits starch and glycogen into residual polysaccharides, e.g., maltose and dextrin
Cellulase	Splits cellulose into various carbohydrate fragments without the production of glucose
Lactase	Splits lactose to glucose and galactose
Maltase (alpha glucosidase)	Splits maltose into two glucose units
Sucrase (invertase or saccharase)	Splits sucrose to glucose and fructose
Esterases	
Simple esterase	Splits esters of lower alcohols and fatty acids
Lipase	Converts fats into glycerol and fatty acids
Phosphatase	Converts phosphoric acid esters into phosphate and alcohol
Cholinesterase	Hydrolyzes acetylcholine into choline and acetic acid
Lecithinase	Splits lecithin into diglycerides, choline, and phosphate
Pyrophosphatase	Splits pyrophosphate linkages, liberating orthophosphate
Proteinases (endopeptidases)	Act on interior peptide bonds of proteins, breaking off large peptide chains
Pepsin	Converts proteins to proteoses and peptones
Trypsin	Converts proteins, proteoses, and peptones to polypeptides and amino acids
Chymotrypsin	Same as trypsin
Rennin	Converts casein to paracasein
Papain	Converts proteins, proteoses, and peptones to polypeptides and amino acids
Bromelin	Same as papain
Peptidases (exopeptidases)	Act on peptide bonds adjacent to a free amino or carboxyl group
Aminopeptidase	Acts on peptide bond adjacent to the free amino group of polypeptides, forming simpler peptides and amino acids
Carboxypeptidase	Acts on peptide bond adjacent to a free carboxyl group, liberating an amino acid
Dipeptidase	Acts on certain dipeptides, yielding individual amino acids

Continued.

---

*A partial listing. There are many classifications of enzymes, based chiefly on the names of substrates on which they act and on the type of chemical reaction catalyzed. A new system of enzyme nomenclature was developed in 1961 by the Commission on Enzymes of the International Union of Biochemistry. This new system classifies enzymes into six major divisions, each with 4 to 13 subclasses. Each enzyme is assigned a code number consisting of four digits, the first digit being the major class to which the enzyme belongs. The following are the six major classes of enzymes and their explanations:

Oxidoreductases	Enzymes catalyzing oxidation-reduction between a pair of substrates
Transferases	Enzymes catalyzing the transfer of a group, other than hydrogen, between a pair of substrates
Hydrolases	Enzymes catalyzing hydrolysis of a variety of compounds by water
Lyases	Enzymes catalyzing reactions involving removal of a group by mechanisms other than hydrolysis, leaving double bonds
Isomerases	Enzymes catalyzing interconversion of optical, geometric, or positional isomers
Ligases	Enzymes catalyzing the linking together of two molecules, coupled with the breaking of a pyrophosphate bond

Summary of enzymes—cont'd

Name and class	Action
Nucleases	
Polynucleotidase	Acts on nucleic acids, liberating oligo- and mononucleotides
Nucleotidase	Acts on nucleotides, forming nucleosides and phosphoric acid
Nucleosidase	Acts on nucleosides, forming carbohydrate and purine or pyrimidine bases
Amidases	
Arginase	Splits arginine to ornithine and urea
Urease	Splits urea to carbon dioxide and ammonia
Asparaginase	Splits NH_2 from asparagine
Glutaminase	Splits NH_2 from glutamine
Transferases	Transfer groups from one substrate to another
Transaminase	Transfers amino groups of certain amino acids to alpha keto acids
Transacylase	Transfers acetyl group, reversibly
Transphosphorylase	Transfers phosphate groups from one compound to another
Transmethylase	Transfers methyl groups
Oxidoreductases	Concerned in biologic oxidations
Dehydrogenases	
Malic dehydrogenase	Converts malic acid to oxalacetic acid
Lactic dehydrogenase	Converts lactic acid to pyruvic acid
Succinic dehydrogenase	Converts succinic acid to fumaric acid
Oxidases	
Cytochrome oxidase	Reversible oxidation-reduction of prosthetic group from ferrous to ferric state, accepting and transferring electrons to oxygen
Xanthine oxidase	Oxidizes hypoxanthine to xanthine, then to uric acid
Phenol oxidase	Oxidizes phenol derivatives to quinones
Tyrosinase	Oxidizes tyrosine to orthoquinone
Catalase	Decomposes hydrogen peroxide, liberating molecular oxygen
Decarboxylase	Removes CO_2 without oxidation from various carboxylic acids
Hydrases	Adds to or removes water from specific substrate
Fumarase	Interconverts malic and fumaric acid
Aconitase	Interconverts citric, *cis*-aconitic, and isocitric acids
Enolase	Interconverts phosphoglyceric and phosphopyruvic acids
Isomerases	Intramolecular rearrangement; e.g., interconversion of aldose and ketose sugars
Phosphoglucose isomerase	Interconverts glucose-6- and fructose-6-phosphate
Phosphomannose isomerase	Interconverts fructose-6- and mannose-6-phosphate

■ APPENDIX K
Summary of endocrine glands

Gland and hormone	Site of action	Physiologic action
Adenohypophysis		
Adrenocorticotropic hormone (ACTH)	Adrenal cortex	Formation and secretion of adrenal cortical steroids
	Adipose tissue	Release of lipid
Follicle-stimulating hormone (FSH)	Ovaries	Development of ovarian follicles; ovulation and estrogen secretion together with luteinizing hormone
	Testes	Development of seminiferous tubules; spermatogenic activity
Luteinizing hormone (LH) or interstitial cell-stimulating hormone (ICSH)	Ovaries	Luteinization; secretion of progesterone
	Testes	Development of interstitial tissue; secretion of androgen
Luteotropic hormone (LTH) or lactogenic hormone; prolactin	Mammary gland	Development and proliferation; stimulation of milk secretion
	Corpus luteum	Functional activity and hormonal secretion
Somatotropic hormone (STH) or growth hormone	General	Growth of epiphyseal cartilages of long bones; anabolic effect on nitrogen, calcium, and phosphorus metabolism; carbohydrate metabolism; anti-insulin and diabetogenic effects
Thyroid-stimulating hormone (TSH)	Thyroid	Development and functional activity of thyroid gland and stimulation of its hormonal secretion
Neurohypophysis		
Oxytocin (pitocin)	Smooth muscle, particularly uterus	Uterine contraction; initiation of labor
	Mammary gland	Promotion of lactation and ejection of milk
Vasopressin (antidiuretic hormone or pitressin)	Kidney tubules	Reabsorption of water
	Arterioles	Increased blood pressure
Pars intermedia		
Melanocyte-stimulating hormone (MSH)	Melanophores	Darkening of skin
Adrenal cortex		
Mineralocorticoids Aldosterone Deoxycorticosterone	General	Water and electrolyte balance
Glucocorticoids Corticosterone Cortisone Hydrocortisone	General	Metabolism of carbohydrate, protein, and lipids; maintenance of circulatory and vascular homeostasis; antitoxic, antiallergic, and antishock activities
Adrenal medulla		
Epinephrine (adrenaline)	Smooth muscle, heart muscle, arterioles	Contraction of most smooth muscle; acceleration of cardiac action; constriction of certain blood vessels; relaxation of intestine; dilation of bronchi
	Liver, muscle	Glycogenolysis
	Adipose tissue	Release of lipid

Continued.

Summary of endocrine glands—cont'd

Gland and hormone	Site of action	Physiologic action
Norepinephrine (noradrenaline)	Arterioles	Constriction of practically all blood vessels; increased peripheral resistance and blood pressure
	Adipose tissue	Release of lipid
Thyroid		
Thyroxine; di- and triiodothyroxine	General	Stimulation of oxygen consumption and rate of metabolism
Parathyroid		
Parathormone	Skeleton, kidney, gastrointestinal tract	Metabolism of calcium and phosphorus; increased calcium absorption; mobilization of bone calcium; phosphate diuresis
Testes		
Androgen	Accessory sex organs	Development, maturation, and normal function; stimulation of seminal vesicles for germ cell formation
Testosterone		
Androsterone	General	Development of secondary sex characteristics; growth; skeletal and muscular development
Ovaries		
Estrogen	Accessory sex organs	Growth and development of the genitalia and mammary glands; maturation and normal cyclic function
Estradiol		
Estrone		
Estriol	General	Development of secondary sex characteristics
Corpus luteum		
Progesterone	Uterus	Induction of progestational changes of the uterine mucosa with increase in vascularity and secretory activity
	Mammary glands	Development of alveolar system
Relaxin	Symphysis pubica	Widening of the symphysis, relaxation of the cervix, and in some animals induction of parturition
Placenta		
Estrogen	Same as ovarian hormone	Same as ovarian hormone
Progesterone	Same as corpus luteum hormone	Same as corpus luteum hormone
Chorionic gonadotropin	Same as LH and FSH	Similar to LH and FSH
Pancreas		
Insulin	General	Utilization of carbohydrates and glycogen formation
	Adipose tissue	Lipogenesis
Glucagon	Liver	Glycogenolysis; increase in blood sugar level
	Adipose tissue	Release of lipid
Gastrointestinal tract		
Cholecystokinin	Gallbladder	Contraction of gallbladder and release of bile
Enterocrinin	Intestinal mucosa	Stimulation of intestinal juice secretion
Enterogastrone	Stomach	Inhibition of motility and secretion
Gastrin	Stomach	Stimulation of gastric juice secretion
Pancreozymin	Pancreas	Secretion of pancreatic juice rich in enzymes
Secretin	Pancreas	Secretion of fluid rich in alkali

■ APPENDIX L

Agencies concerned with nutrition in the United States

Official

United States Department of Agriculture
  Agricultural Research Service
  Economic Research Service
  Federal Extension Service
  Consumer and Food Economics Research Division
  Consumer and Marketing Service
  Cooperative State Research Service
Department of Health, Education, and Welfare
  Children's Bureau
  Food and Drug Administration
  Indian Health Program
  National Institutes of Health
  National Nutrition Program
  National School Lunch Program
  Office of Education
Other governmental agencies
  Agency for International Development
  Bureau of Commercial Fisheries
  Bureau of Indian Affairs
  Federal Trade Commission
  Peace Corps

Foundations

Ford Foundation
Kellogg Foundation
National Vitamin Foundation
Nutrition Foundation, Inc.
Rockefeller Foundation
Williams-Waterman Fund of the Research Corporation

Industry sponsored

American Institute of Baking
Borden Company
Campbell Soup Company
Cereal Institute
Florida Citrus Commission
General Mills, Inc.
H. J. Heinz Company
National Dairy Council
National Livestock and Meat Board
Pillsbury Company
Wheat Flour Institute

Professional organizations

AAAN	American Academy of Applied Nutrition
AAP	American Academy of Pediatrics
ABN	American Board of Nutrition
ADA	American Dental Association
ADA	American Diabetes Association
ADA	American Dietetic Association
AHA	American Heart Association
AHEA	American Home Economics Association
AIN	American Institute of Nutrition
AMA	American Medical Association, Council on Foods and Nutrition
ANA	American Nurses Association
ANS	American Nutrition Society
APHA	American Public Health Association
ASCN	American Society for Clinical Nutrition
ASFSA	American School of Food Service Association
ICAN	International College of Applied Nutrition
IFT	Institute of Food Technologists
NLN	National League for Nursing

Voluntary agencies

American Red Cross
Civic groups
Educational groups
Institutions
Social agencies

Description of selected agencies

AAAN (American Academy of Applied Nutrition). The AAAN is composed of professional and lay persons interested in nutrition, especially as it pertains to the prevention and treatment of diseases. The organization aims to promote and advance by educational means the science and art of nutrition as an integral part of the professions of dentistry and medicine. It also encourages the study of the relationship of nutrition to general medicine and dental practice. It was formerly called the American Academy of Nutrition.

ABN (American Board of Nutrition). The ABN is an organization of physicians qualified to treat nutritional and metabolic disorders and persons having doctorate degrees who work on problems of human nutrition and nutrient requirements. The board establishes standard qualification for persons desiring to be specialists in the field of human nutrition and certifies those who meet the qualifications. To be certified a candidate must have a Ph.D. degree or its equivalent in biologic science or an M.D. degree from an approved school; have completed additional special training in the principles of nutrition and underlying science; have 3 years' experience in the practical aspects of human nutrition; and pass oral and written examinations provided by the board.

ANS (American Nutrition Society). The ANS is an organization of lay persons primarily interested in nutrition. It disseminates to the public information on good health and nutrition supplied by the professional section of the American Academy of Applied Nutrition (AAAN).

FNB (Food and Nutrition Board). The FNB is a division of the National Academy of Sciences/National Research Council. It evaluates nutritional science as it applies to food processing and public health. It is composed of several committees: Amino Acids, Dietary Allowances, Fats in Human Nutrition, Milk, Food Standards, Food Protection, and Protein Malnutrition.

ICAN (International College of Applied Nutrition). The ICAN is an organization of physicians, dentists, veterinarians, and scientists in fields related to nutrition, all having doctorate degrees. Its aims are to stimulate and encourage research in the nutritional aspects of disease, to promote the science and study of nutrition and allied subjects in medical and dental schools and hospitals, and to promote greater interest among physicians, dentists, and specialists in the nutritional aspects of ecology.

■ **APPENDIX M-1**

Methods of research in nutrition: nutritional surveys

Objectives and values of nutritional surveys

The main purpose of a nutritional survey is to assess the nutritional status of a person or population. Specific objectives may be classified into basic research (e.g., to obtain data on specific lesions of nutrient inadequacies or to determine the effects of certain supplements) or applied nutrition (e.g., to motivate a community

to improve food habits or to form some basis for training nutrition workers to serve as a guideline in formulating health programs, etc.).

Techniques used in nutritional surveys

A combination of two or more of the methods listed below is more meaningful than using only one approach since nutritional status is dependent on dietary intake as well as the extent of nutrient utilization in the body.

Dietary survey. Food consumption data help detect inadequate diets and faulty food habits.

Medical history. A record of past and present illnesses, physical condition, etc. helps detect conditioning factors of malnutrition.

Clinical tests. Physical examination for any signs and symptoms suggestive of certain nutrient inadequacies will supplement dietary data in evaluating nutriture.

Instrumental or biophysical tests. Biophysical means are useful in detecting anatomic lesions observed in certain nutrient deficiencies or states of malnutrition. Examples of instruments or apparatuses employed are the biomicroscope, x-ray films, and skin calipers.

Biochemical tests. Biochemical tests are useful in detecting tissue levels of nutrients or metabolites.

For other types of information useful in nutrition studies, see Methods of research in nutrition: biochemical tests, Appendix M-4.

Ten State Nutrition Survey (National Nutrition Survey)

In 1967 Congress authorized a nutritional survey to detect the nutritional and related health problems of the Americans. This was the first comprehensive nutritional survey conducted in the United States. Due to limitations, only ten states plus one city were surveyed: California, Kentucky, Louisiana, Michigan, Massachusetts, New York, South Carolina, Texas, Washington, West Virginia, and New York City. Approximately 40,000 individuals of varying income levels were surveyed. They received a clinical examination that included a medical history, physical examination, anthropometric measurements, x-ray examination of the wrist, dental examination, and hemoglobin and hematocrit determinations. Some selected high-risk groups such as infants, young children, adolescents, pregnant or lactating women, and elderly persons received more detailed biochemical and dietary evaluations. Of the total number surveyed, 53% were 16 years or younger, 30% were from 17 to 44 years old, and 17% were 45 years or older.

The results of the Ten State Nutrition Survey indicated that a large portion of the population was malnourished or in danger of developing nutritional problems. Adolescents, particularly males, and the elderly had the greatest incidence of nutritional deficiencies. Low hemoglobin and hematocrit values were found in all age groups, indicating a high incidence of iron-deficiency anemia. A large number of pregnant and lactating women had low serum albumin levels even though their protein intakes were adequate. Vitamin A nutriture was found to be poor in Spanish Americans and also in the younger age groups. Even though iodine intake was sufficient, goiter was found frequently. Vitamin C intake was found to be low in some males and tended to decrease with age.

■ APPENDIX M-2
Methods of research in nutrition: dietary surveys*†

Methods of obtaining food consumption data of individuals

Estimation by recall. The subject or parent of subject recalls food intake within the last 24 hours (24-hour recall) or longer time. Data obtained are in ordinary servings or household measures. Aids such as food models and various cups, spoons, and glasses may be used. This method is useful in obtaining information on food habits and occurrence of certain food groups. It is easy to obtain data but this method gives a qualitative rather than a quantitative picture of the dietary intake.

Food record. The subject or parent of subject

keeps a day-to-day record for varying lengths of time (usually 3 to 7 days) of all food eaten using common measures. Nutrient intake can be calculated using food composition tables. This method is useful in nutritional surveys or studies of food habits. Accuracy depends on full cooperation of recorder and his ability to correctly estimate quantities of servings.

Dietary history. The history is a combination of the first two methods; subject recalls and keeps food records for a relatively long period of time. This is useful for food habits study or for following progress in nutrition programs, especially of mothers and children.

Weighed intake. The subject or a trained person weighs all foods consumed. Samples may be set aside for analysis or nutrient intake is calculated using food composition tables. This method is time-consuming and is limited to metabolic studies. In nutritional surveys, weighed intake method is sometimes used, depending on the objectives of the study and the degree of accuracy desired.

Methods of obtaining food consumption data by groups of persons

Food account. The recorder keeps a running report of food purchased or produced that enters the household or institution. The length of data collection varies, depending on the complexity of the diet and the aims of the study. This method is simple but the summarizing task is tedious. The food account is useful for checking trends of food purchases by families and institutions.

Food list by recall. The housekeeper or recorder estimates quantities (by weight or measure) of all foods consumed in previous days, usually 3 to 7 days. A complete list of food items is used to aid the subject in recalling data. Nutrients are calculated using food composition tables or key food groups are noted. This method is less tedious for the recorder but needs proper scheduling and well-trained interviewers.

Food record. The recorder weighs food before and after the study period. Day-to-day inventory is taken by weighing all foods that enter the household or institution with or without recording kitchen or plate wastes. Nutrients are calculated using food composition tables. This method tends to be more accurate than the first two methods, but it is costly and time-consuming.

---

*Adopted from USDA and FAO materials.
†The dietary survey as the primary tool of research in nutritional surveys is effective only if the following are observed: accurate recording and accurate weighing or measuring; adequate sampling of foods consumed; accurate application of food composition tables, exchange lists, or other tools for evaluation by the researchers and aides; proper interpretation of results; and correlation of results with other data obtained from clinical, biochemical, and other methods used in nutrition studies.

■ **APPENDIX M-3**

Methods of research in nutrition: clinical tests*

PHYSICAL SIGNS ASSOCIATED WITH MALNUTRITION

General appearance. Apathetic.

Hair. Dry, staring; dyspigmented.

Skin, facial. Seborrhea, nasolabial; seborrhea, other; erythema, folliculosis.

Skin, general. Dryness and scaling; crackled skin; hyperpigmentation; depigmentation; follicular keratosis; perifolliculosis; acne-form eruption; thick, pigmented pressure points; purpura and petechia; bluish red, cold extremites; pellagra-form lesions; "crazy pavement" dermatitis; telangiectasis; redness of palms; nails brittle, flaking, ridging, spoon shaped.

Eyes. Bitot's spots; canthi, fissures; circumcorneal injection; conjunctival infection.

Lids. Blepharitis, follicular hypertrophy.

Lips and mouth. Angular lesions; angular scars; cheilosis; pallor; ulcerations.

Tongue. Papillary atrophy; papillary hypertrophy; magenta color; red tip and/or sides; fissures; erosions or ulcers; serrations and swelling.

Teeth. Caries; edentulous; dentures; fluorosis.

Gums. Marginal redness; marginal swelling; bleeding.

Thyroid. Enlarged (colloid goiter).

Parotid gland. Bilateral enlargement.

Neuromuscular. Calf tenderness; loss of ankle or knee jerks; "burning feet"; motor weakness, paralysis; loss of vibratory sense; loss of positional sense; hypesthesia and anesthesia; tetany.

Skeletal. Posture; frontal or parietal bosses; protuberant abdomen; Harrison's groove; knock-knees; bowlegs; enlarged wrists; enlarged costochondral junctions; flaring ribs; winged scapula; abnormalities of sternum.

Cardiovascular. Hypotension; bradycardia or tachycardia; cardiac enlargement; abnormalities of rhythm; murmurs; cardiac failure.

Liver. Enlarged, nodular.

Symptoms and signs suggestive of deficiencies of certain nutrients

Caloric deficiency. Underweight and underheight; wasting of tissues.

Protein deficiency, adults. Weight loss; wasting of muscles; enlarged liver; edema.

Protein deficiency, infants and children (kwashiorkor). Growth retardation; depigmentation or hyperpigmentation of skin; dyspigmentation of hair; enlarged liver; peevish mental apathy; edema.

Vitamin A deficiency. Night blindness; xerophthalmia; Bitot's spots; dry, scaling skin; follicular hyperkeratosis.

Thiamin deficiency. Burning soles of feet; numbness and tingling of toes; calf muscle tenderness; hyperesthesia or hypesthesia of feet and legs; loss of vibratory sense; absent patellar and Achilles reflexes; motor weakness (squat test); edema; advanced polyneuropathy; beriberi heart disease; Wernicke's encephalopathy; retrobulbar neuritis; central ophthalmoplegia.

Riboflavin deficiency. Photophobia, lacrimation, burning, and itching of eyes; soreness of lips and tongue; circumcorneal injection and corneal vascularization; cheilosis; angular maceration and fissures; glossitis (purplish color, abnormalities of papillae); nasolabial seborrhea.

Niacin deficiency. Soreness and burning of tongue; chronic diarrhea; glossitis (redness, swelling, serrations, abnormalities of papillae); pellagrous dermatitis; mental changes (anxiety, depression, hallucinations, disorientation); encephalopathic states.

Vitamin B$_6$ deficiency. Seborrheic dermatitis; glossitis; angular stomatitis; peripheral neuropathy.

Folic acid deficiency. Weakness and pallor; glossitis (redness, abnormalities of papillae); diarrhea, steatorrhea.

Vitamin B$_{12}$ deficiency. Weakness and pallor; glossitis (redness, abnormalities of papillae); subacute combined sclerosis; peripheral neuropathy.

Ascorbic acid deficiency. Purpura, petechiae, ecchymoses; red, swollen, bleeding gums; perifolliculosis; poor wound healing.

Vitamin D deficiency. Craniotabes; frontal and parietal bosses; enlarged joints (wrists and ankles); Harrison's groove; enlarged costochondral junctions; deformities of sternum; bowlegs or knock-knees; osteomalacia.

Vitamin K deficiency. Hemorrhagic manifestations and jaundice.

Calcium deficiency. Paresthesia; carpopedal spasm; convulsions.

---

*From Goldsmith, G.: Nutritional diagnosis, Springfield, Ill., 1959, Charles C Thomas, Publisher.

Methods of research in nutrition—cont'd

Iodine deficiency. Simple goiter.

Iron deficiency. Weakness and pallor; chronic glossitis, koilonychia.

Magnesium deficiency. Gross muscle tremor; delirium.

Potassium deficiency. Muscular weakness, hypotonia; flaccid paralysis; cardiac or respiratory failure.

Sodium deficiency. Weakness, apathy; anorexia, nausea, vomiting; muscle cramps; peripheral circulatory collapse.

■ APPENDIX M-4

Methods of research in nutrition: biochemical tests

Uses and limitations of the biochemical method

The main purpose of biochemical tests is to help assess the nutritional status of a person or population group. Suboptimal nutriture that cannot be recognized by clinical manifestations can be detected by biochemical tests, using one or more of the techniques listed below. To be an effective tool of research in nutrition, this method depends on accuracy, sensitivity, and reproducibility of a particular analytical technique for a nutrient or its metabolite; proper sampling and collection of urine, blood, tissue, etc.; facilities for transportation, storage, laboratory space, etc.; proper interpretation of results; and availability of reagents, time, trained workers, etc.

Techniques or general types of biochemical tests

Blood level. The concentration of a particular nutrient or its metabolite in the plasma, blood cells, or whole blood is determined and compared with normal levels; this measurement reflects recent nutrient intake. For further details, see Normal constituents of blood, Appendix Q.

Tissue biopsy. Especially useful in experimental animal nutrition, e.g., liver biopsy or whole carcass analysis.

Saturation or load tests. The degree of tissue storage or nutrient depletion is determined. For details, see *Load test* in the text.

Urine level. The amount of nutrient or its metabolic end product excreted in the urine is measured; it reflects immediate past nutrient intake. Examples of data suggestive of certain deficiencies are as follows:

Nutrient or metabolite in urine	Deficient level
N-methylnicotinamide (mg/6 hr)	0.2
Riboflavin (μg/6 hr)	10.0
Thiamin (μg/6 hr)	10.0
Folic acid, after 5 mg folic acid orally (mg)	<1.5
Xanthurenic acid, after 10 gm tryptophan (mg/24 hr)	>50

Summary of information for nutrition studies

Food balance sheet. Gives a gross estimate of agricultural production, soil fertility, extent of food imports and exports, etc. It determines the availability of food.

Socioeconomic data. Supplementary information on purchasing power of families; distribution of available food, lack of knowledge; attitudes, beliefs, habits, etc.

Dietary survey. Gives qualitative and/or quantitative nutrient intakes of a person or group of individuals; detects "unsatisfactory diets." See Dietary survey, Appendix M-2.

Vital and health statistics. Morbidity and mortality data are especially useful in pointing out the vulnerable groups in the population.

Anthropometric measurements. Useful in assessing nutritional status because of the direct effects of nutrients on physical development. See Methods of research in nutrition: nutritional surveys, Appendix M-1.

Clinical methods. Physical signs and symptoms that deviate from a normal healthy picture may indicate certain nutrient inadequacies. See Methods of research in nutrition: clinical tests, Appendix M-3.

Biochemical tests. Deviations from the normal levels of nutrients or metabolites in body fluids or tissues may indicate malnutrition.

■ APPENDIX N

Applications of isotopes in biology and medicine

Isotope	Application
Carbon 13 or 14	Investigative: tracer studies for labeling metabolites, carcinogens, or injected drugs
Chromium 51	Diagnostic: study of blood volume, blood cell life, and cardiac output with radioactive labeled erythrocytes
Cobalt 60	Therapeutic: inexpensive gamma ray therapy and interstitial radiation for malignancies
Deuterium	Investigative: tracer studies and body water determination
Gold 198	Therapeutic: metastasized cancer and other malignant tumors, carcinomas, and lymphomas; chronic leukemia
Iodine 131	Therapeutic: cancer of the thyroid and lungs; hyperthyroidism; severe heart disease
	Diagnostic: study of thyroid and antithyroid activity and drugs; determination of cardiac output, blood plasma volume, and location of brain tumors; fat absorption; pancreatic function
Iron 59	Diagnostic: study of blood volume, iron metabolism, and blood transfusion
Lead 210	Therapeutic: lesions and benign conditions of the eye
Nitrogen 15 or 14	Investigative: tracer studies (metabolism of protein, amino acids, nucleic acids, etc.)
Oxygen 18	Investigative: tracer studies
Phosphorus 32	Therapeutic: chronic leukemia; polycythemia vera; lymphomas; brain tumor
	Diagnostic: determination of blood volume; study of peripheral vascular disease
Potassium 42	Diagnostic: localization of brain tumors; study of potassium metabolism; determination of intracellular fluid volume
Radium 226	Therapeutic: treatment of malignancies by interstitial radiation (cancers of uterine cervix and fundus, urinary bladder, skin, and metastatic cancer of the lymph nodes)
Sodium 24	Diagnostic: study of peripheral vascular disease, sodium metabolism, and extracellular fluid volume
Strontium 90	Therapeutic: benign conditions of the eye, traumatic corneal ulceration, and small lesions
Tritium	Investigative: tracer studies; body water composition

■ APPENDIX O

Dietary management of selected disorders

Adrenocortical insufficiency High protein, high calorie, and high salt diet. To avoid hypoglycemia, serve meals frequently with between-meal feedings. In ACTH therapy, mild sodium restriction is often necessary. Avoidance of salty foods and no added salt on the table is usually sufficient.

Alcoholic liver disease Withdrawal of alcohol and a diet high in protein and vitamins, especially the B complex vitamins. Poor food intake and consequent malnutrition contribute to the fatty liver and alcoholic hepatitis. The objectives of the diet are nutritional rehabilitation, correction of deficiency states, and repair of hepatic and neural damage caused by inadequate nutrition.

Alkaptonuria The exact dietary treatment is not yet known, although restriction of dietary protein to reduce homogentisic acid formation may be of some value.

Allergy Avoid or exclude the offending food allergen from the diet. Take note of forms of food preparation in which the food allergen may be used. When the offending food allergen is not known, one of several test diets for allergy may be used. See *Diet, Rowe's elimination,* in the text.

Anemia, folic acid–deficiency A diet liberal in protein of high biologic value with folic acid and vitamin C supplementation. Emphasis is placed on liver, meats, fish, legumes, deep green leafy vegetables, citrus fruits, and other vitamin C–rich foods. Vitamin C is necessary for the conversion of folic acid to its metabolically active form, folinic acid.

Anemia, iron-deficiency A diet high in iron, protein of high biologic value, and vitamin C for absorption of iron. Foods high in iron include liver, egg yolk, kidney, beef, dried fruits, molasses, and whole-grain cereals.

Anemia, pernicious Vitamin B_{12} in therapeutic doses plus a diet high in protein of good biologic value with iron and vitamin supplementation. A sore mouth or gastrointestinal irritation may necessitate a soft or even liquid diet.

Anemia, protein-deficiency The protein level in the diet should be very high (2.5 to 3.0 gm/kg or approximately 120 to 150 gm/day). Carbohydrate and caloric intake should be high for proper utilization of protein.

Anorexia nervosa It is best not to press food at the beginning, since rejection of food is part of the illness. Serve attractive and palatable meals in small quantities and gradually increase the amount until 3000 or more calories are being consumed. When the patient refuses to eat, it may be necessary to give food by tube feeding.

Arginosuccinic aciduria The exact dietary treatment is not known. Protein restriction with arginine supplementation has been tried.

Arthritis There is no specific dietary regimen as long as the nutritional status of the patient is satisfactory. A reduction in weight is advisable in osteoarthritis to lessen the extra weight placed on weight-bearing joints. On the other hand, patients with rheumatoid arthritis who have lost weight and are malnourished should be given a high calorie, high protein diet. Some sodium restriction may be necessary in ACTH therapy. Patients with a type IV plasma lipid profile may benefit from a type IV diet for hyperlipoproteinemia. See discussion of dietary management of hyperlipoproteinemia.

Ascites Rigid sodium restriction is usually required (250 mg/day in severe cases; 500 mg/

day in milder cases). Diuresis may occur within a few days or weeks. As the fluid retention subsides, the sodium restriction can be liberalized gradually up to 2000 mg/day. See *Diet, sodium-restricted,* in the text.

Atherosclerosis The diet is aimed at lowering serum lipid concentrations. This can be achieved by decreasing calorie intake, restricting cholesterol intake to 300 mg or less per day, and substituting vegetable oils rich in polyunsaturated fats in place of saturated fats. Weight reduction is indicated for the overweight.

Burns A high calorie, high protein, high fluid diet liberal in vitamins, especially vitamin C. Restore fluid and electrolyte balance to prevent shock. Tube feeding may be necessary if the patient is unable to eat or drink.

Calculi Urinary calculi are seldom "pure." They are usually a mixture of several substances such as uric acid, cystine, calcium oxalate, calcium carbonate, and calcium phosphate. Once the stones are formed, no diet is effective in bringing about their dissolution. However, for the predisposed individual, dietary management may help prevent or retard the growth or recurrence of the stones The type of diet depends on the chief component of the stones. Restrict calcium and phosphorus in calcium phosphate stones; maintain an acid urine in magnesium phosphate stones; restrict sulfur-containing amino acids and maintain an alkaline urine in cystine stones; restrict oxalate and calcium intakes in calcium oxalate stones; and maintain an alkaline urine to keep urate stones in solution. A high fluid intake is recommended in all types of stone formation. See *Diet, ash; Diet, calcium-phosphorus–restricted;* and *Diet, oxalate-restricted,* in the text.

Cancer Appetizing food is emphasized since anorexia is common. Cancer in the gastrointestinal tract may require a bland, low fiber diet given in small, frequent feedings. A low residue diet or elemental diet is indicated in cancer of the bowel. A mechanical soft diet consisting of smooth, semisolid foods is indicated in cancer of the esophagus. Tube feeding is often used when there is difficulty in swallowing.

Cardiac diseases Caloric intake is adjusted to bring about weight loss and consequent lowering of blood pressure, slowing of heart rate, and reduction in the work of the heart. Rest is the primary consideration in acute heart diseases such as heart failure or coronary occlusion. Even fluids are restricted during the first few days. With improvement, soft and easily digested foods are gradually introduced in small amounts as tolerated. Sodium intake is restricted to 500 mg in edema and then maintained at 1000 to 1500 mg/day once edema disappears. In ischemic heart disease involving hypercholesterolemia and atherosclerosis the fat in the diet should be predominantly of the polyunsaturated type; cholesterol and saturated fats are restricted. In chronic heart condition, three small meals with between-meal feedings are recommended to avoid strain on the heart. Constipation should be avoided and maintenance of normal or slightly below normal weight is desirable. Sodium may be mildly restricted (2000 mg/day) to prevent edema.

Celiac disease A gluten-restricted diet high in calories and protein (6 to 8 gm/kg body weight) with mineral and vitamin supplementation to correct nutritional deficiency states resulting from impaired absorption. In infants with severe diarrhea, immediate administration of fluid and electrolytes is necessary. Fat is restricted in the milk formula. Simple carbohydrates and fruits and selected starches, such as corn, rice, arrowroot, cassava, and potato, supply the remaining calories. The restriction in gluten intake should be regarded as a permanent diet in this condition. See *Diet, gluten-free,* in the text.

Cerebral palsy A high calorie diet (up to 4000 calories) for the athetoid type or those who are constantly in motion and are often underweight and a low calorie diet for the spastic type or those who are prone to obesity because of limited activity. Vitamins, especially the B complex, and mineral supplements are usually needed. Tube feeding may be indicated when there is difficulty in swallowing.

Cholecystectomy After surgery, give a low fat diet for a month or longer and then gradually increase fat intake as tolerated. The amount of fat tolerated varies with individual patients. Avoid excessive intake of bulky, rich, and fatty foods in one meal.

Cholecystitis A low fat bland diet is indicated. Restriction in fat intake will prevent stimulation of gallbladder contraction. In acute cases, nothing is given orally for 24 hours or more.

Then a clear liquid diet is given for 2 to 3 days, and the diet is progressed to one low in fat (20 to 30 gm/day) and restricted in coarse fiber. In chronic cholecystitis a moderate intake of fat (40 to 50 gm/day) is indicated to promote the flow of bile and induce drainage of the biliary tract. Weight reduction is desirable for the overweight.

Cholelithiasis When stones form an obstruction or the gallbladder is inflamed, give a low fat diet to decrease gallbladder contraction and lessen the pain. A moderate fat intake is desirable if the gallbladder is sluggish or "lazy" to stimulate its contraction and prevent stagnation of bile. It is unlikely that restriction of cholesterol in the diet has any appreciable effect on reducing cholesterol stones. Weight reduction is indicated for the overweight.

Cirrhosis A high calorie, high protein, high carbohydrate diet with a moderate amount of fat and plenty of vitamins, especially B complex vitamins. The objectives of dietary treatment are to promote healing and regeneration of liver tissue and prevent fat stasis and formation of fibrous tissues. Allow 2 gm protein/kg desirable body weight and 300 to 350 gm carbohydrate to spare protein. Protein should be immediately curtailed in impending coma. Restrict sodium to 500 mg or less if ascites and peripheral edema are present, and avoid fibrous and coarse foods if esophageal varices are present. Alcohol is not allowed.

Citrullinemia The exact dietary treatment is not known. Protein restriction is recommended to control blood ammonia.

Cleft palate Inability to suck adequately presents a problem. In the newborn a medicine dropper or a plastic bottle and a soft nipple with an enlarged hole may be used. Milk can be squeezed a little at a time in coordination with the infant's chewing motions. When starting solid foods, pureed baby foods may be mixed with milk in the bottle or diluted with milk and spoon-fed.

Colostomy Start with a clear liquid diet and progress gradually to one low in residue. Then give soft and short-fibered foods as tolerated. A high calorie, high protein intake will speed up recovery and prevent weight loss.

Constipation Diet is not a cure but provides relief or comfort to the patient. In atonic constipation a high fiber diet will stimulate peristalsis, provide bulk to the intestinal contents, and help retain water in the feces to facilitate bowel movement. Emphasis is placed on liberal intakes of whole-grain cereals, raw fruits, and vegetables. In spastic constipation a low fiber diet will prevent undue distention and stimulation of the bowel. See *Diet, fiber modified,* in the text.

Coronary heart disease Weight reduction and/or maintenance of desirable weight by an appropriate combination of physical activity and caloric intake is desirable. Specific dietary advice varies with the nature of the blood lipid profile. For details, see discussion of the dietary management of hyperlipoproteinemia.

Cystathioninuria Large intakes of pyridoxine (vitamin B_6) seem beneficial. A commercial powder preparation low in methionine and cystine has been used.

Cystic fibrosis A high calorie, high protein, low fat diet supplemented with fat-soluble vitamins. A pancreatic enzyme preparation (e.g., pancreatin and Cotazym) should be taken at each meal and even with snacks to compensate for the pancreatic deficiency. For infants a half skim milk formula is suggested. Several formulated milk preparations high in protein and low in fat are available commercially. (See Proprietary foods: composition, features, and uses, Appendix P-1.) As much fat as can be tolerated should be given as determined by the number and bulk of stools and the presence of abdominal discomfort. If fat has to be severely restricted, MCT oil may be used to increase fat intake. During the acute stage, starch is often not well tolerated. Give only simple carbohydrates. Generous salt intake may be necessary to replace sodium losses in sweat. As the condition improves, fat and starchy carbohydrates are gradually introduced and adjusted to the individual's tolerance.

Cystinuria A high fluid intake is desirable to dilute the urine. An alkaline-ash diet is sometimes prescribed. See *Diet, ash,* in the text.

Diabetes mellitus The most important dietary consideration is control of total caloric intake to attain or maintain desirable weight. This means weight reduction for the overweight and weight increase to achieve desirable weight for the underweight, especially the young diabetics who are insulin dependent. Individualizing the diet to specific needs of the patient is essential. A more liberal intake of carbohydrate (up to 60% of calories) in the form of polysaccharides may be allowed. However, ingestion of concentrated simple sugars should be minimized to avoid hyperglycemic peaks. Limitation in intake of saturated fat and cholesterol is recommended to reduce the predisposition to the development of atherosclerotic disease. Also important is regular spacing of meals to avoid intermittent hypoglycemia, particularly among those receiving insulin therapy.

Diabetic coma Immediate treatment consisting of insulin, electrolytes, and fluids is essential. In severe ketoacidosis, fluid and electrolyte administration must usually be intravenous. A 5% glucose solution is given as hyperglycemia and glycosuria subside. If there is no vomiting, salty broth and tea may be given, followed by fruit juices and other liquids.

Diarrhea Food is withheld for 12 to 24 hours and fluids and electrolytes are given to prevent dehydration. As the stools are formed, small amounts of food may be gradually introduced. In infants, give a half-strength formula low in carbohydrate and fat or use a special proprietary milk preparation such as Probana or Nutramigen. The addition of 5% to 10% apple powder, banana flakes, or pectin-agar mixture may hasten the development of formed stools. In adults, start with simple foods such as broth, tea, and toast. Gradually introduce foods low in residue and build up to a normal diet as the condition improves.

Disaccharide intolerance Exclude the poorly tolerated disaccharide from the diet and replace with utilizable carbohydrate. Supplementation with the deficient enzyme is beneficial in the initial stage. The enzyme deficiency is apparently compensated for in later years.

Diverticular disease The main therapeutic goal is to increase the caliber of the stools and distend the bowel wall. Thus the low residue diet is not recommended, except during acute phases of diverticulitis, ulcerative colitis, or infectious enterocolitis when the bowel is markedly inflamed. Initially, clear liquids or an elemental diet may be given. The diet may gradually progress to a regular diet. However, it is still advisable to avoid excessive intake of raw fruits and vegetables because of their mild laxative effect. Excessive intake of spices such as pepper and chili pepper should also be avoided. A bulk-forming agent such as methyl-cellulose is beneficial in initiating normal colonic function and regular bowel action.

Dumping syndrome Dietary management consists of small dry meals given at frequent intervals with liquids taken between meals (usually 30 to 45 minutes after meals). The diet should be high in protein, moderate in fat, and low in carbohydrate. Foods that have a strong osmolar effect such as sugars, sweets, and jellies are omitted. Artificial sweeteners may be used. Milk and dishes containing milk frequently precipitate symptoms and hence should also be omitted or limited. It is important to rest before meals, eat slowly, chew well, and relax after meals.

Dysentery During the acute stage, give only clear liquids in the form of broth, tea, and thin gruel. Gradually add strained fruit juices and boiled milk as tolerated. When the condition improves, nonirritating foods low in fiber may be gradually added to the diet.

Dyspepsia No simple dietary rule can be set down. Food should be adequate, well cooked, not too spicy, and served in a relaxed atmosphere. It is best to eat small meals at a time. In majority of cases, dyspepsia is of nervous origin and disappears once the psychoneurotic cause is removed. If due to organic causes, a soft diet low in fat may be beneficial.

Emphysema A soft, high calorie diet is usually indicated. Patients experience difficulty in eating breakfast and are short of breath after a night's sleep. Give concentrated foods in small, frequent feedings. Avoid fibrous fruits and vegetables and tough meats that will require much chewing.

Enteritis A high calorie, liberal protein, low fiber diet with vitamin and mineral supplementation. Moderately restrict fats (25% of calories) in regional enteritis with malabsorption steatorrhea. In severe cases, strict fat restriction (as low as 10% of calories) may be necessary. The use of MCT oil is desirable in such cases.

Epilepsy As a rule, a normal diet for the individual's age and activity is prescribed when drug therapy is used. However, the ketogenic diet is still valuable in the control of some specific types of seizures that do not respond to drug therapy alone. To produce a state of ketosis, a ketogenic-antiketogenic ratio of 3:1 or 4:1 is maintained. To obtain this, carbohydrate is drastically reduced and the bulk of calories is taken from fat. Protein is maintained at normal levels. A typical 1800-calorie ketogenic diet would have a nutrient distribution of 50 gm protein, 30 gm carbohydrate, and 170 gm fat. The regimen is instituted with a starvation period of 3 to 5 days. Nothing is given orally except for small amounts of water until the patient has lost about 10% of his weight and/or his urine reveals marked acidosis. The use of medium-chain triglycerides (MCT oil) is found to be more effective than dietary fats in inducing ketosis. It also allows more carbohydrate, making the diet more palatable. A typical MCT-ketogenic diet has a calorie distribution of 60% MCT oil, 10% dietary fat, 10% protein, and 20% carbohydrate.

Fever and febrile conditions The diet should be high in calories, protein, carbohydrate, salt, and fluid. Recommended intakes are 3000 to 3500 calories to meet increased energy needs due to higher basal metabolic rate; 100 to 120 gm protein to replace nitrogen losses and tissue destruction characteristic of febrile conditions; 300 to 350 gm carbohydrate to replenish depleted glycogen stores and spare protein; and 10 to 15 cups of liquid per day, preferably as salty broths, fruit juices, and milk, to replace fluid lost through perspiration and to facilitate elimination of toxins through increased urination. The consistency of the diet varies with the condition. In acute fever it may be necessary to give a full liquid diet. With recovery, progress the diet to soft and then regular consistency. Frequent small feedings are better tolerated than large meals.

Fracture A high calorie, liberal protein diet with mineral and vitamin supplementation. Important nutrients to consider are protein, for bone matrix formation; calcium and phosphorus, for deposition in bone; vitamin D, for efficient utilization of calcium; and vitamin C, for intercellular cementing substance.

Galactosemia Give a galactose-free diet. Milk and milk products are not allowed. Nonmilk formulas are available commercially for infants. For details, see *Diet, galactose-free,* in the text. See also Proprietary foods: composition, features, and uses, Appendix P-1, for nonmilk preparations.

Gastrectomy Small but frequent feeding of easily digested foods. The progression of the diet varies with the extent of gastric resection and tolerance of the patient for food. The usual progression consists of hourly feeding of 60 to 90 ml water on the first day, clear liquids on the second day, and full liquids on the third day. Starting on the fourth day, soft and easily digested solid foods chosen from stage III of the progressive bland diet are gradually introduced. As the patient improves, six small feedings of soft, low fiber foods are given, keeping the carbohydrate intake relatively low. Mineral and vitamin supplements are needed because of impaired absorption.

Gastritis During the acute stage, food is restricted for 24 to 48 hours to rest the stomach. For relief of thirst, small amounts of water or bits of crushed ice may be given. Food is progressed until the patient can take a soft diet. In chronic gastritis, stage IV of the progressive bland diet given in small, frequent feedings may be used initially, with progression to greater amounts and wider variety of foods as tolerated by the patient. Some restrictions in fat intake may be beneficial, as fat depresses gastric acid production and motility. Alcohol is to be avoided.

Glomerulonephritis Sufficient calories must be supplied by carbohydrate and fat to spare protein and reduce breakdown of endogenous or body protein. Salt intake is restricted to 500 to 1000 mg in the presence of edema and high blood pressure, and fluid intake is restricted to 500 to 700 ml when there is oliguria. Protein restriction is indicated only when there is nitrogen retention. Allow 0.2 to 0.3 gm/kg body weight (about 15 to 20 gm protein) of high quality protein supplied chiefly by egg and milk protein. As the condition improves, protein intake is gradually increased until a normal allowance is taken. In chronic glomerulonephritis, normal protein intake of 0.9 to 1.0 gm/kg body weight is sufficient to maintain nitrogen balance. There is no sufficient evidence that a high protein diet is useful and will make up for losses in the urine. Sodium intake is restricted in the presence of edema.

Gluten-induced enteropathy Elimination of wheat, oat, rye, barley, and buckwheat from the diet. See *Diet, gliadin-free,* in the text.

Glycinuria Protein restriction with arginine and pyridoxine supplementation may be beneficial. The exact dietary treatment is not known.

Glycogen storage disease A high protein diet given in small, frequent feedings. The use of corticosteroids in the control of hypoglycemia may require mild sodium restriction.

Gout Weight reduction for the obese is beneficial. The diet should be high in carbohydrate to increase urate excretion and low in fat, since fat inhibits excretion of uric acid. During acute gouty attacks, some physicians prescribe a diet restricted in purine. Alcoholic drinks should be avoided. Therapy by drugs has largely replaced rigid purine restriction in the diet. Patients with increased plasma triglyceride concentrations may benefit from the type IV diet for hyperlipoproteinemia. See *Diet, purine-restricted,* in the text. See also discussion of the dietary management of hyperlipoproteinemia.

Hartnup disease A liberal protein intake (90 to 120 gm/day) with niacin and pyridoxine supplementation has been recommended.

Heartburn A soft diet given in six small meals. Avoid excessive intake of alcohol. Also avoid spices, gas-forming vegetables, rapid eating, and large meals.

Hemorrhoids A low fiber diet is indicated to provide comfort for the patient. A high fluid intake (8 to 10 glasses) is also desirable to avoid constipation and to reduce possible irritation from too much roughage. Irritants such as highly seasoned foods, relishes, and harsh laxatives should be avoided. After hemorrhoidectomy, progress the diet from clear liquids to full liquids without milk and then to the low residue and soft diets until the patient is fully recovered.

Hepatic coma The basic principle of the diet is to avoid tissue protein catabolism and to reduce ammonia production. It is not always necessary to reduce protein intake. Initial treatment may be directed at reducing the intestinal production of ammonia by bacteria. When antibiotic therapy is not sufficient or effective, it may be necessary to restrict dietary protein. The level of protein restriction may range from 0 (protein free) to between 0.2 and 0.3 gm/kg body weight. Protein restriction should be used for as short a time as possible because it is important in healing the liver tissue. As the condition improves, increase the protein intake by 10 to 20 gm daily until a normal allowance is consumed. Provide sufficient calories from carbohydrate and fat (1800 calories or more) to keep body tissue breakdown to a minimum. See *Diet, protein modified,* in the text.

Hepatitis A high calorie, liberal protein, high

carbohydrate, and moderate fat intake. The objectives of the diet are to aid in the regeneration of liver tissue and to avoid further injury to the liver. A high calorie intake of 3000 to 4000 calories will counteract weight loss and assist in maximum utilization of protein. A liberal protein intake of 90 to 110 gm/day or an allowance of 1.5 to 2 gm/kg is sufficient for regeneration and maintenance of liver tissue. A carbohydrate intake of 300 to 400 gm daily will protect the liver against injury, ensure a large glycogen reserve for liver function, and spare protein. Recent investigations reveal that fat intake may be liberalized as long as carbohydrate and protein intakes are adequate. Give the diet in liquid or semiliquid form during the acute phase of the disease, gradually progressing the diet to a soft and eventually a regular diet as the condition improves. Frequent small feedings are better tolerated than three large meals.

Hiatus hernia Small, frequent feedings to prevent gastric distention. Avoid eating 2 hours before retiring.

Hypercholesterolemia Weight reduction for the obese, reduction in cholesterol intake to 300 mg or less, moderate restriction in fat, and replacement of saturated fats with those containing polyunsaturated fatty acids. See *Diet, cholesterol-restricted, fat-controlled,* in the text. See also the discussion of the hyperlipoproteinemia type II diet.

Hyperinsulinism Carbohydrate in the diet should be drastically reduced (75 to 125 gm/day) to minimize the production of insulin. A high protein intake (120 gm or more) is recommended; fat furnishes the remaining calories. The diet is calculated using the food exchange lists, and the day's food allowance is divided into three meals with equal distribution of carbohydrate, protein, and fat. In planning meals, bread and starchy carbohydrates are ordinarily omitted. Milk, fruits, and vegetables supply the prescribed carbohydrate. Artificial sweeteners may be used.

Hyperlipoproteinemia Five types of diets have been recommended by the National Institutes of Health, depending on the particular lipoprotein fraction that is elevated in the blood. These diets are summarized below.

Type I The diet is aimed at restricting the intake of dietary fat to a minimum level (35 gm or less daily) to keep blood triglycerides low and prevent abdominal pain associated with the ingestion of dietary fat. The intakes of carbohydrate, protein, and cholesterol are not restricted. Alcohol is not recommended. All separable fats and oils are eliminated and only lean, trimmed meat is used. Meat is restricted to 5 ounces cooked weight per day. Additional protein should come from skim milk, fruits, and vegetables. To increase fat intake, 30 to 40 gm of medium-chain triglycerides may be prescribed. The medium-chain triglycerides are absorbed directly into the portal system and transported to the liver without chylomicron formation.

Type II The diet involves lowering the intake of cholesterol to 300 mg or less per day, restricting the intake of saturated fats, and increasing the use of vegetable oils and margarines high in polyunsaturated fatty acids to give a P/S ratio of about 2. All foods high in cholesterol are eliminated and the desired P/S ratio may be achieved by consuming 2 teaspoons polyunsaturated fat or oil per ounce of cooked meat. Calories, carbohydrate, and protein are not restricted. Alcohol may be used with discretion.

Type III Initially, a weight reduction diet if necessary and then maintenance of desirable weight. Carbohydrate and fat intake are controlled to contribute 40% of calories from each. Protein intake is high at 20% of calories. Sugars and concentrated sweets are to be avoided and polyunsaturated fats are preferred to saturated fats, although the P/S ratio is not emphasized. Cholesterol is restricted to 300 mg or less per day. Alcohol is limited to two servings per day in exchange for a serving from the bread or cereal group.

Type IV Weight reduction to attain desirable body weight, followed by a maintenance diet restricted in carbohydrate and alcohol (excess of either tends to increase endogenous triglyceride concentrations). Protein and fat intakes are not limited, although saturated fats should be restricted and replaced with polyunsaturated fats. Cholesterol is only moderately restricted to 300 to 500 mg/day, with an allowance of 3 egg yolks/week or the substitution of 2 ounces of organ meats or cheddar cheese for an egg. Because of its caloric content and its effect on blood triglycerides, the total amount of alcohol is limited to two servings per day, which should be taken as a substitute for bread.

Type V After weight reduction, a maintenance diet is prescribed with the following modifications: restricted and modified fat, controlled carbohydrate, and moderately restricted cholesterol (300 to 500 mg/day). Alcohol is not recommended. Fat is computed at 25% to 30% of total calories (50 to 85 gm/day). It is best to keep the level of fat in the diet as low as possible. A fat allowance of 1 gm/kg body weight is a safe intake. The P/S ratio is not emphasized. However, polyunsaturated fats are recommended in preference to saturated fats. Carbohydrate is about 50% of total calories. Because of restricted fat and carbohydrate intakes, the protein intake is higher than the normal intake (20% to 25% of calories or an allowance of 1.5 gm or more/kg body weight).

Hypertension Weight reduction for the overweight is desirable. Strict sodium restriction (200 to 250 mg/day) is the best dietary regimen for lowering blood pressure. The diet, however, is unpalatable, difficult to follow, and requires about a month or longer before noticeable improvement may be seen. The use of antihypertensive drugs combined with mild sodium restriction (1500 to 2000 mg/day) has become the cornerstone of therapy. See *Diet, sodium-restricted*, in the text.

Hyperthyroidism A high calorie, liberal protein and carbohydrate diet with calcium, phosphorus, and vitamin D and B complex supplementation. The basic aim of the diet is to compensate for the increase in basal metabolic rate (3500 to 4000 calories) and nitrogen metabolism (90 to 120 gm protein). A high carbohydrate intake will replenish depleted liver glycogen storage. Vitamin D is essential for the utilization of calcium and phosphorus, and the B complex vitamins are needed for the increased caloric intake and high basal metabolic rate.

Hypoglycemia Mild hypoglycemic reactions to insulin disappear following ingestion of fruit juice or candy. In the fasting type of hypoglycemia, as seen in Addison's disease, liver disease, and hypopituitarism, a high carbohydrate intake with between-meal feedings is recommended. Restrict carbohydrate intake in

stimulative or functional hyperinsulinism. Insulin secretion by the pancreas is stimulated by carbohydrate foods.

Hypokalemia Dietary supplementation with natural foods may suffice in mild cases. Food sources rich in potassium include bananas, tomato juice, citrus fruits and juices, prunes, and potatoes.

Hypothyroidism Reduce caloric intake because of reduction in basal metabolic rate (30% to 40% below normal). Dietary aim is to control increase in weight.

Ileitis In the acute stage prescribe an elemental diet or the minimal residue diet with mineral and vitamin supplementation. Progress the diet to one low in residue and then to a low fiber, high protein diet as the condition improves. Resume the normal diet as soon as tolerated.

Indigestion Eat slowly and find time to relax after meals. Avoid overeating, especially foods that are bulky and difficult to digest.

Irritable colon A soft diet with high fluid intake is suitable. Sometimes it is necessary to begin the dietary treatment with a bland, low residue diet. An elemental diet may be used during the acute stage. Gradually introduce fiber but select those foods that are soft and nonirritating to the mucous membrane of the intestinal tract. The use of bulking agents may be necessary to avoid constipation. Emphasize high fluid intake, good habits of personal hygiene, relaxation, and freedom from nervous upsets.

Jaundice A high calorie, high protein, low fat diet with mineral and vitamin supplementation (especially calcium, iron, and vitamin K). Fortification of the diet with bile salts will help correct poor fat absorption.

Kwashiorkor Protein in the form of skimmed milk is commonly prescribed. An initial allowance of 2 to 5 gm protein/kg body weight is necessary. Sufficient carbohydrate and calories are needed to spare protein and correct weight loss. After a week, a mixed diet may be given in addition to milk. Mineral and vitamin supplementation should correct the other nutritional deficiencies.

Lactose intolerance Omit lactose and all sources of lactose. For infants give Nutramigen, Sobee, or Mullsoy and gradually introduce foods that do not contain milk and added lactose. For details, see *Diet, lactose-free*, in the text.

Leucine-induced hypoglycemia Restrict leucine

309

to 150 to 230 mg/kg body weight. Protein-rich foods are restricted, particularly milk and eggs, until tolerance to these foods is established. Sugars and other readily absorbable carbohydrates should be avoided. Ingestion of small amounts of carbohydrate (about 10 gm) 30 to 40 minutes after each meal will help counteract the hypoglycemic effect of leucine.

Liver diseases A diet high in protein, carbohydrate, and calories with vitamin supplementation, particularly fat-soluble vitamins. Alcohol is not allowed. Sodium intake should be restricted in ascites, and protein is curtailed in hepatic coma. Foods should be soft and low in fiber in the presence of bleeding esophageal varices. See the recommended diets for ascites, cirrhosis, hepatitis, and hepatic coma.

Malabsorption syndrome Feeding of medium-chain triglycerides is effective in alleviating the steatorrhea associated with a variety of malabsorption syndromes such as cystic fibrosis, pancreatitis, sprue, and gastrectomy. During the initial phase of the treatment, patients are usually maintained on a liquid formula emulsion containing 45% carbohydrate, 15% protein, and 40% fat of the medium-chain triglyceride type. Intake of dietary fats is restricted to the amount found in 1 egg and 4 ounces of lean meat, fish, or poultry. For additional protein, use skim milk, egg white, legumes, and cereal products. A product made with sodium caseinate and MCT is available commercially (Portagen). Medium-chain triglycerides may be mixed with salad dressings, fruit juices, and fried and sauteed foods.

Malaria A high calorie, high protein, high fluid intake with vitamin supplementation. During an acute attack with chills and fever, the diet outlined for acute febrile condition is suitable. Frequently the liver is enlarged and liver function is impaired. Diet indicated for liver disease is beneficial. See the discussions of the dietary recommendations for fever and febrile conditions and liver diseases.

Maple syrup urine disease A diet restricted in leucine, isoleucine, and valine. A preparation with reduced levels of these amino acids may be made from acid hydrolyzed casein. Give small amounts of milk to aid growth.

Marasmus Dietary management depends on the presence of complications such as dehydration, electrolyte imbalance, vitamin deficiencies, and infections. Fluid and electrolyte imbalance should be corrected promptly. Oral or parenteral administration of glucose solution provides immediate energy. After a day or two, give skim milk as the basic food and gradually add solid foods as tolerated. Provide sufficient protein of good quality and adequate calories to bring about greater nitrogen utilization. Vitamin and mineral supplements are needed.

Mental illness Dietary management must be individualized. The basic dietary aim is to maintain good nutritional status while providing security and pleasurable satisfaction from food. Among the feeding problems one will encounter are the following: (1) a depressed patient loses interest in food; (2) an overactive patient will not sit long enough to eat; (3) the delusional patient may develop fears and suspicions about his food; (4) an emotionally insecure patient may indulge in overeating for personal satisfaction; (5) patients with anorexia nervosa are difficult to feed; and (6) patients undergoing shock therapy may need a high caloric intake.

Myocardial infarction Restrict sodium intake (1000 to 2000 mg/day) and initially give a liquid diet. As the patient improves, progress the diet to a soft and eventually a regular diet.

Nephritis Basic dietary objective is to reduce the work of the kidneys by minimizing the rate of excretion of waste products, especially urea and salt. The diet also aims to prevent edema caused by retention of water and salt, prevent uremia caused by retention of nitrogen, and adjust body electrolytes, especially sodium, potassium, and chloride. Fluid intake should approximate measured output plus 500 ml for insensible loss. Sodium restriction is necessary (1000 to 2000 mg/day) during the acute phase of edema formation and hypertension. Protein intake need not be restricted unless renal failure develops. Give high quality protein and adequate calories to ensure positive nitrogen balance.

Nephrosclerosis Weight reduction is recommended for the obese to lessen the work of the circulatory system. Dietary considerations in the management of atherosclerosis should also be noted. Unless there is nitrogen retention, allowance for protein is generally normal.

Nephrotic syndrome The basic dietary objective is to replace protein (albumin) lost from the plasma into the urine. Provide high protein foods of good biologic value (about 120 to 150 gm/day). Calorie and carbohydrate intake should be high to ensure efficient utilization of protein. Sodium is restricted to 1000 to 2000 mg/day in the presence of edema. A more severe sodium restriction would present problems in planning a diet high in animal protein foods, especially if the patient does not like low sodium milk.

Obesity Reduce caloric intake below the total energy requirement and permit a rate of weight loss satisfactory to both the physician and the patient. Protein allowance must be normal or slightly higher to keep the patient in nitrogen equilibrium and to enhance water elimination. Dividing the total food allowance into small portions at frequent intervals (six to eight meals a day) gives better results than planning a diet around three meals a day. Reduction in salt intake may be necessary for patients who are not losing weight because of water retention. For the resistant obese patients, some physicians recommend a few days of fasting before starting on a reducing regimen. The ketosis and anorexia resulting from fasting precipitate the weight loss. The application of behavior therapy or behavior modification to promote changes in dietary eating habits has been tried with some degree of success. The key to a successful weight reduction program is patient education. He must change his basic eating habits and learn to maintain his desirable weight through the years.

Pancreatic insufficiency The condition is generally relieved by pancreatic enzyme preparation. The diet should be low in fat with the bulk of the calories coming from concentrated forms of carbohydrate such as sugars, jellies, and sweets. Use of medium-chain triglycerides (about 3 to 4 tablespoons/day) will increase fat and calorie intake. Provide adequate amounts of tender meats and restrict fruits and vegetables to the ones low in fiber content.

Pancreatitis The basic dietary aim is to rest the pancreas by restricting foods that will stimulate it to action. In the acute stage, nothing is given orally. Then the diet is progressed from a clear to a full liquid diet and eventually to a bland, low fat diet as the condition improves. Medium-chain triglycerides are usu-

ally well tolerated. Divide the meals into six small feedings per day.

Parkinson's disease A low protein intake of good quality protein (0.5 gm/kg or about 35 gm/day) tends to potentiate and stabilize the therapeutic effects of levodopa. High protein intakes tend to cancel the therapeutic effects of levodopa and lower the capacity to work. Pyridoxine (vitamin B_6) also reverses the therapeutic effect of levodopa. Doses as small as 10 to 25 mg of pyridoxine may be sufficient to produce this effect.

Peptic ulcer Dietary restriction in the treatment of gastric or duodenal ulcer is now minimal. The current emphasis is on size and frequency of feeding and liberalization of choice of foods. Only those foods known to cause distress are avoided. Except for alcohol, caffeine, pepper, and chili, most foods can be tolerated. The conservative and traditional dietary regimen is planned on a progressive five-stage diet, starting with the hourly feeding of milk and gradually adding soft and smooth foods that are considered to be chemically, mechanically, and thermally nonirritating. For more information, see *Diet, bland,* and *Diet, progressive bland,* in the text.

Pernicious vomiting In severe cases, give nothing orally for 24 to 48 hours. Glucose solution is generally administered intravenously. As vomiting becomes less severe, toast, crackers, jelly, and other simple carbohydrate foods may be given as tolerated. Give fluids between meals and avoid or limit fluid intake with meals. Gradually resume the normal diet but restrict fat if not tolerated.

Phenylketonuria The only treatment is restriction of the phenylalanine content of the diet. Since phenylalanine is required for normal growth and protein synthesis, management of the disease consists of supplying just the required amount so that there is no excessive accumulation in the blood. The daily phenylalanine requirement ranges from 15 to 25 mg/kg body weight, with children over 5 years requiring the lower value, infants the upper value, and 2- to 5-year-old children the medium value. The initial phenylalanine prescription serves only to assess phenylalanine tolerance. Dietary management must be individualized and adjusted as required. Since phenylalanine naturally occurs in protein foods (average of 5% phenylalanine), the diet calls for a special proprietary milk formula containing small amounts of phenylalanine (Lofenalac). This may constitute 85% to 100% of the diet, depending on the age of the child. For the newborn a small amount of milk is mixed with the formula to furnish the phenylalanine requirement. Solid foods are introduced at the usual ages and in the usual texture. Subtract the phenylalanine allotment in the special milk formula from the total phenylalanine requirement. The difference is the amount of phenylalanine to be given in solid foods.

Poliomyelitis During the acute febrile stage the same dietary considerations as in any acute febrile condition are indicated. A high calorie, high protein, and high vitamin liquid or semisolid diet is needed to compensate for the rapid tissue destruction. Difficult dietary management is met in bulbar poliomyelitis where there is failure or difficulty in swallowing food and the possibility of choking or aspiration. This often necessitates initial feeding by the parenteral route, followed by tube feeding. When the patient is able to swallow, give small amounts of clear liquids. Milk and cream are not well tolerated, as they produce mucus. As the patient improves, supplement the liquid diet with small amounts of soft, easily digested foods. The tube feeding is decreased proportionately as the oral intake is increased.

Psoriasis A diet restricted in the amino acid taurine has been tried. Several investigations point out that animal protein foods, particularly seafoods, influence the course of the disease and that psoriasis seems to be an error in taurine metabolism. For details, see *Diet, taurine-restricted,* in the text.

Pyelonephritis An acid-ash diet may be beneficial to increase the acidity of the urine and inhibit bacterial growth. Cereals and animal protein foods give an acidic residue. The intake of basic-forming foods such as milk, fruits, and vegetables should be limited.

Refsum's syndrome A diet restricted in phytanic acid has been recommended. See *Diet, phytanic acid–restricted,* in the text.

Regional enteritis Nutritional deficiencies may be present because of malabsorption. Weight loss may be helped by a diet containing medium-chain triglycerides, which are more readily absorbed. Hypoproteinemia due to loss of protein from the gut requires a high protein diet. Vitamin supplementation, particularly vitamin B_{12}, is necessary.

Renal calculi See the discussion of dietary management of calculi.

Renal failure Dietary management in acute renal failure includes the following: (1) restriction of fluid intake to a volume equivalent to urine output plus extrarenal losses, including an allowance of 400 ml/day for insensible water loss; (2) sodium restriction (500 mg/day) to improve edema and hypertension; (3) potassium restriction because of limited ability to excrete potassium; (4) restriction of protein to 20 gm/day to reduce urea nitrogen retention; and (5) provision of sufficient calories (1800 calories or more) to prevent breakdown of body tissues. The protein in the diet should be of high biologic value and preferably supplied by egg and milk. Special proprietary products such as Controlyte, Cal-Power, Hycal, and low protein wheat starch are good sources of calories low in protein. In chronic renal failure, dietary protein intake is determined by the degree of renal impairment and function. This may range from 20 to 40 gm/day. After hemodialysis has been started, the daily protein intake may be increased to 60 to 65 gm, or a normal allowance of 0.9 gm/kg body weight. Protein restriction may not be necessary after successful renal transplant. The sodium and potassium restrictions vary with individual patients. These may range from 1000 to 2000 mg/day.

Rheumatic fever The full liquid diet is suitable during the acute phase. The diet is increased gradually to a soft diet and eventually to a regular diet high in vitamin C, protein, and calories to recover weight loss. Restrict sodium if there is fluid retention.

Sprue syndrome A high protein intake (120 gm/day) with elimination of gluten from wheat, oat, rye, and barley. Carbohydrate and fat are given as tolerated. Substitution of medium-chain triglyceride for dietary fats greatly improves the steatorrhea associated with sprue. Minerals (especially calcium and iron) and vitamins (especially folic acid and vitamin B_{12}) are needed to correct nutritional deficiencies that accompany the disorder. Use low fiber foods during the initial stage of the disorder.

Dietary management of selected disorders—cont'd

Surgical conditions The objectives of dietary management are to improve the nutritional state of the patient in preparation for the stresses of surgery, to help hasten recovery, and to maintain good nutrition in the postoperative period.

Preoperative diet Prescribe a high protein, high calorie intake. Since obesity is a hazard in surgery, a low calorie diet is indicated for the overweight with a moderate intake of carbohydrate to build up glycogen reserves needed during surgery. The night before surgery, all foods are withheld after supper through the following morning to empty the stomach.

Postoperative diet Immediately after surgery, nothing is given by mouth for several hours; glucose solution is given intravenously. Depending on the patient's condition, the diet is progressed from the clear liquid to the full liquid, the soft, and finally the regular diet. In surgery of the colon a low residue diet or an elemental diet is initially given. Soft and low fiber foods are gradually added as tolerated. For patients who cannot be fed orally, nourishment is given by tube feeding or by parenteral means. Gastric intubation is indicated for those who are unable to swallow due to extensive mouth, head, neck, or esophageal surgery. As soon as the patient regains his appetite, a high calorie, high protein diet with plenty of fluids will hasten replacement of protein and glycogen stores, correct electrolyte and water imbalance, restore losses from bleeding, and shorten the time required for wound healing.

Tonsillectomy After surgery give cold liquids such as bland fruit juices, plain sherbet, and ginger ale. Milk and ice cream are not well tolerated because they produce mucus. On the second or third day, soft and smooth foods such as soft cooked eggs, strained cereals, and plain puddings may be given. Resume the regular diet as soon as tolerated by the patient.

Tuberculosis The diet should supply liberal amounts of protein (90 to 110 gm/day), minerals, and vitamins. Maintenance of desirable body weight is also important. Calcium is necessary for calcification of tuberculous lesions, and iron is needed if there has been hemorrhage from the lungs. Important vitamins to consider are vitamin C for wound healing, vitamin D for efficient utilization of calcium, B complex vitamins to stimulate appetite, and vitamin B_6 to counteract the polyneuritis associated with INH therapy.

Typhoid fever Give a high calorie, high protein liquid diet during the acute stage. Gradually add soft foods low in fiber content to prevent intestinal irritation. Frequent small feedings are recommended to avoid overloading the stomach.

Tyrosinemia A diet restricted in phenylalanine and tyrosine is recommended.

Ulcerative colitis A diet high in protein and calories with vitamin and mineral supplementation. In the acute stages, use an elemental diet or the minimal residue diet to avoid undue irritation to the colon. As soon as tolerated, give a bland diet high in protein, preferably in six small feedings. Only heavy roughage need be avoided.

Undernutrition It is dangerous to force-feed severely undernourished individuals. Skim milk, fed in small amounts, is probably the best food at the start. As the person begins to recover, give small amounts of easily digested foods. Gradually increase the amount until a full meal can be eaten.

Underweight The basic dietary aim is to increase body weight. Theoretically, an excess of 500 calories/day results in a weekly gain of 1 pound. Give a high calorie, high protein diet with snacks between meals. Supplement with B complex vitamins to stimulate the appetite.

Uremia Protein is restricted to 15 to 20 gm/day supplied mainly by 1 egg and 4 to 6 ounces of milk. Provide sufficient calories to prevent breakdown of body tissues. Calories should come from fats, sugars, low protein fruits and vegetables, and special low protein, high calorie proprietary products. See *Diet, minimal protein,* under *Diet, protein modified,* and *Diet, Giordano-Giovannetti,* in the text.

Wilson's disease Restrict the intake of copper to 1 mg/day or less. See *Diet, copper-restricted,* in the text.

Proprietary foods: composition, features, and uses

Name of product	Percent composition			Special features and uses
	CHO	Pro	Fat	
Alacta	44	31	25	Half skim milk powder, high in protein and moderately low in fat; used for low birth weight infants or those with digestive disturbances (Mead Johnson.)
Bremil	43	9	48	Nonfat milk with butterfat replacement (corn, coconut, and peanut oils) and added lactose; in liquid and powder form; vitamins added; iron in powder only; for routine infant feeding (Borden.)
Carnalac	49	14	37	Whole milk with added lactose and vitamins; liquid only; for routine infant feeding (Carnation.)
Casec	0	95	5	Dried calcium caseinate derived from skim milk curd and lime water; a high protein, high calcium formula for premature infants or those with gastrointestinal disorders
Codelid	83	17	0	Elemental food containing chemically defined amino acids, sucrose, vitamins, and minerals; residue free and fat free (Schwarz/Mann.)
Compleat B	48	16	36	Ready-to-use blenderized tube-feeding formula containing nonfat milk, sucrose, corn oil, and pureed beef, vegetables, fruit, and added vitamins and minerals; 1 calorie/ml (Doyle.)
Controlyte	57	0	43	High calorie dietary supplement prepared from cornstarch hydrolysate and added vegetable oil; provides calories in protein-electrolyte restricted diets (Doyle.)
Dextri-maltose	100	0	0	Carbohydrate formula modifier. Contains maltose and dextrins obtained by hydrolysis of cornstarch (Mead Johnson.)
Dryco	44	31	25	Half skim milk formula with added vitamins; high in protein and low in fat (Borden.)
Enfamil	41	9	50	Nonfat milk with added corn and coconut oils, lactose, and vitamins; also available with iron; for routine infant feeding (Mead Johnson.)
Ensure	54	14	32	Lactose-free liquid nutritional product for tube or supplemental feeding; contains caseinate and soy protein isolates, corn syrup, sucrose, corn oil, and added vitamins and minerals (Ross.)
Flexical	61	9	30	Low residue elemental diet made from casein hydrolysates, sucrose and corn syrup, soy and MCT oil, and added vitamins and minerals (Mead Johnson.)
Formil	42	10	48	Cow's milk with partial butterfat replacement (corn and coconut oil) and added lactose and vitamins; also available with added iron; for routine infant feeding (Pet.)
Formula 2	48	15	36	Ready-to-use blended food for tube feeding; contains nonfat milk, beef, egg yolk, corn oil, and strained vegetables, fruit, cereal, and added vitamins and minerals (Cutter.)

Proprietary foods: composition, features, and uses—cont'd

Name of product	Percent composition			Special features and uses
	CHO	Pro	Fat	
Gevral	27	68	5	High protein, low fat nutritional supplement with added vitamins and minerals; relatively low in sodium (Lederle.)
Hycal	98	< 1	< 1	Low protein, low electrolyte, high carbohydrate liquid product made with demineralized glucose; ready-to-serve as a drink or dessert topping; available in four fruit flavors (Beecham-Massengill.)
Isomil	40	12	48	Milk-free formula made with soy protein, soy and corn oils, corn sugar, sucrose, and added vitamins and minerals; for milk-sensitive infants (Ross.)
Jejunal	90	9	< 1	Minimal residue elemental diet consisting of chemically pure amino acids, simple carbohydrates, trace of safflower oil, and added vitamins and minerals; in powder form as beverage, broth, or pudding (Johnson & Johnson.)
Klim	30	20	50	Whole milk powder with added vitamins and minerals; for routine infant feeding (Borden.)
Lactum	46	16	38	Cow's milk with added corn sugar and lactose, vitamins, and minerals; for routine infant feeding (Mead Johnson.)
Lambase	50	15	35	Hypoallergenic formula for infants sensitive to milk; made with meat protein (lamb heart), corn oil, sucrose, corn sugar, and added vitamins and minerals (Gerber.)
Lipomul— Oral	0	0	100	Creamy white emulsion containing 10 gm corn oil/15 ml; source of fat when extra calories are needed; rich in polyunsaturates (Upjohn.)
Liprotein Powder	10	33	57	High protein, high fat, low carbohydrate dietary supplement in powder form with added vitamins; for use in milk drinks to increase calories and protein (Upjohn.)
Lofenalac	50	15	35	Low phenylalanine product for infants and children with phenylketonuria; chemically treated casein hydrolysates to remove phenylalanine and supplements of methionine, tryptophan, and tyrosine; added corn oil, mixed carbohydrates, vitamins, and minerals (Mead Johnson.)
Lonalac	30	21	49	Low sodium product prepared from casein, coconut oil, lactose, and added vitamins and minerals; for persons requiring low sodium milk (Mead Johnson.)
Lytren	0	0	0	Oral electrolyte formula to replace water and electrolyte losses (Mead Johnson.)
Meat Base	29	20	51	Hypoallergenic formula for infants sensitive to milk; made with meat protein (beef heart), sesame oil, sucrose, and added vitamins and minerals (Gerber.)

Continued.

Name of product	Percent composition			Special features and uses
	CHO	Pro	Fat	
Meritene	46	24	30	High protein dietary supplement for oral or tube feeding; made with nonfat milk, corn syrup, vegetable oil, sodium caseinate, sucrose, and added vitamins and minerals; in liquid or powder form (Doyle.)
Modilac	48	14	38	Skim milk with corn oil, mixed carbohydrates (lactose and corn syrup), and added vitamins and iron; for routine infant feeding (Gerber.)
Mull-soy	44	26	30	Hypoallergenic formula made from soy protein, soy oil, and added sugar, vitamins, and minerals (Borden.)
Nutrament	54	25	21	High protein dietary supplement for oral or tube feeding; made with nonfat milk, soy oil, sodium caseinate, sucrose, vitamins, and minerals; in liquid and powder form (Drackett.)
Nutramigen	50	15	35	Hypoallergenic formula for infants sensitive to milk and lactose; contains casein hydrolysate, corn oil, sucrose, arrowroot starch, vitamins, and minerals; in powder form only (Mead Johnson.)
Nutri-1000	40	13	47	High fat nutritional supplement for oral or tube feeding; made with skim milk, soy and coconut oils, sucrose, vitamins, and minerals; in liquid form (Syntex.)
Olac	44	20	36	High protein milk formula with butterfat replacement (corn oil) and added corn sugar and vitamins A, D, and E; in liquid and powder form; for low birth weight infants unable to tolerate butterfat (Mead Johnson.)
Pedialyte	0	0	0	Oral electrolyte mixture for maintenance of body fluid and electrolyte balance; for infants and children with diarrhea (Ross.)
Portagen	46	14	40	Sodium caseinate with MCT oil, corn oil, corn syrup solids, sugar, vitamins, and minerals; for persons with malabsorption and fat intolerance; virtually lactose free (Mead Johnson.)
Precision-LR	90	9	< 1	Nutritionally complete low residue food for oral and tube feeding; made with egg white solids, maltodextrin, sugar, vegetable oil, vitamins, and minerals; available in four fruit flavors (Doyle.)
Pregestimil	51	13	36	Protein hydrolysate formula containing glucose, MCT oil, vitamins, and minerals; for infants with malabsorption problems; in powder form (Mead Johnson.)
Probana	47	24	29	Cow's milk with added casein hydrolysate, glucose, banana powder, and lactic acid; fortified with vitamins A and D; for infants with diarrhea, cystic fibrosis, and celiac syndrome (Mead Johnson.)
Prosobee	40	15	45	Milk-free formula made with soy protein isolate, soy oil, corn sugar, sucrose, and added iron, vitamins, and minerals; for infants sensitive to cow's milk (Mead Johnson.)
Protein Milk	22	30	48	Whole-milk curd and nonfat milk with added lactic acid and sodium lactate; a high protein acidified milk for use in celiac syndrome, cystic

Proprietary foods: composition, features, and uses—cont'd

Name of product	Percent composition			Special features and uses
	CHO	Pro	Fat	
				fibrosis, and other gastrointestinal disturbances; in powder form (Mead Johnson.)
Protenum	50	45	5	High protein, low fat supplement; nonfat dry milk, calcium caseinate, dextrose, cocoa, vitamins, and minerals (Mead Johnson.)
Protinal	42	56	2	High protein, low fat dietary supplement to correct protein deficiency; contains refined soya and corn, sugar, nonfat dry milk, vegetable oil, and calcium (National.)
Similac	41	11	48	Skim milk with added lactose, corn and coconut oils, iron, and vitamins; in liquid and powder form; for routine infant feeding (Ross.)
Similac PM 60/40	43	9	48	Mixture of electrodialyzed whey and nonfat milk, corn and coconut oils, lactose, minerals, and vitamins; 60% lactalbumin and 40% casein in protein; for infant feeding (Ross.)
S-M-A Formula S-26	43	9	48	Mixture of partially demineralized whey and nonfat milk, vegetable oils (corn, coconut, and soy), oleo oil, lactose, vitamins, and minerals; in liquid and powder form (Wyeth.)
Sobee	46	19	35	Milk-free formula made from soy protein, soy and coconut oils, sucrose, corn sugar, and added vitamins and minerals; for persons with lactose intolerance and milk sensitivity (Mead Johnson.)
Somagen	15	85	0	Concentrated protein and B vitamin supplement; nonfat milk with yeast, liver, vitamins, and calcium; relatively low in sodium (Upjohn.)
Soyalac	54	12	36	Milk-free formula made of soy protein, soy oil, corn sugar, sucrose, and added vitamins and minerals; in liquid and powder form; for milk sensitivity and lactose intolerance (Loma.)
Sustacal	55	24	21	High protein nutritional supplement for oral or tube feeding; made with skim milk, sugar, soy fat, sodium caseinate, corn syrup, vitamins, and minerals; in liquid and powder form (Mead Johnson.)
Sustagen	55	24	20	Complete nutritional supplement for oral or tube feeding; made with whole and skim milk, calcium caseinate, maltose, dextrin, and added vitamins and minerals (Mead Johnson.)
Vivonex-100	91	9	1	Elemental diet low in residue consisting of synthetic amino acids, safflower oil, simple sugars, vitamins, and minerals; in powder form and six flavors; for patients with reduced absorptive ability; also available as Vivonex-100 HN with twice the nitrogen content as the standard formula (Eaton.)
W-T low residue food	91	8	1	Elemental diet low in residue consisting of chemically defined amino acids, safflower oil, dextrin, vitamins, and minerals; in powder form and four flavors; for nutritional support of patients with reduced absorptive capacity (Warren-Teed.)

■ APPENDIX P-2

Protein food mixtures*

Product	Country	Composition
Aliment de sevrage	Senegal	Millet flour, peanut flour, skim milk powder, sugar, vitamins A and D, and calcium
Arlac	Nigeria	Peanut flour, skim milk powder, salts, and vitamins B_1, B_2, B_{12}, and D
Bal-ahar	India	Mixed wheat flour, vegetables, defatted oil seed flour, vitamins, and calcium
CSM	United States	Maize (precooked), defatted soybean flour, skim milk powder, $CaCO_3$, and vitamins
FAP	Morocco	Fish protein concentrate
Fish flour	Chile	Fish flour, butter, lactose, sucrose, cornstarch, vitamins, and minerals
Fortifex	Brazil	Maize, defatted soybean flour, vitamins A, B_1, and B_2, DL-methionine, and $CaCO_3$
Incaparina	Guatemala	Maize, cottonseed flour, vitamin A, lysine, and $CaCO_3$
	Colombia	Same plus defatted soybean flour
	Mexico	Same with defatted soybean flour instead of cotton-seed flour
Indian multipur-pose food (MPF)	India	Peanut flour, chick-pea flour, vitamins A, B_1, and B_2, and $CaCO_3$
Lactone	India	Groundnut flour, skim milk powder, wheat and barley flour, vitamins, and calcium
Laubina	Lebanon	Wheat, chick-pea, sesame, skim milk, minerals, vitamins A, B_1, B_2, and D, and niacin
Prolo	United Kingdom	Soya flour, DL-methionine, minerals, vitamins A, B_1, B_2, and niacin
Pronutro	South Africa	Maize, skim milk powder, peanut, soybean, fish protein concentrate, yeast, wheat germ, vitamins A, B_1, and B_2, niacin, sugar, and iodized salt
Protone	United Kingdom, Congo	Maize, skim milk powder, yeast, vitamins, and minerals
Saridele	Indonesia	Dry soya, sugar, vitamins B_1, B_{12}, and C, and $CaCO_3$
SM	Ethiopia	Teff, peas, chick-pea, lentils, and skim milk powder
Superamine	Algeria	Wheat, chick-pea, lentils, skim milk powder, sugar, and vitamin D
Supro	East Africa	Maize or barley flour, *Torula* yeast, skim milk powder, salt, and condiments

*Compiled from the following sources: Manocha, S. L.: Malnutrition and retarded human development, Springfield, Ill., 1972, Charles C Thomas, Publisher; Robson, J. R. K.: Malnutrition. Its causation and control, New York, 1972, Gordon & Breach, Science Publishers, Inc., vol. 2.

■ APPENDIX Q
Normal constituents of blood*

Physical measurements

Specific gravity	1.025-1.030
Reaction	pH 7.37-7.45
Bleeding time	1-5 minutes
Coagulation time, venous blood (Lee-White method)	4-12 minutes
Prothrombin time, plasma (Quick method)	14-18 seconds
Sedimentation rate (Wintrobe)	
Men	0-9 mm/hour
Women	0-20 mm/hour

Hematology

Cell volume	39%-50%
Cells, differential count	
Lymphocytes	25%-35%/mm³
Monocytes	4%-10%/mm³
Neutrophils	50%-65%/mm³
Eosinophils	0.5%-4%/mm³
Basophils	0%-2%/mm³
Erythrocytes (RBCs)	4.2-5.5 mil/mm³
Leukocytes (WBCs)	5-10 thousand/mm³
Thrombocytes (platelets)	150-300 thousand/mm³
Reticulocytes	0.5%-2% red cells
Hematocrit (vol% red cells)	
Men	40%-54%
Women	37%-47%
Hemoglobin	
Adults	
Men	14-17 gm/100 ml
Women	12-15 gm/100 ml
Children (varies with age)	10-18 gm/100 ml
Volume, whole blood	70-100 ml/kg
Total protein, serum	6-8 gm/100 ml
Albumin, serum	4-5.5 gm/100 ml
Globulin, serum	1.3-2.7 gm/100 ml
Albumin/globulin ratio	1.8-2.5
Ceruloplasmin, plasma	15-30 mg/100 ml
Fibrinogen, plasma	0.2-0.4 gm/100 ml

Nitrogen constituents

Amino acid nitrogen, blood	4-8 mg/100 ml
Ammonia, blood	40-70 μg/100 ml

Continued.

*Compiled from the following sources: Cecil, R. L., et al.: A textbook of medicine, Philadelphia, 1955, W. B. Saunders Co.; Cooper, L. F., et al.: Nutrition in health and disease, Philadelphia, 1958, J. B. Lippincott Co.; Goldsmith, G. A.: Nutritional diagnosis, Springfield, Ill., 1959, Charles C Thomas, Publisher; Goodhart, R. S., and Wohl, M. G.: Modern nutrition in health and disease, Philadelphia, 1964, Lea & Febiger; Harper, H. A.: Review of physiological chemistry, Los Altos, Calif., 1963, Lange Medical Publications; Harrow, B., and Mazur, A.: Textbook of biochemistry, Philadelphia, 1966, W. B. Saunders Co.; Proudfit, F. T., and Robinson, C. H.: Normal and therapeutic nutrition, New York, 1961, Macmillan Inc.; White, A., Handler, P., and Smith, E. L.: Principles of biochemistry, New York, 1964, McGraw-Hill Book Co.

Ammonia, serum	0.15-0.30 mg/100 ml
Creatine	0.2-0.9 mg/100 ml
Creatinine	0.8-2 mg/100 ml
Nonprotein nitrogen, blood	20-40 mg/100 ml
Urea nitrogen, blood	10-20 mg/100 ml
Urea, blood	20-35 mg/100 ml
Uric acid, blood	2.5-5 mg/100 ml
Amino acids	
Amino acids, total	35-65 mg/100 ml
Alanine	3.0-3.7 mg/100 ml
Alpha-aminobutyric acid	0.2-0.4 mg/100 ml
Arginine	1.2-1.9 mg/100 ml
Asparagine	0.5-0.7 mg/100 ml
Aspartic acid	0.01-0.07 mg/100 ml
Cysteine and cystine	1.1-1.3 mg/100 ml
Glutamic acid	0.4-1.2 mg/100 ml
Glutamine	5-12 mg/100 ml
Glycine	1.3-1.7 mg/100 ml
Histidine	0.8-1.5 mg/100 ml
Isoleucine	0.7-1.3 mg/100 ml
Leucine	1.4-2.3 mg/100 ml
Lysine	2.5-3.0 mg/100 ml
Methionine	0.3-0.4 mg/100 ml
Ornithine	0.6-0.8 mg/100 ml
Phenylalanine	0.7-1.0 mg/100 ml
Proline	1.8-3.3 mg/100 ml
Serine	1.1-1.2 mg/100 ml
Threonine	1.2-1.7 mg/100 ml
Tryptophan	1.0-1.2 mg/100 ml
Tyrosine	0.8-1.5 mg/100 ml
Valine	0.4-3.7 mg/100 ml
Carbohydrates	
Glucose	
Nelson-Somogyi	70-100 mg/100 ml
Folin-Wu	80-120 mg/100 ml
Fructose	6-8 mg/100 ml
Glycogen	5-6 mg/100 ml
Hexoses	70-105 mg/100 ml
Hexuronates (as glucuronic acid)	0.4-1.4 mg/100 ml
Pentose, total	2-4 mg/100 ml
Lipids	
Cephalin	0-30 mg/100 ml
Cholesterol, serum	
Total	150-240 mg/100 ml
Esters	100-180 mg/100 ml
Cholesterol, free	50-60 mg/100 ml
Fats, neutral	150-300 mg/100 ml
Fatty acids, serum (total)	350-450 mg/100 ml
Fatty acids, free	8-30 mg/100 ml

Lecithin	100-200 mg/100 ml
Lipids, serum (total)	450-850 mg/100 ml
Phospholipids, serum (total)	230-300 mg/100 ml
Plasmalogen	7-8 mg/100 ml
Sphingomyelin	10-50 mg/100 ml

Blood gases

CO_2-combining power	50-65 vol%
	21-28 mEq/L
CO_2 content	
Serum	50-70 vol%
	21-30 mEq/L
Whole blood	40-60 vol%
	18-27 mEq/L
CO_2 tension	38-40 mm Hg
O_2 capacity, whole blood	16-27 vol%
O_2 content	
Arterial blood	15-23 vol%
Venous blood	10-16 vol%
O_2 saturation	
Arterial blood	94%-96%
Venous blood	60%-85%
O_2 tension	95-100 mm Hg

Minerals

Base, serum (total)	145-155 mEq/L
Calcium, serum	9-11 mg/100 ml
	4.5-5.5 mEq/L
Chlorides, serum	355-376 mg/100 ml
	100-106 mEq/L
Copper	130-230 μg/100 ml
Iodine	
Total	8-15 mEq/L
Protein-bound	4-8 μg/100 ml
Iron, serum	80-180 μg/100 ml
Magnesium, serum	2-3 mg/100 ml
	1.6-2.4 mEq/L
Phosphate	1.6-2.7 mEq/L
Phosphorus, inorganic, serum	3-4.5 mg/100 ml
	1-1.5 mEq/L
Potassium, serum	16-20 mg/100 ml
	4-5 mEq/L
Sodium, serum	310-340 mg/100 ml
	136-145 mEq/L
Sulfates, inorganic, serum	2.5-5.0 mg/100 ml
	0.5-1.5 mEq/L

Vitamins

Ascorbic acid	
Serum	0.4-1.0 mg/100 ml
White blood cells	25-40 mg/100 ml

Continued.

Folic acid	3.4 μg/100 ml
Riboflavin	20 μg/100 ml
Thiamin	3.4 μg/100 ml
Vitamin A	40-120 IU/100 ml
Vitamin B_6, xanthurenic acid excretion after 10 gm tryptophan	30 mg/day
Vitamin B_{12}	350-750 μg/100 ml
Vitamin D, alkaline phosphatase	5-15 Bodansky units
Vitamin E, serum tocopherol	
Adults	1.0-1.2 mg/100 ml
Infants	0.23-0.43 mg/100 ml
Vitamin K, prothrombin time	10-15 seconds
Organic acids	
Acetoacetic acid	0.8-2.8 mg/100 ml
Alpha-ketoglutaric acid	0.2-1.0 mg/100 ml
Citric acid	1.4-3.0 mg/100 ml
Lactic acid	8-17 mg/100 ml
Malic acid	0.1-0.9 mg/100 ml
Pyruvic acid	0.4-2 mg/100 ml
Succinic acid	0.1-0.6 mg/100 ml
Ketone bodies	0.3-2 mg/100 ml
Enzymes	
Amylase, serum	80-180 Somogyi units/100 ml
Lipase, serum	450-850 mg/100 ml
Phosphatase, alkaline	
Bodansky	1-4 units/100 ml
Gutman	3-10 units/100 ml
King-Armstrong	8-14 units/100 ml
Shinowara	2-8 units/100 ml
Phosphatase, acid	
Bodansky	0.5-2 units/100 ml
Gutman	0.5-2 units/100 ml
King-Armstrong	1-5 units/100 ml
Shinowara	0.1-1 units/100 ml
Miscellaneous	
Bicarbonate	24-30 mEq/L
Bilirubin, serum (total)	0.2-1.4 mg/100 ml
Direct	0.1-0.2 mg/100 ml
Indirect	0.1-0.6 mg/100 ml
Carotenoids	60-180 μg/100 ml
Icterus index, serum	4-7 units
Taurine	0.4-0.8 mg/100 ml

■ APPENDIX R
Normal constituents of urine

Specific gravity	1.008-1.030
Reaction	pH 5.5-8.0
Volume	1000-1500 ml/24 hours
Total solids	55-70 gm/L
Organic constituents	
Acetone (ketone) bodies	0.003-0.015 gm/24 hours
Ammonia	0.4-1.0 gm/24 hours
Bile	None
Creatine	None (0-0.2 gm/24 hours)
Creatinine	1.0-1.5 gm/24 hours
Hippuric acid	0.1-1.0 gm/24 hours
Indican	0.004-0.020 gm/24 hours
Nitrogen, total	10-17 gm/24 hours
Protein (albumin)	None (0-0.015 gm/24 hours)
Purine bases	0.006-0.014 gm/24 hours
Sugar	None (in some persons, 0.002-0.003 gm/ 24 hours after a heavy meal)
Sulfate, organic	0.06-0.2 gm/24 hours
Urea	20-35 gm/24 hours
Uric acid	0.5-0.8 gm/24 hours
Inorganic constituents	
Calcium	0.1-0.3 gm/24 hours
Chloride (as NaCl)	10-15 gm/24 hours
Iron	0.001-0.005 gm/24 hours
Magnesium	0.15-0.30 gm/24 hours
Phosphorus	2.0-2.5 gm/24 hours
Potassium	1.5-2.5 gm/24 hours
Sodium	2.0-5.0 gm/24 hours
Sulfur, total	1.5-3.0 gm/24 hours

■ APPENDIX S
pH values of various body fluids

Aqueous humor of eye	7.4
Blood serum	7.35-7.45
Cerebrospinal fluid	7.35-7.45
Feces	7.0-7.5
Gallbladder bile	5.4-6.9
Gastric juice, pure	About 0.9
Hepatic duct bile	7.4-8.5
Intestinal juice	7.0-8.0
Milk	6.6-6.9
Pancreatic juice	7.5-8.0
Saliva	6.35-6.85
Skin, intracellular, various layers	6.2-7.5
Tears	7.4
Urine	4.5-7.5

■ APPENDIX T

Common prefixes, suffixes, and combining forms

Prefixes

a, an	without; as avitaminosis
ab	away from; as abnormal
ad	near, toward; as adrenal
ana	upward; as anabolism
anti	against; as antibiotic
auto	self; as autodigestion
bio	life; as biology
calor	heat; as calorimeter
cata	downward; as catabolism
chole	bile, gall; as cholagogue
chroma	color; as chromatosis
co	together; as coenzyme
di	two, double; as diplopia
dis	ill, negative; as disease
dys	bad, difficult; as dyspepsia
ec	outside; as ectopic
encephal	brain, skull; as encephalogram
endo	inside; as endogenous
exo	outside; as exogenous
hemo	blood; as hemopoiesis
hyper	above, excessive; as hyperacid
hypo	below, little; as hypofunction
im	not; as immature
in	not; as incurable
inter	between; as interstitial
intra	within; as intravascular
meta	change; as metaplasia
necro	dead; as necrosis
para	beside; as paravertebral
peri	around; as pericardium
post	after; as postmortem
pre	before; as prenatal
syn	union, together; as synthesis

Suffixes

algia	pain; as neuralgia
ase	enzyme; as amylase
cide	kill; as bactericide
clysis	drenching; as venoclysis
cule	small; as molecule
cyte	cell; as erythrocyte
ectomy	cut off; as appendectomy
emesis	vomiting; as hematemesis
emia	blood; as anemia
esthesia	sensation; as anesthesia
ism	condition; as alcoholism
itis	inflammation; as appendicitis
lysis	destruction; as hemolysis
malacia	softening; as osteomalacia
oma	tumor, swelling; as adenoma
opsy	to view; as biopsy
osis	condition; as tuberculosis
pathy	disease of; as neuropathy
penia	poverty; as leucopenia
phagia	to eat; as polyphagia
phil	to love; as basophil
phobia	fear of; as photophobia
pnea	breath; as hyperpnea
poiesis	to produce; as hemopoiesis
ptysis	to spit; as hemoptysis
rrhea	to discharge; as diarrhea
tomy	to cut; as vagotomy
trophy	growth; as hypertrophy
uria	urine; as glucosuria

Combining forms

adeno	gland; as adenoma
arthro	joint; as arthrology
cephalo	head; as cephalocaudal
colo	colon; as colostomy
costo	rib; as costochondral
cysto	bladder; as cystogram
cyto	cell; as cytoblast
derma	skin; as dermatology
entero	intestines; as enterocolitis
erythro	red; as erythrocyte
gastro	stomach; as gastrointestinal
glossa	tongue; as glossitis
hemato	blood; as hematology
hepato	liver; as hepatomegaly
hetero	mixed; as heterogenous
hydro	water; as hydrolysis
hystero	uterus; as hysterogram
ileo	ileum; as ileostomy
iso	equal; as isocaloric
kerato	horny; as keratoderma
leuko	white; as leukocyte
lith	stone, calculus; as cholelith
macro	large; as macrocyte
mal	ill or bad; as malnutrition
mega	enlarged; as hepatomegaly
micro	small; as microorganism
myo	muscle; as myoglobin
nephro	kidney; as nephrosis
neuro	nerve; as neurology
oligo	few, scant; as oligosaccharide
ophthalmo	eye; as ophthalmology
opia	sight, vision; as myopia

Common prefixes, suffixes, and combining forms—cont'd

osteo	bone; as osteoporosis
oto	ear; as otoscope
pan	all, every; as pandemic
path	disease; as pathogenesis
phago	to eat; as phagocytosis
phlebo	vein; as phlebotomy
poly	many; as polysaccharide
procto	anus; as proctoscopy
proto	first; as protoplasm
psycho	mind; as psychology
pulmo	lung; as pulmonary
pyelo	kidney, pelvis; as pyelonephritis
pyo	pus; as pyorrhea
rrhage	excessive flow; as hemorrhage
sclero	hard; as arteriosclerosis
thio	sulfur-containing; as thiochrome

■ APPENDIX U

Common abbreviations on patients' charts

a	ante; before
$\overline{aa}$	each; of each
Abd	abdominal; abdomen
ac	ante cibes; before meals
ad lib	ad libitum; as desired; as needed
Adm	admission
AF	artificial
A/G	albumin-globulin
AHD	arteriosclerotic heart disease
AID	acute infectious disease
alb	albumin
ALK	alkaline
amt	amount
AP	anterior-posterior
APC	arterial premature contraction
approx	approximately
Aq	aqua; water
ARF	acute rheumatic fever
ASA	aspirin; acetylsalicylic acid
ASHD	arteriosclerotic heart disease
as tol	as tolerated
B	born; basophils
Ba	barium
bid	bis in die; twice daily
bilat	bilateral
BM	bowel movement
BMR	basal metabolic rate
BP	blood pressure
BPH	benign prostatic hypertrophy
BR	bed rest

BRP	bathroom privileges
BSL	blood sugar level
BSP	bromosulfonphthalein
BUN	blood urea nitrogen
$\overline{c}$	cum; with
C	centigrade
Ca	carcinoma; cancer; calcium
cap	capsule
cath	catheterize
cbc or CBC	complete blood count
cc	cubic centimeter
CC	chief complaint
CCF	cephalin-cholesterol flocculation
CCU	coronary care unit
cd	cane die; daily
CHF	congestive heart failure
chr	chronic
ck	check
Cl	chloride
cm	centimeter
CNS	central nervous system
CO_2	carbon dioxide
Cpd or Comp	compound
CRF	chronic renal failure
C & S	culture and sensitivity
CSF	cerebrospinal fluid
CV	cardiovascular
CVA	cerebral vascular accident
CVP	central venous pressure
Cw	crutch walking
d	daily
DBW	desirable body weight
D & C	dilatation and curettage
Diag or Dx	diagnosis
dil	dilute
disc or D/C	discontinue
Disch	discharge
DL	danger list
D_2O	deuterium or heavy water
DOA	dead on arrival
DOS	day of surgery
DPM	discontinue previous medication
DPT	diphtheria, pertussis, tetanus inoculation
dr	dram; drachm; 3.8 gm
DR	delivery room
D/S	dextrose and saline
DSD	dry sterile dressing
DT	delirium tremens
DW	distilled water
e	et; and

Common abbreviations on patients' charts—cont'd

E or EOS	eosinophils	hx	hospitalization; history
ECG or EKG	electrocardiogram	ibid	same as before
		Ict Ind	icterus index
ED	emergency department	ICU	intensive care unit
EDC	expected date of confinement	I & D	incision and drainage
EEG	electroencephalogram	i.e.	that is
e.g.	for example	IM	intramuscularly
Elix	elixir	Imp	impression
ENT	ear, nose, and throat	int	internal
ER	emergency room	I & O	intake and output
ESR	erythrocyte sedimentation rate	IPPB	intermittent positive pressure breathing
etc	and so forth		
EUA	examine under anesthesia	irrig	irrigation
exp	expired	IU	international unit
Expl Lap	exploratory laparotomy	IV	intravenously
ext,	external	IVP	intravenous pyelogram
extr	extract	IVSD	intraventricular septal defect
F	father; female; Fahrenheit	K	potassium
FBS	fasting blood sugar	kg	kilogram
FeSO$_4$	ferrous sulfate	KUB	kidney, ureter, and bladder
FH	family history; fetal heart	L	liter
Fib	fibrillation	lat	lateral
FLD	fluid	LBBB	left bundle branch block
FTT	failure to thrive	liq	liquid
FUO	fever of unknown origin	LLL	left lower lobe
Fx	fracture	LLQ	left lower quadrant
GA	gastric analysis	LMP	last menstrual period
GB	gallbladder	LP	lumbar puncture
GBD	gallbladder disease	LR	labor room
GBS	gallbladder series	LUL	left upper lobe
GC	gonococcal count	LUQ	left upper quadrant
GE	gastroenteritis	lym	lymphocyte
GI	gastrointestinal	lytes	electrolytes
GIT	gastrointestinal tract	m	minim
gm	gram; 15.43 grains	M	mother; monocyte; male
gr	grain	M et N	mone et nocte; day and night
gtt(s)	gutta; drop(s)	mcg	microgram
GTT	glucose tolerance test	mec	meconium
GU	genitourinary	mEq	milliequivalent
Gyn	gynecology	mg	milligram
h	hour	MGW	magnesium sulfate, glycerine, and water enema
hb, Hg, or Hgb	hemoglobin		
		MI	mitral insufficiency; myocardial infarction
hct	hematocrit		
HCVD	hypertensive cardiovascular disease	ml	milliliter
hem	blood	MO	mineral oil; month
HO	house officer	MOM	milk of magnesia
H$_2$O	water	M & R	measure and record
HNV	has not voided	MS	mitral stenosis; multiple sclerosis
HPN	hypertension	n	nocte; night
HR	heart rate	Na	sodium
hs	hora somni; at bedtime	NaCl	sodium chloride

Common abbreviations on patients' charts—cont'd

NDF	no diagnostic findings		pp	postprandial; postpartum
neg	negative		PPD	purified protein derivative
N/G or NG	nasogastric		pr	per rectum
nil	nothing		prn	pro re nata; whenever necessary
no or #	number		prog	prognosis
NP	neuropsychiatry		PSP	phenolsulfonphthalein
NPH	isophane insulin (neutral protamine Hagedorn)		pt	patient
			PT	physical therapy
NPN	nonprotein nitrogen		PTA	prior to admission
NPO	nil per os; nothing by mouth		PTB	pulmonary tuberculosis
NS or NSS	normal saline solution		pu	peptic ulcer
NSR	normal sinus rhythm		PWB	partial weight bearing
N & T	nose and throat		PZI	protamine zinc insulin
NTG	nitroglycerin		q	quaque; every
NWB	no weight bearing		qd	quaque die; every day
O	oral		qh	quaque hora; every hour
O₂	oxygen		qid	quater in die; four times a day
OB	obstetrics; occult blood		ql	quantum libit; as much as desired
od or OD	oculus dexter; right eye		qn	quaque nocte; every night
oint	ointment		qns	quantity not sufficient
OM	omne mone; every day		qod	every other day
ON	omne nocte; every night		qoh	every other hour
OOB	out of bed		qon	every other night
OOR	out of room		qs	quantum sufficiat; quantity sufficient
O & P	ova and parasites		R	respiration rate; rectal
OPD	outpatient department		RAI	radioactive isotope
ophth	ophthalmology		RBBB	right bundle branch block
OR	operating room		RBC	red blood cell
Orth(o)	orthopedics		re	concerning
os or OS	oculus sinister; left eye		RHD	rheumatic heart disease
OT	occupational therapy; old tuberculin		RLQ	right lower quadrant
ou	both eyes		R/O	rule out
oz	ounce		RR	recovery room; respiratory rate
p	post; after		rt or R	right
P	pulse; phosphorus		RUQ	right upper quadrant
PA	posterior anterion (x-ray film)		Rx	treatment; take
PAF	paroxysmal atrial fibrillation		s̄	without
Pap smear	Papanicolaou smear		"S"	service patient
PAT	pregnancy at term		SAH	subarachnoid hemorrhage
path	pathology		sbs	soft brown stool
PBI	protein-bound iodine		sc	subcutaneous
Pc	post cibum; after meals		SCD	surgical cut down
PE	physical examination		sed rate	sedimentation rate
PH	past history		sgs	soft green stool
PI	present illness		sibs	brothers and sisters
PID	pelvic inflammatory disease		sig	sign; let it be labeled
PKU	phenylketonuria		S & O	salpingo-oophorectomy
PM	postmortem		SOB	short of breath
PMI	post myocardial infarction		Sol	solution
PMP	previous menstrual period		spec	specimen
po	per os; by mouth; orally		sp gr	specific gravity
Post	posterior		s̄s̄	one half

Common abbreviations on patients' charts—cont'd

SSE	soapsuds enema
Staph	staphylococcus
stat	immediately
Strep	streptococcus
syr	syrup
sys	soft yellow stool
Sx	symptoms
Sy	syphilis
t or tsp	teaspoon
T	temperature
T or tbsp	tablespoon
T & A	tonsils and adenoids
tab	tablet
TAH	total abdominal hysterectomy
tbc or TBC	tuberculosis
TBW	total body weight
TCR	turn, cough, and rebreathe
temp	temperature
tid	three times a day
TP	total protein
TPR	temperature, pulse, and respiration
tr or tinct	tincture
Trach	tracheostomy
TTT	thymol turbidity test
TURP	transurethral prostatectomy
TWE	tap water enema
U	unit
ung	ointment
URI	upper respiratory infection
USP	*United States Pharmacopoeia*
UTI	urinary tract infection
V	ventricular
vd	void
VD	venereal disease
via	by way of
viz	namely
VNS	visiting nurse service
vol	volume
VP	venous pressure
VPC	ventricular premature contraction
VS	vital signs
WA	when awake
Wass	Wassermann
WB	weight-bearing
WBC	white blood count; white blood cell
WNL	within normal limits
wt	weight
x	times
x-match	cross match

Miscellaneous

♂	male
♀	female

+	positive
−	negative
0	nothing
$\overline{i}$	one
<	less than
>	greater than
∴	therefore
~	similar to

■ APPENDIX V
Weights and measures

1 teaspoon	=	60	drops
		5	milliliters
		5	grams
1 tablespoon	=	3	teaspoons
		15	milliliters
		15	grams
		½	ounce
1 cup	=	16	tablespoons
		240	milliliters
		240	grams
		8	fluid ounces
1 quart	=	2	pints
		4	cups
		960	milliliters
1 peck	=	2	gallons
		8	quarts
1 ounce	=	2	tablespoons
		30	grams
		⅛	cup
1 kilogram	=	2.2	pounds
		1000	grams
		1	quart
1 dessert spoon	=	2	teaspoons
		10	milliliters
		10	grams
1 pint	=	2	cups
		480	milliliters
		480	grams
		16	fluid ounces
1 gallon	=	4	quarts
		16	cups
		½	peck
1 bushel	=	4	pecks
		8	gallons
1 pound	=	16	ounces
		454	grams
		2	cups

Weights and measures—cont'd

To convert ounces to grams, multiply the ounces by 30 (or 28.35).

To convert grams to ounces, divide the grams by 30 (or 28.35).

To convert pounds to kilograms, divide the pounds by 2.2.

To convert kilograms to pounds, multiply the kilograms by 2.2.

Abbreviations

bu	bushel
c	cup
gal	gallon
gm	gram
kg	kilogram
L	liter
lb	pound
mg	milligram
ml	milliliter
oz	ounce
pk	peck
pt	pint
qt	quart
tbsp or T	tablespoon
tsp or t	teaspoon

Milliequivalent weight (mEq)

The milliequivalent weight of an element is the atomic weight divided by the valence. To convert milligrams (mg) to milliequivalents (mEq), divide the atomic weight in milligrams by the milliequivalent weight of the element, as in the following formula:

$$\text{Milliequivalents (mEq)} = \frac{\text{Atomic weight}}{\text{Milliequivalent weight}}$$

To convert milliequivalent (mEq) to milligrams (mg), multiply the milliequivalent value by the milliequivalent weight of the element, as in the following formula:

$$\text{Milligrams (mg)} = \text{Milliequivalents} \times \text{Milliequivalent weight}$$

Milliequivalent weights of some elements

Na	23
K	39
Cl	35.5
Mg	12
P	15.5
Ca	20

Thus, 1 mEq Na = 23 mg
 1 mEq K = 39 mg